Food for Healing

RACHEL CHARLES has written several books, including *Mind, Body and Immunity*, also published by Cedar. The subject of nutrition has fascinated her for more than twenty years and she has studied the topic in depth, furthering her scientific knowledge at the Institute for Optimum Nutrition and becoming a member of the Society for the Promotion of Nutritional Therapy. Her own health problems, in particular the menace of cancer, prompted the initial interest, but she now uses her knowledge to assist her clients. As a practising psychotherapist, her special area of concern is the way that nutrients affect mood, thought and indeed the whole chemistry of the brain.

She was brought up in the Lake District and received her degree from Bristol University. Before training as a Psychosynthesis counsellor and psychotherapist, she spent several years in publishing. Now she combines her therapy practice with writing and lives with her husband in the peace and quiet of rural Suffolk, where they have a beautiful organic garden. Otherwise spare moments are spent music-making, for she is also an accomplished cellist.

Also by Rachel Charles
and available in Cedar

Mind, Body and Immunity

RACHEL CHARLES

Food for Healing

How to prevent and cure
common ailments
with nutritional therapy

Illustrations by John Fulcher

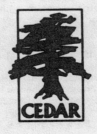

CEDAR

To all those dedicated researchers and
health-care professionals who have dared
to question the traditional assumptions
about food and dietary habits, out of a
genuine desire to help prevent and cure
disease without resorting to the
unnecessary use of drugs.

A Mandarin Paperback
FOOD FOR HEALING

First published in Great Britain 1995
as a Cedar Original
This edition published 1996
by Mandarin Paperbacks
an imprint of Reed International Books Ltd
Michelin House, 81 Fulham Road, London SW3 6RB
and Auckland, Melbourne, Singapore and Toronto

Copyright © Rachel Charles 1995
The author has asserted her moral rights

Illustrations © John Fulcher 1995

The charts on pages 22 and 23 are taken
from *The Food Scandal* by Caroline Walker and
Geoffrey Cannon and published by
Century Publishing Co. Ltd. 1984

All rights reserved. No part of this book may be
reproduced or transmitted in any form or by any
means, electronic or mechanical, including
photocopying, recording, or by any information
storage and retrieval system, without the written
permission of the Publisher, except where permitted
by law.

ISBN 0 7493 2411 2

Phototypeset by Intype, London
Printed and bound by
Cox & Wyman Ltd, Reading, UK

1 3 5 7 9 10 8 6 4 2

Contents

Acknowledgements

Firstly, thanks must go to Sarah Hannigan, formerly of Cedar Paperbacks, who provided the original inspiration for this book and helped to nurture it during its early stages.

Heartfelt thanks are due to John Fulcher, my husband, not only for providing the superb line drawings, but also for being a constant source of encouragement and support throughout the many months spent researching and writing *Food for Healing*. He also willingly acted as 'guinea pig', expressing honest opinions about a number of the recipes.

I am particularly grateful to my sister, Mary Pratt, M.A. (Oxon), M.Sc., who gave up a half-term holiday to read through my manuscript and check it in detail, subsequently making very valuable comments and suggestions.

The Institute for Optimum Nutrition kindly allowed me to use their specialist library of books and journals, offering friendly hospitality and a constant supply of much-appreciated herb teas.

Those who so generously described their case histories must remain anonymous, but their stories have made a major contribution to the book, and I am much obliged to them.

Author's Note

If you feel unwell or are concerned about your health in any way at all, always consult your doctor in the first instance. There are sound scientific reasons for the recommendations made in this book, but response to nutrients can vary from person to person according to the individual's own biochemistry. If you wish to switch to a different diet, or to take nutritional supplements, therefore, make sure you are carefully monitored by a fully qualified professional nutritional therapist or consultant. Also read the words of caution concerning some supplements in chapter 3.

Case histories illustrate the value of nutritional therapy in particular instances (although names have been altered to preserve confidentiality). However, many different factors can contribute to any one disorder and suggested treatments need to be tailored to suit each patient. A good nutritionist will spend at least an hour with a client during the initial consultation, asking many questions, to ensure that all special requirements are met. There may therefore be a variation between your best route back to health and the corresponding case history described in the book.

Introduction

This kitchen was unique. A hefty slab of polished oak, its edges left rough-hewn, served as work-top and dining table combined and visitors perched on high stools to eat. This was fine as long as the houseboat remained securely on the sand-bank, but as soon as the tide lifted it from the bottom of the Chelsea Reach, putting fork or spoon to mouth took some concentration. Jo assured us that eating with such care was excellent for the digestion, allowing time for the nutrients to be absorbed into the bloodstream and do their vital rebuilding and repair work. Moreover the gentle rocking of the boat created a relaxed and soothing ambiance that was certainly kind to the stomach.

Lunch was simple but delicious: watercress soup, followed by a crisp salad with jacket potato filled with cottage cheese and flavoured with spring onions, then raspberries and yoghurt for afters. As we ate, Jo gave us a detailed account of the vitamins and minerals contained in the food and what they would do for us. I was fascinated: calcium and vitamin A in the watercress (good for bones and vision); vitamin C in the green peppers and raspberries (to keep colds at bay); potassium in the jacket potatoes and spring onions (essential for proper functioning of nerves and muscles); more calcium in the cottage cheese and yoghurt as well as complete protein which provides the basic building materials for our muscles, skin and hair and other parts of our bodies.

The other guest, a newly qualified doctor called Robert, was showing more interest in the Klimt print hanging by the porthole of a loving couple, limbs entwined, painted in exotic, shimmering colours. He yawned, having worked long hours at the hospital. 'You don't want to bother your heads with vitamins and minerals,' he said. 'As long as you stick to an average diet, you will get all you need.'

This casual comment caused a sudden eruption from Jo. He launched into a tirade against the vices of white bread and white sugar, both of which grab nutrients from the body in order to be metabolized, because all their natural goodness has been refined out of them. He then added a thing or two about saturated fats from meat which clog up the arteries and lead to heart disease. He was a committed vegetarian. He asked the young doctor if he had studied nutrition at medical school and Robert replied:

'We're trained to recognize deficiency diseases such as rickets, but these are very rare now because, as I said, the nation as a whole is well nourished.' Then he warned us that vegetarians can suffer from anaemia and lack of protein. I could not resist pointing out that Jo was hardly fading away on his diet. On the contrary, his energy levels were high, his skin clear and his gaze was almost unnervingly direct from strangely yellow-flecked blue eyes.

The doctor had to get back to the hospital for another long stint on duty. He thanked Jo for the lunch and departed saying jokingly, 'Bangers and mash tonight. Delicious!' Clearly, there was no hope of converting him to healthier eating habits.

The year was 1970. I did not realize it then, but Jo's attitude to food was well ahead of his time. Links between diet and degenerative diseases are now well proven and vegetarianism has at last been accepted as beneficial, but in those days giving up meat was generally met with utter derision. Over the years, the medical profession and government have grudgingly come to admit that the high-

2

meat, high-dairy-produce diet promoted after the Second World War has not been in the best interest of the nation's health. In the short term, deficiency diseases were eradicated, but in the long term, disorders of middle age have reached epidemic proportions.

Jo had a number of small bottles on the work-top. He took one or two pills from each, totalling about seven, of different shapes and colours, and then swallowed the lot. I gasped. Pills to me at that time meant drugs. He saw my concern: 'Don't worry, they're pure nutrients. They can only do me good.'

'Do you really need all of these?' I asked, torn between his sincere belief in the wonderful power of vitamins and the young doctor's approach which, after all, was backed by the bulk of medical opinion. He beckoned me up the steps to his sitting room. It had been built directly on to the deck and enjoyed a panoramic view of the river, where the activities of passing boats were an endless source of fascination. He took a book from a shelf. 'Read,' he said.

I flopped on to a large cushion, which was covered in a richly coloured hand-woven material, and opened the pages. It was *Let's Eat Right to Keep Fit* by Adelle Davis, an American nutritionist. She had plenty to say about the healing powers of food supplements, but it was the subject of breakfast that immediately grabbed my attention. She recommended the inclusion of protein for a gradual release of energy to meet the demands of the morning and only a light meal in the evening when activities are probably less demanding. This way energy is available when you need it and you are less likely to put on weight by sleeping on a full stomach. I had been troubled for years by listlessness and fainting around mid-morning, combined with blurred vision and headaches. My doctor had assured me that it was due to low blood pressure, which in any case is healthy, and I would just have to put up with the effects. He never asked me what, if anything, I ate for breakfast. I resolved

3

to follow Adelle's advice and improve my eating habits. At the very least no harm could result and at best the fainting might be cured.

At that time, I had no idea I was suffering from hypoglycaemia or low blood sugar, and it took me years to discover the name of this condition. With Jo's encouragement I replaced the cornflakes with sugar-free muesli made from jumbo oats well soaked in skimmed milk or orange juice, adding fresh fruit and nuts with a little live yoghurt on top. That was always followed by something substantial, such as a fish cake, scrambled eggs or cheese on wholemeal toast. My dizziness disappeared as if by magic, and what a simple cure! By eating moderately in the evening I was hungry enough first thing the next day to consume a nutritious breakfast. As a result my blood glucose remained steady for several hours while digestion was taking place, rather than rising quickly and then dropping dramatically after the cornflakes and sugar, causing the fainting and disturbed vision.

These debilitating symptoms had been seriously affecting my work and my mood for a long while. Suddenly to find myself full of vigour and in good humour all morning was both a relief and a revelation. After that Jo and I spent many hours sprawled on his gently swaying deck under the leafy pot plants studying nutrition and testing the efficacy of this or that vitamin or mineral. I no longer cared if people called me a crank. Adelle had found a dedicated follower.

Chapter 1

The Story of Vitamins

One of the most terrifying infections ever to attack the human race was the bubonic plague, or Black Death, which started in the East and spread along the trade routes to Europe in the late 1340s carried by the fleas of rats. The devastation was appalling. Probably one-quarter of the population was wiped out, about 24 million people. Ships floated helplessly around the seas, entire crews having perished, while on land crops and animals withered and died from lack of attention and in the towns residents were too frightened to visit their neighbours, knowing only of their demise from the stench of their rotting corpses. The symptoms were swollen glands in the groin or armpits, followed by black spots, the sure sign of imminent death. Families wondered what they could have done to deserve such fearful punishment, but penance and prayers were in vain.

An eyewitness account from Giovanni Boccaccio, author of *The Decameron*, who lived in the city of Florence, helps us to understand the cruel suffering caused by this disease, which no known remedy could alleviate. While some thought it was the result of bad air, others realized that it was passed from one person to another and the only solution was for the healthy to band together and live in seclusion. They also instinctively felt that good food might help to keep the plague at bay: '(They) lived a separate and secluded life . . . avoiding every kind of luxury, but eating and drinking very moderately of the most delicate viands and the finest wines, holding converse with none but one another'. Some of these wealthy lords and ladies were lucky enough to survive, as were the inhabitants of a few English villages who followed similar tactics. These people clearly understood the principles of contagion and knew from experience that a fresh, simple diet kept them healthy, but science had not yet taught them that nutrients in high-quality food help to boost immunity.

Essential to life

We have to scrutinize the history of the mid-eighteenth century before finding someone who attempted to prove that certain foods have disease-preventing, life-preserving qualities. James Lind, a British naval surgeon, had to deal with thousands of cases of scurvy, which killed more sailors during wartime than the actual combat. Conditions at sea were grim for ordinary seamen, who had living quarters that were damp, dark and low. Food consisted of salted beef, gruel made from brackish water, and hard biscuits which had to be sharply knocked before eating to get rid of the weevils. A piece of mouldy cheese might occasionally add a little variety. There were no fresh vegetables or fruit. It seems hardly surprising that during a long voyage men started to get sick. The first signs of scurvy were flaking skin and bleeding from the gums, with teeth eventually falling out. Internal haemorrhages caused large bruises and weakness of the limbs and, if this occurred in a vital organ, death inevitably followed, often lingering and painful.

Lind heard that Dutch seamen had apparently kept themselves healthy some 200 years previously by taking citrus fruits with them on long voyages. He decided to carry out an experiment. After dividing twelve scurvy-ridden sailors into pairs, he gave each a different, commonly used treatment: the first had a quart of cider each day, the next had 25 drops of dilute sulphuric acid three times daily, the third had half a pint of seawater with the same frequency, the fourth received two spoons of vinegar instead, while the fifth pair had a herbal mixture and the sixth had two oranges and one lemon daily for six days. This last pair made such a good recovery that they were used as nurses for the others, who, with the exception of the cider pair, deteriorated steadily.

Lind had no idea that the special healing nutrient was vitamin C. Indeed, he still wondered whether the disease could be due to a poison. Despite the success of his treatment it was another forty years before the British Admiralty adopted regular doses of lemon or lime juice as a preventive measure, wiping out scurvy and doubling its fighting force at the same time. Since then British sailors have been referred to as 'Limeys'.

*

In 1830 a new invention was introduced by a man named Müller to assist in the production of food: it was the steel roller wheat mill for the refining of flour. Sadly, it did not lead to a healthier diet, for the daily bread was no longer rich in vitamins B and E and the minerals zinc, calcium, potassium, iron and magnesium; these had all been extracted along with the bran and germ of the wheatgrain. During this period white sugar had become more freely available, especially after 1874 when the tax on it was lifted. People began to suffer from deficiency diseases caused by the removal of essential nutrients through these refining processes.

In the East, communities whose staple food was rice suffered similarly after polishing became popular, a process that removed the husk with the vitamin-rich embryo. The disease beriberi had a devastating effect on the Imperial Fleet in Japan, crippling almost 40 per cent of the men. It presents itself in two forms: in the 'dry' type the nerves connected to the limbs are damaged so that the patient is unable to walk properly; in the 'wet' type the heart muscle becomes weak and flabby and the legs and abdomen swell from the leakage of fluid into the tissues. Eventually paralysis sets in and death results from heart failure. This fearsome malady has a simple cause: lack of thiamin (vitamin B_1). When patients are given this nutrient, improvement is dramatic. But it was not until the end of the nineteenth century that the connection was made.

A young Dutch physician and pathologist, Christian Eijkman, went to Java to try and get to the bottom of beriberi, believing it to be caused by a bacterium. In 1890, while working in his laboratory, he noticed that the chickens which he kept for experiments were ailing: their wings drooped and their walking became erratic and feeble. Some collapsed altogether and others seemed unable to eat. His diagnosis was polyneuritis, remarkably like that suffered by the beriberi victims. Yet it was another seven years before he eventually proved that the disease was due to feeding the chickens on polished, rather than natural, brown rice. Even so, he maintained that the polyneuritis was probably a result of the action of intestinal microorganisms rather than a missing nutrient.

It took two biochemists, a Polish-American named Casimir Funk and a Briton, Frederick G. Hopkins, to develop the theory of vitamin-deficiency diseases. By 1912 Funk had tried, but not succeeded, in isolating the anti-beriberi ingredient from discarded rice polishings. Believing that it probably belonged to a group of chemical compounds termed 'amines', he named it 'vitamine', meaning 'amine essential to life'. A few years earlier Hopkins had studied the effect of diet on rats and concluded that foods contain essential factors that are vital for the healthy growth and maintenance of the body. He termed them 'accessory food factors' to distinguish them from the 'basic food factors' which had already been identified as carbohydrates, fats, proteins, minerals and water.

*

8

Despite growing awareness that food contained special protective, life-enhancing factors, deficiency diseases were widespread in the early part of the twentieth century. In northern latitudes children's bones sometimes failed to calcify properly and these poor little creatures limped about with bow-legs or knock-knees. They often had defective teeth, deformed ribs, or even badly shaped skulls. The folk remedy of cod livers seemed to be effective, as was sunlight, but this was often in short supply. Doctors began to understand the importance of calcium and phosphorus for young bones during the years when they were developing, but it took a little longer to comprehend the role of vitamin D which aids calcium absorption. This is present in cod livers and it is created in the skin on exposure to ultraviolet light.

Cod-liver oil had also been recommended as a treatment for the children's eye disease xerophthalmia by a Japanese doctor, M. Mori. It is appropriately termed 'dry eye', for the tear glands cease to function and the surface of the eyeball becomes opaque. If infection follows, as it generally does, blindness can occur. This debilitating disorder struck Danish children in particular during the First World War. At that time most of their butter was being exported and local people were fed on margarine instead. When it was shown that butter cured the condition, exportation was limited and Danish children grew up with healthier eyes. Later it was demonstrated that both butter and cod-liver oil contain vitamin A, essential for good vision. Subsequently butter became known as a 'protective' food.

In the southern states of America until 1937 a particularly pathetic complaint afflicted poor people in rural areas, whose staple diet was corn and fat meat. This was pellagra. Symptoms included sores on the skin and tongue, diarrhoea and vomiting, loss of appetite, headaches, depression and finally dementia. Haggard and emaciated, the malnourished victims often ended up in a mental hospital. The experiment that clearly proved they were suffering from a deficiency disease took place in a prison: volunteers ate the food of the local poor and after several months, as expected, signs of pellagra began to appear. When yeast, milk, cheese and liver were given to them also, the symptoms vanished. Niacin, or nicotinic acid, had been identified as a constituent of yeast extract as early as 1912, but it was another quarter of a century before the medical profession made the link with communities prone to pellagra, finally realizing that this essential B vitamin (B_3) was lacking in their diet.

It was also a long time before vitamin C was isolated in a crystalline form from the adrenal gland of an ox by the Hungarian-born scientist Albert Szent-Györgyi. He gave some of this sugar-like substance to the English chemist W. N. Haworth, who defined its structural formula. They named the substance ascorbic acid (from 'antiscorbutic' or anti-scurvy) and in 1937 they received the Nobel Prize for their discovery and synthesis of vitamin C.

Pioneers of vitamin therapy

During the next two decades, medical science was dominated by the development of the so-called 'miracle drugs' of antibiotics, steroids and tranquillizers. The speed with which many of these can act has certainly been impressive and drug companies have spent millions on research, patented the new remedies and made millions more on their sale. Nutrients, however, being substances naturally occurring in our food, cannot be patented, so that no single company can claim exclusive right to their production. Needless to say, there is little incentive to fund scientists to make further investigations into their efficacy and this has generally been left to individual enthusiasts.

One such was Dr William Kaufman who lived in Connecticut. Many of his patients suffered from arthritis and he was all too aware of what little he could do to alleviate this painful disease. He decided to try high doses of vitamins; after all, they could cause no harm and might prove to be beneficial. After some experimentation, he found that the very vitamin that cured pellagra (vitamin B_3) could also be used in its amide form (i.e. nicotinamide) as a remedy for arthritis, if taken in high doses under careful supervision.

In Virginia, Dr Frederick Klenner had had some startling successes with megadoses of vitamin C and published a paper entitled 'The treatment of poliomyelitis and other viral diseases with vitamin C'. These other maladies included serious infections such as hepatitis as well as commonly occurring colds and cold sores. He claimed that the vitamin actually killed the viral organisms, but it is now believed that it helps to boost elements of the immune system which in turn fight the invading virus. He administered huge doses of the vitamin, from 30 to 100g daily, by injection, according to the patient's tolerance and the severity of the illness.

Dr Linus Pauling, winner of the Nobel Prize for chemistry, helped to lend credibility to such theories. In 1960 he proposed the phrase 'orthomolecular nutrition' to describe how disease might be eradicated by giving the body the right ('ortho') molecules so that it can heal itself. Together with a Scottish surgeon, Ewan Cameron, he found that even cancer patients could be helped with doses of around 10g of vitamin C per day.

Treatment of physical and mental disorders through correct nutrition is not a new idea. As long ago as AD 390 Hippocrates declared: 'Let food be your medicine and medicine be your food'. Yet only during the last decade has nutritional therapy increasingly gained recognition as a valuable, virtually risk-free way of preventing and curing disease. Private colleges have opened up to train aspiring therapists, professional associations have been formed and registers of practitioners are kept (see Addresses at the end of the book).

*

If you have a medical problem, always consult your doctor in the first instance, but try to find one who is sympathetic to vitamin therapy, then you can work together to regain your health. Remember, however, that using nutrients to correct long-term deficiencies which have resulted in disease can take some weeks. You will be working in cooperation with natural processes so that your body has the best possible chance to heal itself, generally a gradual procedure. Do not expect overnight miracles! In the long term, however, your patience will be well rewarded. At the same time you will be sure that the therapy is treating the root cause of your health problem, unlike many doctor's prescriptions which concentrate on banishing symptoms. Moreover, many drugs are really selective poisons that can have damaging side-effects. A recent television documentary suggested that between 10 and 20 per cent of all hospital admissions are due to modern medical practices. Nutrients, on the other hand, when taken in balanced proportions, can only do your body good.

Dr Carl Pfeiffer, an American psychiatrist and expert on the chemistry of the brain, told a colleague: 'Good nutritional therapy is the medicine of the future. We have already waited too long for it.'

Chapter 2

How Balanced is Our Diet?

No one can deny the wonders of twentieth-century medicine, with its mass inoculation programmes that have conquered frightening diseases such as smallpox, diphtheria,
tetanus, polio and measles, while antibiotics can successfully treat tuberculosis, typhoid fever and other conditions
created by an invasion of bacteria. Amazing, too, are
advances in surgery, aided by high-tech diagnosis, providing ever more reliable information about the state of each
part of the body. We marvel at the creation of minute
cameras able to pass inside an artery and photograph a
blockage, or of an electron scanning microscope that can
magnify a single bacterium some 40,000 times.

Yet, ironically, many of these sophisticated techniques
would not even be necessary if only we looked after ourselves better and kept disease at bay with regular exercise,
lower stress levels and nutritious food. Now that childhood
infectious illnesses are under control, together with the
most serious vitamin-deficiency diseases, we need to revise
our commonly held views on nutrition in the light of the
current epidemic of maladies of middle age, many of which
are the result of a poor diet.

What is good for us?

In the 1970s messages about food were becoming increasingly confusing and contradictory. In Britain a new

Education Act in 1971 under Margaret Thatcher declared that children over seven years were no longer entitled to free milk and she earned the nickname 'Milk Snatcher'. Even rickets began to reappear, especially among Asian communities. At the same time food manufacturers were spending heavily on advertising their sweet, sticky, refined, processed, additive-impregnated concoctions and the Butter Information Council was desperately maintaining that natural dairy products were healthier than margarine. On the instigation of the then Minister for Health, Sir Keith Joseph, the National Advisory Committee on Nutrition Education (NACNE) was set up to 'provide simple and accurate information on nutrition' and to work towards 'slow change'.

Meanwhile in America, former presidential candidate George McGovern was chairing a committee of the Senate which was putting together a report called *Dietary Goals for the United States*. It was published in 1977 and stated, 'Our diets have changed radically within the past 50 years, with great and very harmful effects on our health. Too much fat, too much sugar or salt, can be and are linked directly to heart disease, cancer, obesity and stroke, among other killer diseases.' Dr Mark Hegsted, chief scientific advisor to the committee, added, 'The diet we eat today was not planned or developed for any particular purpose. It is a happenstance related to our affluence, the productivity of our farmers and the activities of our food industry.' Despite the huge uproar that ensued, a second edition of the report set out aims for a healthy diet consisting of more whole grains, legumes, fresh fruit and vegetables that were high in fibre, vitamins and minerals and low in saturated fats, sugars and salt. If the nation changed to such a diet, it was estimated that 250,000 deaths a year from heart disease would be averted together with a saving of $10,000 million for treatment. In addition, children's intelligence would

14

increase by about 10 IQ points and there would be a 5 per cent increase in work productivity.

Back in Britain the NACNE committee had come to similar conclusions, but was having a rough ride. Statements such as 'the consensus of medical opinion is that the population should not be consuming the type of diet currently eaten in Britain' and 'the plan for action should be to change the eating habits of the nation as a whole, not [as officially hoped] merely the habits of those who were already ill or "at risk" ' were given a cold reception by the government and the British Nutrition Foundation. Funded by the food industry, including Rank Hovis McDougall, who then shared 85 per cent of the white bread market with Allied Bakeries and made 75 per cent of the table salt, and Tate & Lyle, who monopolized the importation of refined sugar, the BNF attacked the first draft of the NACNE report, saying that there was no justification to cut sugars and alcohol. In response to the second draft, which had the backing of the World Health Organization, representatives of the Foundation said that to follow the recommendations of the McGovern and NACNE reports by cutting fats and sugars 'would require major changes in eating habits resulting in a diet of doubtful palatability' and 'would have far-reaching economic implications world-wide'.

After 'intense commercial pressures to maintain sucrose intakes', the NACNE committee presented a third draft. By now it was 1983. In this draft, short-term, easily achievable goals – such as simply to cut consumption of confectionery and soft drinks – were set out, equivalent to only one-third of long-term recommendations 'while food manufacturers are making their more important reductions'.

Clearly, business and medical science had collided head on, while the government was not prepared to take responsibility for the nation's health, even though in America death rates from heart disease were already beginning to drop in response to the targets of the McGovern report.

15

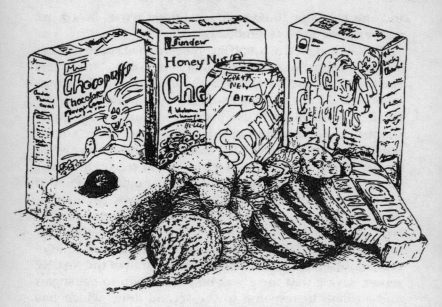

Foods such as these are very high in refined carbohydrates and saturated fats, but low in naturally occurring nutrients, providing mainly empty calories. Artificial preservatives and colourings are often included. Children brought up on 'junk food' will suffer many health problems and never achieve their full potential.

Ten years on, the situation in the UK was no better: 'Junk food diet led to scurvy' reads a headline in the *Guardian* of 3 March 1993. The copy continues: 'A 14-year-old Ulster girl whose diet was mainly cola, chocolate, hamburgers and crisps developed scurvy, the bane of seamen two centuries ago, it emerged yesterday. The girl's doctor said he had heard of four or five cases of the disease among western teenagers.' This poor creature was not just so severely short of vitamin C that she had developed a potentially fatal sickness long thought to have been eradicated, but her atrocious diet supplied so little nourishment that both her body and her mind are likely to be stunted for ever. Children brought up on white bread, biscuits, ice cream

16

and other confectionery will never have the chance of achieving their full potential.

In 1984 a survey of 1,000 small children was carried out by the University of Bristol, which reported: 'There are many malnourished children in the project samples, some of whom suffer continual illnesses, which are treated by strong drugs or hospitalization.' The director of the project, Dr Walter Barker, said, 'Most of the children from poor households, and many of the better-off children, were eating a poor diet, high in sugars and low in whole foods. This can lead to retarded brain growth.'

What has been done in the past decade to remedy this appalling situation? The answer is: virtually nothing. Why not? The answer to that is lack of political will and that the big food-manufacturing companies are busy lining their pockets, while those who eat their sugar- and fat-infested products carry on lining their arteries. Worse, despite the fact that the British government is now aware of the damage a high-fat diet can cause, it persists in subsidizing only full-fat milk used by schools rather than the healthier skimmed milk, simply because the EU butter mountain is, at the time of writing, 168,000 tonnes high. It is hardly surprising that British teeth and hearts remain the unhealthiest in the world.

Food of the hunter-gatherers

Human bodies have not evolved to be able to cope with the amount of saturated fat that we commonly consume in the West from meat and dairy products, nor with refined sugar that offers only empty calories. Nor can they survive well on highly refined, processed foods that are depleted of vital nutrients and provide insufficient fibre. To understand what foods are most naturally the best for us we need to take a look at our forebears, who, for two million years or more, had a way of life that revolved around gathering plants, nuts and berries and hunting small game. It is only relatively recently, in the last few thousand years, that people have led a settled existence tied to agriculture.

Despite high infant mortality, the hunter-gatherers were so successful that they gradually spread out of Africa into many other parts of the globe, learning how to adapt to different climates and conditions. So what were their lives like? Archaeological evidence is sketchy, but mobile groups that live by gathering and hunting still exist in remote areas and give us a good idea how well they survived. For example, the bushmen of south-west Africa subsist entirely on wild food, yet their choice of menu is astonishing. As many as 84 edible plants are available, although they tend to prefer around one-third of these, and 54 different animals can be hunted. All in all these provide a very wide range of nutrients, and of course everything is eaten fresh and generally raw before the vitamins deteriorate. The mongongo nut is the staple of the diet and is an excellent food, providing five times the amount of calories of cooked rice and twice the protein of beef. Deficiency diseases are non-existent and one in ten people live to beyond 60 years of age, gaining high status in the group.

As for leisure time, they enjoy more of this than anyone in an industrialized country could possibly dream of. Needless to say, work-induced stress is completely unknown. The women, who do the gathering, spend not more than three hours a day at this task; often one is sufficient. The men's hunting work is carried out in intensive spurts, perhaps a week at once followed by two or three weeks' rest. Food is plentiful and would have been even more so in primitive times, needing little effort to find and involving at the most six miles of walking on one expedition. Single people are exempt from foraging and, since they rarely marry at under 20 years of age, they have many years of freedom to enjoy before settling down and producing children. Material objects have small value in a mobile society and therefore little time is spent in producing them.

The planting and tending of crops, with all the extra work that these involve, hold no attraction for hunter-gatherers: 'Why should we plant when there are so many mongongo nuts in the world?' asked one bushman of an anthropologist. Leisure activities and ceremonies, however, are of great importance.

Hunting is very much a hit-and-miss affair with low success rates, especially with primitive weapons. The main emphasis of the diet, therefore, is on plant food with the occasional addition of insects, snails and small game caught in traps. The quality of this meat is far removed from the intensively bred, factory-farmed creatures that are dished up on our plates. These are pumped with hormones, force-fed an unvaried diet designed only for weight-gain, and cramped together in small pens with no space to run around. Thus, fat, unhealthy animals are fed to fat, unfit people. And the kind of fat produced is harmful in that it is high in saturates and low in beneficial polyunsaturates. This is a very different kind of meat from the flesh of wild game, which comes from a lean, fit animal fed on a nutrient-rich, unpolluted diet, and the fat that there is (only about 4 per cent as opposed to 30 per cent in domestic cattle) is proportionally higher in polyunsaturates.

Tropical diseases such as malaria, yaws and sleeping sickness must have affected primitive people but, because the forest was dense and the population as a whole very low, tribes would rarely come into contact with one another so that spread of infections would be restricted. Moreover, mothers breast-fed their babies for years which ensured that they started life with plenty of healthy antibodies in their immune systems, ready to fend off any invading organisms.

Settled communities

After the introduction of agriculture the situation was very different. According to Jared Diamond, a physiologist at

19

the University of California, this was 'the worst mistake in the history of the human race'. It is likely that babies were weaned earlier on grain mash, so that women's fertility was no longer naturally suppressed by extended lactation. Not only were farmers ploughing up the land of the hunter-gatherers, but they were out-breeding them. At the same time their crowded living conditions, restricted diet and long working hours left their bodies scraggy and more prone to sickness, while tooth decay was common. Lives were brief.

Archaeological evidence shows that when agriculture took over in the areas now called Greece and Turkey at around 4000 BC, men became shorter by as much as 7 inches (18cm), leaving them with a height of about 5ft 3 in (1.6m), and women lost some 5 inches (12.7cm), dropping to 5ft 1in (1.5m). Indeed, modern Greeks and Turks have still not regained the stature of their healthy hunter-gatherer ancestors. As communications increased with the building of roads and the opening up of trade routes, so humans became threatened with diseases to which they had little or no natural immunity.

The fall from Paradise

In this sense, then, humans have truly fallen from Paradise, or rather they have themselves systematically destroyed the environment which was once so rich and life-sustaining, providing them with all their needs. Instead of learning from their mistakes they have continued to exploit the natural resources of the world, more recently adding insult to injury by causing widespread pollution through the dumping of toxic chemicals and the degradation and poisoning of agricultural land through soil erosion and heavy use of pesticides.

This, then, is our inheritance. Rather than walking several miles a day to collect a wide variety of fresh, vitamin-rich, natural foods, sluggish modern humans climb

20

into their cars, drive to the supermarket and pile their trolleys high with packaged items adulterated with artificial additives or pesticides, many of which have sat on the shelves for extended periods, having long since lost much of their natural goodness through age, processing, canning or refining.

Humans can carry on for just so long on an inadequate intake of nutrients, but then succumb to serious illness: women with poor absorption of calcium in their middle years will later suffer from osteoporosis; people low in the trace element selenium are more likely to develop cancer; those deficient in iron will suffer from anaemia, and so on. The NACNE report lists many medical conditions that are diet-related, as follows:

Over-consumption	Under-nutrition	Resulting disease
fats	fibre	cancer of large bowel (colon)
	fibre	constipation
fats, sugars		diabetes[1]
	fibre	diverticular disease
fats, sugars	fibre	gall-bladder disease[1]
fats		heart disease[1]
fats, salt		high blood pressure[1]
	fibre	irritable bowel syndrome
fats, sugars	fibre	overweight, obesity
fats, salt		strokes
sugars		tooth decay

[1] also associated with overweight and obesity

21

From this it can be deduced that too much saturated fat causes diseases of the heart and blood vessels, while too little fibre leads to disorders of the alimentary tract. The list continues:

Over-consumption	Under-nutrition	Resulting disease
alcohol		cirrhosis of the liver
	folic acid	neural tube defects in babies
	vitamin D	osteomalacia[2]
	vitamin D	osteoporosis[2]

[2] also caused by lack of exercise

Accumulated scientific evidence also points to the following:

Over-consumption	Under-nutrition	Related disease
fats		angina
fats, sugars (?)		cancer of the breast
fats (?)		cancer of the pancreas
salt		cancer of the stomach
	fibre	piles
sugars (?)		kidney stones
fats (?), sugars(?)	fibre (?)	ulcer of intestine
fats (?), sugars (?)	fibre (?)	ulcer of stomach
	fibre	varicose veins

In addition, the bulk of evidence points to diet as a factor in the following, but these are not included in the NACNE report:

Over-consumption	Under-nutrition	Related disorder
	fibre	appendicitis
	essential fats (?)	arthritis
additives		eczema[3]
alcohol		foetal alcohol syndrome
sugars		gout
	fibre (?)	hiatus hernia
additives		hyperactivity[3]
sugars		hypoglycaemia[4]
additives		migraine & allergies[3]
	essential fats (?)	multiple sclerosis(?)
	essential fats (?)	rheumatoid arthritis (?)

[3] can also be caused by cereals, cow's milk and other foods.
[4] can also be caused by other foods.
? evidence still regarded by some medical scientists as speculative.

These lists are by no means comprehensive, but perhaps they will help to convince anyone who remains sceptical that the average Western diet is damaging in the long term and, in the short term, can leave people feeling below par. The truth is that the human body, with its 60 trillion cells, needs just the right nutrients each day in the right quantities in order to achieve optimum health. It is staggering that our bodies, neglected and abused as they are, get by as well as they do.

A sickly, high-fat diet

Let us take a closer look at this typical diet which, according to many (ill-informed) doctors, is still supposed to be 'balanced' and to provide us with all that we need for good health and long life! What do most Westerners eat for breakfast, if they bother to have any at all? Packaged cereals (many of which consist of 48 per cent sugars) with milk and more refined sugar sprinkled over, followed by white bread, butter and marmalade or jam. This is generally swilled down with a cup of instant coffee, probably with more milk and even more white sugar. So far the person has eaten at least 1oz (30g) of refined sugar. Then there is, say, $\frac{1}{2}$oz (15g) of saturated fat in the butter, at least as much again in the $\frac{1}{2}$ pint (275ml) of milk that is likely to be used. All of the natural fibre that would have been available in the sugar cane or sugar beet and in the wheat has been removed in the refining processes, together with all the vitamins and minerals from the sugar and nearly all from the wheat, although, with a bit of luck, 4 nutrients out of about 24 might have been returned to the white flour in synthetic form. Because these foods have been so denuded of nutrients, the body now has a hard task to metabolize them and has to filch vitamins stored for other essential purposes, such as cell repair work. Vitamin B_1, in particular, is necessary for the metabolism of glucose and therefore serious deficiency of this vitamin can result, which in extreme cases can cause heart failure.

This person, then, has started the day with a high energy intake in terms of fat and refined carbohydrates, with an added caffeine boost from the instant coffee, and in about 45 minutes, when the glucose enters the bloodstream, there will be a feeling of well-being. This will last only a short while, until the blood-sugar level drops, and a craving will set in for a snack. If the calories are not used up with physical exercise of some sort they will accumulate, most likely around the abdomen or thighs. As for the saturated fat consumed, this may well be on its way to lining the blood vessels around the heart, storing up trouble for the future.

Is there anything good about this breakfast? Yes, there is calcium in the milk and butter, but then if the milk were skimmed and the butter omitted the person would still gain calcium without the risks posed by the fat. There is also some protein in the dairy products, but probably not enough to provide a good start to the day. The vitamin A in the dairy foods is certainly important, but there are other safer sources, such as apricots. The packaged cereal will no doubt boast plenty of added nutrients, but unless it is specifically a high-bran product it will certainly be low in roughage. We have already seen from the NACNE report how many diseases a poor intake of dietary fibre is connected with.

Our typical person has now reached the coffee break and is desperate for more sugar and fat, probably in the form of biscuits, especially chocolate-coated ones, also for another caffeine boost. Excessive coffee drinking is associated with a number of disorders, including fibrocystic breast disease, infertility and higher cholesterol levels. However, the fresh consumption of calories will see the average working Westerner through the rest of the morning until lunchtime. Perhaps the next port of call will be the local fast-food place or pub. The most likely choice here will be white bread sandwiches or rolls filled with, say, ham, and a can of soft drink or a pint of beer. The protein in the ham is, of course, beneficial, but unfortunately it comes with a high sodium content (some 2 to 3 per cent) and saturated fat – more trouble for the heart. Processed meats and cheeses also contain N-nitroso compounds, known carcinogens linked with brain tumours. Most people do not realize that when they buy a fizzy drink they are paying for water, sugar, colouring and flavouring, plus sodium citrate: in other words, empty calories yet again. Such drinks rarely contain any real value for money in the form of natural fruit juice. The beer would provide very small quantities of vitamins and minerals but also a large amount of calories; one pint (570ml) would probably constitute 6 per cent of the day's allowance.

Bloated from the beer, constipated from the lack of roughage, short on vitamins and with teeth rotting from the accumulated sucrose, our typical person may wonder why the afternoon seems such an effort and is likely to have an overwhelming desire to nod off. To rectify this, another cup of coffee with milk and extra sugar is consumed. Tea time is welcomed with a sigh of relief: more caffeine, milk and sugar and another dollop of fat from the cake or biscuits together with yet more refined flour and sucrose, which will drain the body of its depleted resources of nutrients just to metabolize them.

Time to knock off and our unfit friend is anxious to rush home to dinner, probably the best source of nutrients of the day. But the metabolism faces another challenge: the menu consists of packet tomato soup, followed by beef sausages, chips and peas, and apple pie with plenty of custard for pudding. The taste buds will be deceived by the flavour-enhancers into believing that the tomato soup is delicious, but close scrutiny of the list of ingredients will reveal that it consists mainly of fats, sugars and sodium in different forms, plus a good dose of 'E' numbers. Any vitamins from the tomatoes will have long since disappeared during the process of turning them into a powder. However, the manufacturers will be happy because sugar and salt are cheap and they also increase shelf life – and thus profit.

Regulations governing the content of sausages are such that producers can get away with including as little as 22.5 per cent real lean beef or 29 per cent lean pork. The rest consists of, guess what, saturated fat and a wonderful mixture of gristle, sinew and rind preserved with sodium and once again coloured and flavoured to deceive the eye and tongue.

The chips, alas, will have lost some of their mineral content along with the potato peelings, although the oil (let's hope it is fresh vegetable oil) will have added some back. A trace of vitamin C may remain and healthy potassium, but only if the potatoes were fresh and not processed, forced into regular shapes, impregnated with fat and then frozen to create the 'oven ready' variety.

At last the body is offered some vitamins from the peas, C and A and traces of B complex, that is if they were frozen rather than canned, and a little dietary fibre. There may even be a few nutrients left in the cooked apples, but the pastry is, once again, high in fat and sugar with more of the same in the custard, plus colouring thrown in for good measure. Soft drinks will probably accompany this meal, followed by another cup of tea or coffee with the usual milk and sugar. Additives present in fizzy drinks have often been linked with hyperactivity in children and an assortment of allergies.

At the end of the day, full of fats, sugars, refined flours, caffeine and plenty of additives, our typical person is likely to fall asleep on a full stomach, so those excess calories will now turn into blubber.

Malnutrition is rife

This, then, is the 'balanced diet' that our over-fed, under-nourished Westerner is likely to consume, apparently continuing to give most people, including many doctors, the illusion that we are all bouncing with good health! In 1978 an extremely disturbing report was published in the USA, the Nationwide Food Consumption Survey, which revealed widespread malnutrition throughout all socio-economic groups, although the wealthy were slightly better nourished than the poor. It reported that one-third of Americans were low in vitamins A and C and iron, while as many as one-half were deficient in vitamin B_6, calcium and magnesium. The definition of deficiency used was an intake of less than 70 per cent of the Recommended Daily Allowance (RDA) of that particular nutrient. In other words, there were many others in the study who were consuming less than the RDA, but counted as not deficient for the purposes of the survey.

More than 20,000 individuals were tested and only 3 per cent were declared free of the most common symptoms of malnutrition. For one of the most affluent nations in the world, this is indeed a shocking result. The reason is that half of everything eaten in America is processed convenience food which has lost most of its natural health-giving properties.

Food for lasting health

So what can we do to correct this alarming situation and improve our health and the quality as well as the quantity of our lives? Quite simply we can heed the wisdom of our hunter-gatherer forebears. Most of their protein came from plant sources, with infrequent lean meat from trim game and fish caught in lakes and rivers. Translated into our terms this means cutting back drastically on all meats, especially the fatty ones such as pork and beef. Occasional lean lamb and free-range poultry is fine, and fish is a rich source of protein that is high in polyunsaturates but free of saturated fat. However, think of any meat as the accompaniment to the vegetables, rather than vice versa.

On five days of the week substitute a plant protein such as beans, lentils or nuts. Give up your full-fat milk and cream and swap to skimmed milk or, better still, fortified soya milk. Start your day like our ancestors, with fruit, nuts and berries, with the addition of whole grain flakes in the form of muesli. Cut back on tea and coffee, ban all soft drinks and gradually replace them with herb teas and fresh fruit juices. Do not add salt to food and learn to cook without it; it is so bad for the blood vessels. If you desperately miss that flavour then replace with Losalt, Biosalt or Ruthmol which have the correct balance of potassium with the sodium. Ban all white sugar – you do not need it! Use the slower-acting malt syrups (made for example from brown rice), or a little honey instead; apple juice works well in desserts. Eat a raw salad every day with a variety of ingredients. Eat plenty of vegetables, just lightly steamed. Instead of butter, use margarine that is not hydrogenated (see under 'Fats' in the next chapter). Never eat white bread; wholemeal is now easily obtainable and is an excellent food. Have brown rice and wholemeal pasta often. Replace sweet snacks and puddings with fresh fruit. Try not to use raising agents in cakes as they kill off B vitamins. Avoid all processed 'convenience' foods and refrain from opening tins whenever possible.

Do I hear you groan? Do you protest that you are far too busy to follow such a diet? Of course it is very difficult to make changes to eating habits and you will need to do this gradually. Encourage yourself with the thought that every little improvement helps. Remember that you will actually do less baking and cooking as you change to fresh fruit and raw salads. It is true that vegetarian meals can be time-consuming to prepare and of course fresh vegetables have to be washed, but it is also fun to create new dishes – there are plenty of ideas for recipes in chapter 20 – and wholesome food always tastes wonderful.

Whatever is wrong with canned food? you may enquire. It is generally heat-treated at high temperatures which destroys nutrients. For example, tinned salmon contains less than half the B_6 of fresh. Spinach that is canned has lost 82 per cent of its manganese and 80 per cent of its pantothenic acid. Beware, too, of those hidden additives, especially salt, sugar and starch which are often, quite unnecessarily, included in tins. Then there may be lead contamination from the seam. Freezing can also be harmful, damaging especially vitamins E and B_6, so do not freeze bread, which, if wholemeal, is likely to be your main source of vitamin E.

Suppose, then, that our average Westerner changes to this healthy diet, what are the benefits? First of all, muesli for breakfast supplies vitamins and minerals from the uncooked grain flakes (e.g. jumbo oats), the dried and fresh fruits (say, sultanas, banana and apple), and nuts and seeds (such as almonds, hazelnuts and sunflower seeds) as follows: **vitamins** A, B_1, B_2, B_3, B_6, C, E, biotin, folic acid, pantothenic acid; **minerals** calcium, chlorine, copper, iron, magnesium, phosphorus, potassium, sodium, sulphur and zinc. A sprinkling of wheatgerm will also provide manganese and the important trace element selenium. Then there will be protein in the skimmed milk or soya milk and in the nuts and seeds. The content of saturated fat and cholesterol is very low, but healthy oils (both monounsaturated and polyunsaturated) are found in the nuts and seeds. The dietary fibre content is excellent. Sweetness is provided naturally in the form of fructose; there is no need to add refined sugar.

Instead of white bread, our healthy eater has wholemeal, which again provides natural roughage to keep the bowels in good order. It also gives all the B vitamins and vitamin E and all the important minerals mentioned above, plus protein and carbohydrate. Beneficial polyunsaturated fats are available in the unhydrogenated margarine. Instead of jam, our wise person will use dark tahini or perhaps peanut butter as a spread for extra protein, vitamins and minerals. Tahini comes from Greece and consists of crushed sesame seeds. Even better, time will have been allowed for a proper second course of, say, a fish cake and mushrooms. The protein from the fish will keep the person going all morning, so there will be no craving for sticky snacks. And mushrooms are rich in B vitamins and potassium, while potatoes will add more vitamin C.

Lunch offers a further opportunity for raw food in the form of a salad which, if put together from fresh, organically grown ingredients, will supply immunity-boosting vitamin C. Green peppers and tomatoes are the classic sources, but by adding a handful of crisp alfalfa sprouts and a few uncooked broccoli florets our healthy eater's intake will increase by more than 100mg. Grated carrot will contribute that other important antioxidant, beta-carotene, which helps protect against cancer. Raw dark-green vegetables, shredded red cabbage or beetroot will all provide folic acid, essential for healthy blood cells and the construction of DNA, the 'blueprint' of life. Cooking these will almost halve the availability of this crucial B vitamin. Any vegetables, as well as lettuce, are all fine means of acquiring minerals, including potassium and calcium. For protein, the heart-conscious person will select avocado and walnuts to lower cholesterol, while French dressing made from a plant oil is the easiest way to ensure sufficient vitamin E in the diet – another wonder nutrient for the cardiovascular system.

By now the healthy eater's body tissues will be very happy indeed, having been granted all the nutrients essential for their care and repair. The white cells of the immune system will also be flourishing, ready to fend off any unwanted invaders in the form of bacteria or viruses. This person will be full of energy for the afternoon and will look marvellous, with bright eyes and clear skin. The brain, too, will feel alert having received the minerals it needs to operate efficiently – more of this in chapter 16. The day was started so well with a nourishing breakfast that there is no need to have a heavy dinner in the evening. Perhaps a vegetable-and-bean casserole with brown rice followed by fresh fruit will appeal. Once again, this is very low in fat but high in dietary fibre and essential nutrients.

For a summary of this health-giving diet and recipes, see chapter 20.

A lesson learned the hard way

The overall effect of a change in diet such as this has to be experienced to be believed. In 1986, after ignoring the needs of my body for many years through the demands of a high-stress job, I was shocked to find myself with breast cancer. Statistics were frightening: one-third dead within five years and two-thirds eventually succumb. Was there any way of improving my chances of staying within the surviving group?

A visit to the Cancer Help Centre at Bristol set me on the right track and reminded me of all those wise things I had learned from Adelle Davis and my friend Jo so many years previously. Unfortunately, when convenience foods are so readily available, it is all too easy to fall into lazy habits and, despite knowing better, this is what I had done. Rather than crying over my own stupidity, I decided to focus my efforts on making changes – permanent ones this time – and an important part of my new programme was a fresh, wholefood diet similar to the one described here, with the addition of some carefully chosen supplements. Knowing that my immune system was receiving all the right nutrients to help fight off any remaining cancer cells, my confidence in my chances of survival gradually improved and I began to feel less panic-stricken about a premature death. At least I was doing everything I could to help myself, so no longer felt like the hapless victim of a very frightening illness.

Of all the other benefits from my change in diet, one of the most unexpected has been a noticeable alteration in mood. Previously prone to extended periods of depression, I now wake up in the morning feeling light-hearted and cheerful, only succumbing to moments of gloom when there are obvious external reasons for these. Another surprise has been the experience of looseness in my limbs, as if my joints have been well lubricated. Then there is a sensation of lightness; I never put on weight on this low-fat diet, even though I sometimes eat like a horse! And my energy levels are marvellous. In other words I am no longer just getting by, just surviving; I am truly *alive*! Does this sound too good to be true? Not at all; there are sound physiological reasons for these changes, which I now understand and would like to share with you.

Chapter 3

The Vital Nutrients

Roll back your sleeve and take a moment to look at your arm. What you will see first of all is your skin, which appears to form a continuous covering over the flesh and bone beneath. You will of course notice the hairs, while closer inspection will reveal the pores. Examined under a microscope you would be able to observe the smallest living unit that exists on earth, probably measuring only $\frac{1}{10}$ to $\frac{1}{100}$mm across – the cell. Scientists define the word 'living' as something that can both reproduce and regulate itself. Sixty trillion or so of these living entities make up the human body and groups of them have varying functions to create a staggeringly complex but orderly being. An electron scanning microscope will divulge even more: the cytoplasm from which the living cell is constructed, and inside that the nucleus, or centre, of the cell, within which the thread-like chromosomes may be identified. Further probing by a method such as X-ray diffraction will disclose great numbers of atoms, the most minute units of matter that can take part in chemical reactions. These are approximately one-hundred-millionth of a centimetre across.

Atomic theory tells us that each atom consists mainly of empty space, in which there are tiny particles of electrically charged energy, constituting a central nucleus (made up of positively charged protons) and even smaller negatively charged electrons revolving around it in rings. To give you an idea of the distance between these, imagine that the nucleus is the size of a squash ball, in which case the revolving electrons at the outer edge of the atom would be hundreds of metres away. Thus, perceiving the skin of your arm as a continuous covering is only an illusion; it is really discontinuous and consists largely of empty space!

The nature of an element is determined by the number of its protons and electrons, hydrogen, the lightest, having only 1 of each, whereas chlorine has 17 of each. Atoms are able to combine with each other to form compounds. For example, ordinary table salt is a combination of the elements sodium and chlorine: atoms of sodium have combined with atoms of chlorine to form the compound sodium chloride.

The most basic element to all living matter is carbon, which has the special ability to combine with itself and create large molecules. Eighteen per cent of a human consists of carbon. The other three most important elements in humans are oxygen, hydrogen and nitrogen. Two atoms of hydrogen can combine with one of oxygen to form water (H_2O), constituting about 62 per cent of our bodies. Imagine carbon atoms formed into a chain, and on to this are added atoms of hydrogen and oxygen in different proportions to create carbohydrates and fats respectively. Proteins are constructed out of all four elements, sometimes with the inclusion of sulphur and phosphorus.

In order to maintain life, therefore, we need carbohydrates, fats, protein and water, together with the essential vitamins and minerals which act as catalysts to assist with important chemical reactions. We are not aware that these are taking place inside us all the time; indeed they happen within every cell. The word 'metabolism' generally describes these chemical changes.

Cells either divide to make new ones (we make literally millions of these every day), or else they may become specialized to form, say, muscle cells with the ability to contract, or nerve cells that can conduct electricity and pass on messages from the brain, or perhaps immune cells that fight off disease. In order to release energy and do their jobs effectively, it is vital that they have just the right nutrients – and nearly all of these come from the food we take in, combined with the oxygen we breathe. Without food, oxygen and water, cells very quickly die. With less than they really need, they become sickly. If the input of essential nutrients is even marginally below the ideal requirements, then they will underperform. So be good to your cells; give them what they need and they will serve you well.

If you take another look at the fluorescent screen of your electron microscope, you will be able to see the cytoplasm, which is like a thick liquid, and within that you will notice tiny particles of food in the form of droplets of oil or granules of starch or proteins. So how does the food get inside the cell? After being broken down by the digestive system (see chapter 6), the nutrients enter the bloodstream and are thus carried to all parts of the body through a marvellous system of arteries and fine capillaries. The outer covering or membrane of each cell is semi-permeable, so the nutrients are able to pass through this selectively. Equally, waste matter passes out.

Within each cell you will also see up to 100 egg-shaped structures between one and four microns in length (a micron is one-millionth of a metre) called mitochondria. With the help of enzymes, the mitochondria are able to release energy from the food, which in turn drives other chemical reactions, or is used for movement or to keep the body warm. In other words each mitochondrion is like a miniature battery, ready charged to release energy rapidly on demand.

At the centre of the cell is the nucleus, which regulates the chemical changes that take place. It therefore gives the cell its identity determining whether it will be a blood cell or a kidney cell or a brain cell and so on. It also initiates cell division. When this happens, the thread-like chromosomes which reside in the nucleus become visible and along these are the genes which carry all our inherited characteristics in the chemical from which they are constructed, DNA or deoxy-ribose-nucleic acid.

Carbohydrates

Carbohydrates from our diet give us the most readily available source of energy. One gram will provide up to 17kJ (kilojoules) of energy. To give you an idea how much that is in terms of what we need, eight hours of sleep will use up 2,400kJ just to keep the heart beating, the lungs breathing, the body warm, the brain functioning at an unconscious level and the various chemical changes taking place that support life; this is known as our basal metabolism.

There are two sorts of digestible carbohydrates: simple and complex. The more complex they are, the longer they take to digest and the more slowly the energy is released. The simple carbohydrates consist of sugars: sucrose from sugar cane and beet, glucose and fructose from fruits and honey, maltose which is found in beer, and lactose from milk. All of these are easily digested and enter the bloodstream rapidly to provide quick energy sources.

It takes approximately 7lb(3kg) sugar cane to make 1lb (0.5kg) refined sugar, while a large beet will yield just one teaspoon. In order to extract our table sugar, therefore, most of the natural plant material is taken away, including all its fibre and all of its naturally occurring vitamins and minerals. All that is left are empty calories in the form of sucrose; no nourishment is provided. This is the problem. Nature never intended us to eat such stuff, yet the average Westerner consumes around 2lb (1kg) of this concentrated sickliness per week. Our bodies are not biologically adapted to cope with it and the consequences include all sorts of metabolic problems in addition to tooth decay and obesity. And do not be misled into believing that brown sugar is better for you; a lot of it is simply white dyed brown with caramel.

If we take in more energy than we need in the form of simple carbohydrates, then the body will store it as glycogen in the liver for later conversion into glucose, or as fat under the skin and around the abdomen. This is why sugar causes obesity. To obtain just one teaspoon of sucrose, you should really be munching your way through a whole beet! It would take you a very long time to put on fat this way, if at all. We were never meant to saturate ourselves with the sort of concentrated doses of energy that sugar provides. Of course it makes us fat. Take your sugar in the form that nature intended, from fruits.

Weight gain, however, does not generally occur with the other sort of carbohydrates – the complex ones. These are very good for us and are found in whole cereals (such as wholemeal flour and brown rice), peas, beans and lentils, and potatoes. You can eat all of these knowing that they are nourishing you well and providing you with a well-regulated and gradual release of energy.

There is yet another form of carbohydrate: dietary fibre. Although this is not a nutrient as such, it is now considered to be very important for our health. Basically it is made up of the structural cell walls of plants consisting largely of cellulose. Humans do not produce or take in enzymes that can digest cellulose, so this roughage reaches the intestine without having been absorbed by the body. The colon contains various beneficial bacteria that can utilize some of the plant cell walls and produce some fatty acids from them. However, most importantly, the roughage adds bulk to the waste matter here, which speeds it on its way through the gut, so preventing the accumulation of unhealthy bacteria. It also helps the contents of the intestine to retain water, which softens the stools. This way constipation is avoided, along with many other diseases of the bowel, some very serious, such as cancer of the colon.

Fats

Fats and oils (often referred to as 'lipids' by scientists) are also used by the body to provide energy. The problem here is that one gram of fat gives us more than twice the amount of energy (37kJ) as the same weight of either carbohydrates or protein. Needless to say, if the energy is not quickly utilized it will be stored as fat in our own bodies. Thus we are more than twice as likely to put on weight if we eat fats rather than other foods.

Yet our cells need lipids for the creation and maintenance of part of their membranes. Fatty acids are available in two forms: either saturated, mainly from animal sources (the hard sort), or polyunsaturated, chiefly found in fish and plants (liquid or soft at room temperature). Of the second group linoleic and linolenic are necessary for the maintenance of our bodies and these are called essential fatty acids (EFAs) or occasionally vitamin F. They cannot be made inside us, so we must obtain them from food, mainly from vegetable seed oils, for example safflower seed and linseed. Ideally they should constitute a minimum of 2 per cent of our total calories, equivalent to four tablespoons of sunflower seeds daily. Signs of deficiency include dermatitis, wounds that are slow to heal and hair loss.

Our bodies are able to make all other essential lipids from carbohydrates and proteins. We do not need saturated fats from animals at all. In fact we are far better off without them, since long-term intake results in serious degenerative diseases, especially of the cardiovascular system. Like sucrose, all they give us are empty calories without nourishment. Worse, they put a strain on our bodies trying to deal with them and raise our blood cholesterol to damaging levels; polyunsaturated fatty acids (PUFAs) have the reverse effect. Fat from meat, therefore, is best avoided.

Hydrogenation

The war between margarine manufacturers and butter producers continues to wage. So which really is the best for us? We all know how delicious real butter is, scraped on to warm toast, or dripping through hot crumpets. But the sad fact is that butter is composed of the saturated fat that our bodies are happier and healthier without. So does this mean that margarine is preferable? Not necessarily.

In order to solidify the plant oils, they are put through a process called hydrogenation, which turns them into transfatty acids; in other words they lose the beneficial properties of the unadultered oils. Indeed the transfatty acids have a similar effect on our bodies as saturated fats. Some of the better-quality margarines contain small amounts of pure oils that have been added back, which are of a little value, but the best margarines of all are those that have not been hydrogenated. You will almost certainly have to take a trip to your local health food store to find these. Have a close look at the tub and make sure it reads 'non-hydrogenated' before buying it.

Proteins

We have to take in protein from our diet to build our own body structures, such as muscle and bones, and to act as transport systems in the blood, as well as to cover our internal organs and tissues in the form of skin. Several types are needed for parts of our cells, including the membranes, mitochondria and chromosomes. Proteins can also be used for energy, in which case they release about the same amount as carbohydrates.

The molecules of proteins are formed from chains of substances called amino acids. The precise arrangement of these determines what sort of protein it is. When we eat proteins, our digestive system breaks them down into their basic amino acids, and then our cells put them back together again in a different order to form the proteins that they need. Cells, in their amazingly clever way, can also swap amino acids and thereby change one kind of protein into another.

There are eight amino acids that we cannot do without and which our own bodies cannot manufacture. We must therefore take in all of these on a regular basis from our diet. If even one is missing, the effectiveness of the others will be lowered, since they work in cooperation with each other. These are: leucine, isoleucine, lysine, methionine (and its relative cystine), phenylalanine, threonine, tryptophan and valine; a ninth, histidine, is essential for infants.

The amount of protein necessary depends on our general state of health, our size and age: growing young people require more than sedentary adults. The recommended daily allowance (RDA) in the UK is set at 72g for a moderately active young man, although a recent report from the World Health Organization suggests only 0.57g per kg of body weight, or about 40g for a 70-kg (11-stone) man; US recommendations are 10 to 15 per cent higher than this. We almost certainly eat far too much. In fact a survey in Germany connected cancer of the pancreas with excess protein consumption.

Contrary to popular belief, the very best source of protein is the soya bean, which contains more than twice as much as meat without the saturated fat. Substituting textured soya protein or tofu or tempeh for your meat portion will therefore give you the protein you require without harming your heart and other body systems.

If you choose proteins of animal origin, including lean meat, poultry, fish, eggs, milk and cheese, they will contain all the essential amino acids, and for this reason they are sometimes termed 'complete' proteins. This unfortunately gives the impression that they are better for you than plant proteins, which are sometimes described as 'incomplete'. What it does mean is that you need to select your plant

BEST SOURCES OF PLANT PROTEINS

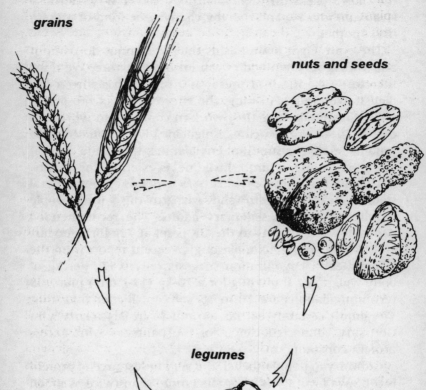

grains

nuts and seeds

legumes

  combination creates high-quality usable protein

 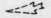 combination generally gives less complete protein, unless legumes are also included

proteins with some care to ensure that you are taking in all eight essential amino acids (EAAs). The main sources of plant protein are: whole grains such as wheat, rice and millet; legumes (beans, lentils, peas); and nuts and seeds. If you combine grains with legumes or legumes with nuts and seeds in the same meal, you can't go wrong. For example rice with beans, or lentil croquettes with a peanut sauce, will each provide you with your eight EAAs. If you combine grains with nuts or seeds, however, also have legumes, such as peas, in the same meal to ensure completion of the protein (see diagram opposite).

Enzymes

If you cut an apple in half and leave it open to the air for a while, it will turn brown. It is the action of enzymes that have brought about this change. If, however, you boil the cut pieces the apple will not go brown because enzymes die if exposed to high temperatures.

Enzymes are proteins that operate as catalysts; in other words they help a chemical reaction to take place, but they are not themselves changed in the process. Indeed they will move on to do another job and many more after that. Without being consciously aware of it, we humans depend on enzymes to release energy from food and keep our cells alive. They are made of protein and they are put together from amino acids inside cells.

Enzymes work in two principal ways: either they assist in the joining up of molecules to form another substance, or they break molecules down into smaller parts. For example two glucose molecules when joined together will form maltose; yet the enzyme in saliva called amylase can break down starch molecules into sugar in a matter of seconds. When enzymes break down glucose (which consists of carbon, hydrogen and oxygen) inside a cell, the waste product carbon dioxide is formed, together with water. During this reaction, energy is released to help drive the cell, to take part in other reactions or to keep the body warm.

From this you will understand what important proteins enzymes are. Without them, many of our biochemical reactions could not take place at all, or only at a very slow pace. Chemical changes that would take days or weeks on their own are brought about in seconds through the presence of enzymes. In order to create these vital substances, our cells need to be fed the correct amino acids, and eight of these, as we have seen, have to come from our food in a reliable supply.

Certain enzymes can be purchased in supplementary form to assist those with poor digestion.

Supplementary amino acids

Amino acids have marvellous healing properties and several are available in the form of supplements, in the same way as vitamins and minerals. Prescribing amino acids for therapeutic use is still relatively new and much research needs to be done, but their importance cannot be over-emphasized. Our cells are able to manufacture more than 100,000 different proteins out of varying chains of amino acids with a very wide range of functions, from the creation of structural parts of the body to assistance with the production of hormones. The following are the most commonly prescribed for particular conditions. It is better to take supplements in their pure form, denoted by the prefix 'L'; 'D' indicates synthetic production. Rather than consuming with meals, swallow them on an empty stomach with water for the best effect. Never take as a substitute for food.

A general amino acid complex supplement may well be helpful when digestion is impaired through illness or old age. Vegans and vegetarians who may be low on some dietary proteins could also benefit.

Caution Never take a single supplement for more than a few weeks without professional advice as this may cause an imbalance with other amino acids. They are not recommended for pregnant women.

L-Arginine. A semi-essential amino acid that stimulates the secretion of the growth hormone, so it is very important for children. It also helps to put on muscle and is therefore often included in body-building programmes.

Dosage Up to 4g daily.

Caution Supplements are not recommended for schizophrenics or anyone with kidney or liver problems. May worsen symptoms of the herpes virus unless taken with at least equal amounts of L-lysine.

Healing qualities Can help cancer patients by inhibiting tumour growth and boosting the immune system. Provides relief for some arthritics. May treat male infertility by normalizing sperm production. Speeds up the healing of wounds.

Sample food sources (in g per 100g) Wheatgerm (5.4), pumpkin seeds (3.71), peanuts (3.37), almonds (2.36), brazil nuts (2.23), dried milk (1.57), pheasant (1.40), turkey (1.37), chicken (1.30), lean beef (1.15), fish (1.14), free-range eggs (0.97), Cheddar cheese (0.93), oat flakes (0.58), yoghurt (0.20), peas(0.05).

L-Cysteine. Made in the body from L-methionine and L-serine, but this process is often hindered by chronic diseases, so useful as a supplement for sick people. Combines with vitamins C and B_1 to protect cells from damage by radiation, or aldehyde found in tobacco smoke or smog, also from the harmful by-products of rancid fats. Stimulates the macrophages in the immune system. Involved in fatty acid metabolism. Prevents low blood sugar by blocking insulin response. It is related to, but not the same as, L-cystine, which is not an antioxidant.

Dosage Begin with 500mg and gradually increase to up to 2g daily. Take with three times the amount of vitamin C.

Caution Not suitable for diabetics.

Healing qualities Clears mucus from the bronchial tissues, therefore greatly assists anyone suffering from bronchitis,

emphysema or TB. Important for strong, thick hair (some 12 per cent is cysteine). Keeps the skin youthful. Together with calcium pantothenate can treat arthritis. May help hypoglycaemics by steadying blood sugar. Detoxifies the system from the effects of alcohol and other ingested poisons.
Sample food sources (as cystine) (in g per 100g)
Wheatgerm (5.4), sesame seeds (0.52), sunflower seeds (0.43), pistachio nuts (0.44), peanuts (0.32), free-range eggs (0.37), free-range chicken (0.30), lean beef (0.20), cottage cheese (0.12), lentil sprouts (0.26), soya beans (0.14).

L-Glutamine. Takes part in many biochemical processes and is found in enzymes and other body proteins. An important energy source for the brain in the form of L-glutamic acid. Also assists in the production of hydrochloric acid in the stomach.

Dosage Up to 2g daily. Best taken with B complex.

Healing qualities Heals peptic ulcers. Reduces alcohol and sugar craving, therefore helpful to people giving up drinking or losing weight. May alleviate some mental disorders and drug dependence.

Sample food sources (as glutamic acid) (in g per 100g)
Wheatgerm (11.22), Cheddar cheese (6.00), almonds (5.62), sunflower seeds (5.35), sesame seeds (4.95), halibut (3.08), free-range poultry (3.00), lean beefsteak (2.84), soya beans (2.79), free-range eggs (1.93), low-fat yoghurt (0.71), corn (0.65), avocado (0.42), jacket potato (0.40), dried figs (0.30), dried peaches (0.24), peas (0.14).

L-Histidine. Widely distributed in body proteins. Involved in the production of histamine, also of gastric juices and neurotransmitters.

Dosage Take with vitamin C. Up to 2g daily; double for rheumatoid arthritis patients.

Caution Not suitable for manic depressives or schizophrenics. Doses in excess of 4g can induce menstruation in women.

Healing qualities Used in the treatment of those with rheumatoid arthritis, who have very low levels of histidine.

Sample food sources (in g per 100g) Wheatgerm (1.88), Cheddar cheese (0.87), pheasant (0.80), lean beefsteak

(0.63), peanuts (0.73), sunflower seeds (0.61), almonds (0.53), free-range chicken (0.60), organic liver (0.54), cod (0.52), soya beans (0.40), free-range eggs (0.37), low-fat yoghurt (0.09).

L-Lysine. Essential for children's growth and development and involved in the repair of tissues and energy production.

Dosage Up to 1,500mg daily in small amounts.

Healing qualities Helps treat herpes simplex, especially if taken with vitamin C. Alleviates migraine, also tiredness and poor concentration.

Sample food sources (in g per 100g) Wheatgerm (4.14), Parmesan cheese (3.28), halibut (1.89), pumpkin seeds (1.69), free-range chicken (1.68), lean beef (1.46), free-range eggs (1.1), peanuts (0.97), soya beans (0.89), almonds (0.63), low-fat yoghurt (0.32), dried figs (0.14), jacket potato (0.14).

Enemy Reduced if heated with sugar.

L-Methionine. A powerful antioxidant, protecting cells from free-radical damage, and helps remove toxic heavy metals from the body. Important for blood proteins.

Dosage Up to 1g. Always take with vitamin B_6 and magnesium.

Caution Doses of 5g or more can cause vomiting.

Healing qualities Used to treat overdoses of paracetamol (but must be taken within 10 hours). Helps to protect against anaemia. May reduce blood cholesterol. Thought to mitigate some symptoms of schizophrenia. Acts as an antihistamine if taken with calcium.

Sample food sources (in g per 100g) Wheatgerm (1.25), Parmesan cheese (0.95), brazil nuts (0.95), sesame seeds (0.89), halibut (0.61), free-range eggs (0.50), free-range chicken (0.47), lean beef (0.41), soya beans (0.18), low-fat yoghurt (0.11).

Enemy Food preservative, sulphur dioxide.

L-Phenylalanine. Involved in the production of adrenaline, dopamine and noradrenaline. Affects blood pressure, oxygen use, blood glucose levels, action of the central nervous system and many metabolic processes.

Dosage 100–500mg daily. Must be taken with vitamins B_6 and C. As D-phenylalanine (DLPA): 750mg three times daily; up to double for pain relief.

Caution Do not use with MAO-inhibitor drugs (antidepressants). Not advised for hypertensives or pregnant women.

Healing qualities Improves the memory and mental alertness. Can treat depression. Useful for slimmers as it controls hunger. As DLPA an effective pain killer, especially if taken with vitamins B_6 and C over a period of time.

Sample food sources (in g per 100g) Wheatgerm (2.68), sesame seeds (1.51), peanuts (1.43), Cheddar cheese (1.31), pistachios (1.01), halibut (0.81), free-range chicken (0.80), lean beef (0.66), soya beans (0.66), low-fat yoghurt (0.20), avocado (0.13).

L-Tyrosine. Made in the body from the essential amino acid L-phenylalanine. Involved in nerve impulses and the control of mood. Neutralizes free radicals.

Dosage Up to 3g daily; double for severe depression over short periods.

Caution Do not take with antidepressants (MAO inhibitors). Not suitable for melanoma patients.

Healing qualities Thought to improve the memory and mental alertness. A proven antidepressant. Reduces symptoms of hay fever.

Sample food sources (in g per 100g) Wheatgerm (2.04), dried milk (2.01), Parmesan cheese (2.00), halibut (0.70), almonds (0.67), pistachios (0.61), free-range chicken (0.66), free-range eggs (0.63), lean beef (0.54), soya beans (0.53).

Enemy The contraceptive pill.

Vitamins: basic facts

Vitamins are chemical compounds that are essential to human life. We simply cannot live without them, even though some are needed in very small amounts. Since we can only manufacture 3 of the 13 known vitamins in our own bodies in sufficient quantities to meet our needs, all the others must be supplied from food. Each has a particular role to play in regulating important chemical reactions through which the body is able to convert food into energy and living tissues. They also work in cooperation with each other, so that a deficiency in one can impair the function of another.

Vitamins are generally divided into two groups by scientists: the fat-soluble ones (A, D, E and K) and the water-soluble ones (B-complex and C). They can be extracted from their natural sources and made into pills or powders for use as supplements, but these in no way replace food; indeed they generally need to be taken with food. Nor are they drugs.

To encourage people to continue buying their supplements, some manufacturers turn them into chewable goodies. I was shocked to see that certain capsules contained the artificial sweeteners aspartame and saccharin as well as hydrogenated vegetable oil, all of which have been linked with health problems. Avoid these sort of confections and purchase supplements that contain just the nutrients you need together with any necessary filler or binder or natural protective coating; these might include calcium phosphate, calcium or magnesium stearate, cellulose, gum arabic, silica or zein, all of which are acceptable. Tablets and capsules should be sugar-free and devoid of any artificial flavourings or preservatives. If you are allergic to gluten, milk (lactose) or yeast, check that these substances are not included.

'Food state' supplements are more readily assimilated by the body, so that lower dosages can be taken. The full chemical names for all the nutrients should be included on the label, together with the actual amount contained in the pill. Some vitamins imported from America are measured in international units (IU) in terms of their biological activity as follows: 1 microgram (mcg) of vitamin A =

3.3IU, 1mcg of vitamin D = 40IU and 67mg of vitamin E (as d-alpha tocopherol) = 100IU.

Essential vitamins required every day in order to maintain health are listed below alphabetically, together with important points about each. The recommended daily allowance (RDA) given is the amount of each vitamin regarded as basic for good health in the average adult. This needs to be adjusted according to body weight, so that children will generally need less except when stated, while pregnant women may need more (their special needs are detailed in chapter 18). Since the amounts differ slightly between countries, the highest has been selected. 'Megadoses' are more than ten times this figure. While the RDA is helpful as a general guide, people vary greatly as to their requirements, depending on their genetic make-up as well as their lifestyle. For example, people under stress will use up far more vitamin C than the RDA, as will those who smoke. Some experts regard the RDAs as inadequate and currently Suggested Optimal Nutrient Allowances (SONAs) are being introduced; figures for these are given below if available.

Fatty meats have not generally been included under 'Sample food sources' if there are others, equally nutritious.

Vitamin A. Found only in animal sources, e.g. egg yolk, milk and liver. Its chemical name is retinol. However, vegans need not worry as several plants contain carotenes, such as carrots and some green vegetables, which the body then converts into vitamin A. In fact water-soluble beta carotene is the best way of taking it, as high doses of retinol in the oily form are stored in the liver and can be toxic if taken in excess.

Vitamin A is essential for the health of the eyes; it actually forms the visual purple, a pigment in the retina, which helps you to see in dim light. So the old saying that carrots help you see in the dark really is true! The vitamin is also vital for the growth of bones and teeth and for the health of the skin, helping to produce mucous secretions that protect against infections. Recent research indicates that carotenoids protect against cancer.

RDA 2,650IU/800mcg (EU and USA). **SONA** 6,600IU. Safe dosage of beta-carotene up to 50,000IU, of retinol up to 5,000IU.

Caution Vitamin A in the oily form as retinol is toxic in high doses and is therefore not recommended as a supplement for lengthy periods.

Healing qualities Can be applied externally to treat skin disorders, such as acne, boils and ulcers. Helps remove age spots. Assists weak eyesight. Aids in the treatment of emphysema and hyperthyroidism. Protective against cancer.

Sample food sources (in mcg per 100g). As retinol: halibut-liver oil (60,000), cod-liver oil (18,000), organic liver (9,300–18,100), fortified margarine (900), butter (750), free-range egg yolk (400), Cheddar cheese (310), salmon (90), mackerel and herring (45). **As carotene:** carrots (12,000), dandelion leaves (8,400), parsley (5,100), spring greens (4,000), sweet potatoes (4,000), dried nori seaweed (3,888), spinach (3,600), watercress (3,000), mangoes (2,334), cantaloup melon (2,000), apricots (1,500), pistachio nuts (1,374), pumpkin (648), tomatoes (600).

Note To obtain retinol equivalents, divide carotene figures by 6.

Enemies High temperatures, especially frying, but survives ordinary cooking; and oxygen (but protected from oxidation by vitamin E); also light. Drying and canning reduce carotene levels in vegetables and fruit.

Vitamin B complex. Was first thought to be a single vitamin, but eight are now identified as being essential for humans, with some others required by animals only. They cannot be stored in the body and need to be replaced daily. They work in cooperation with each other, so that an excess of one can cause a deficiency in another. Any single supplement needs to be balanced with the complete complex, therefore, and B_1, B_2 and B_6 should be supplied in equal amounts.

Vitamin B₁ or thiamin. It is necessary for growth, good appetite and healthy nervous and digestive systems. The body requires it to release energy from carbohydrates. Its removal from foods due to refining causes the fatal disease beriberi; the vitamin now has to be put back into white bread by law.

RDA 1.5 mg (USA). **SONA** 7.1mg. Safe dosage up to 100mg. No known toxicity.

Healing qualities Cures beriberi. Beneficial when anxious or stressed. Important for the muscles and nervous system. Can be used in the treatment of herpes zoster.

Sample food sources (in mg per 100g) Marmite (3.10), spirulina seaweed (3.00), sunflower seeds (2.30), pine nuts (1.25), peas (1.0), dried prunes (0.53), oatmeal (0.50), rye (0.40).

Enemies This vitamin is unstable and destroyed by baking soda when heated, hence the advisability of making cakes without a raising agent. Also destroyed by sulphite preservatives. About 25 per cent is lost in cooking, generally with up to 40 per cent from boiled vegetables, so use that water up in soups and sauces. Some loss through food processing and storage.

Vitamin B₂ or riboflavin. This vitamin is important for growth and for healthy skin and eyes. It helps the body use oxygen efficiently when converting food into energy.

RDA 1.7 mg (USA); slightly more for adolescent males and lactating women. **SONA** 2mg. Safe dosage up to 100mg. No known toxicity. Note that urine may turn yellow with extended high doses, but this is harmless.

Healing qualities Alleviates sore or cracked mouth, swollen lips or tongue and scaly skin around the ears and nose. Eye fatigue can be helped especially if sensitive to light. Generally good for the skin, nails and hair.

Sample food sources (in mg per 100g) Marmite (11.0), brewer's yeast (4.25), lamb's liver (4.40), lamb's kidney (2.30), spirulina seaweed (3.70), nori/laver seaweed (1.34), dried parsley (1.23), almonds (0.92), cream cheese (0.73), wheatgerm (0.72), goat's milk (0.63), wild rice (0.63), free-range eggs (0.47).

Enemies Destroyed by light, therefore do not leave your milk on the doorstep unless it is put in a dark container. Leaches into cooking water, so save that vegetable stock. Like B_1, destroyed by baking soda.

Vitamin B_3 or niacin; also nicotinic acid, niacinamide and nicotinamide. Especially important for normal brain function and the health of the nervous system, for conversion of carbohydrates into energy and also for the synthesis of the sex hormones, as well as insulin, cortisone and thyroxine. The body can make its own niacin with the assistance of the amino acid tryptophan, but only if vitamins B_1, B_2 and B_6 are present.

RDA 19mg (USA); 20mg adolescent males and lactating women. **SONA** 25mg. Safe dosage up to 1,000mg as nicotinamide or 100mg as nicotinic acid. Toxic at three times these amounts. Tingling and flushing may occur, but these are not harmful.

Caution Diabetics and people with peptic ulcers or damaged liver, or with glaucoma are advised not to take megadoses of niacin.

Healing qualities Cures pellagra. Promotes healthy digestive system and can alleviate gastro-intestinal problems and sometimes bad breath. Can ease migraine headaches. Increases circulation and reduces high blood pressure and cholesterol. Cuts down vertigo in Ménière's syndrome. Can help to reverse negative personality changes. Good for the skin.

Sample food sources (in mg per 100g) Brewer's yeast (37.50), rice bran (29.80), lamb's liver (15.2), tuna fish (15.0), spirulina seaweed (12.8), turkey (10.0), halibut (9.0), mackerel (8.7), red salmon (5.5), raw mushrooms (4.0), cooked broad beans (3.0), raw peas (2.5).

Enemies Lost in cooking water unless reused, and food processing, but stable to heat. Sulpha drugs, sleeping pills, the contraceptive pill and alcohol all have a negative effect.

Vitamin B_5 Better known by its chemical name, pantothenic acid. Also referred to as panthenol or calcium pantothenate. Involved in carbohydrate and fat metabolism and helps to create antibodies. Essential for functioning of adrenal glands. Important for growth, cell building and a healthy nervous system. This is one of the few vitamins that can be made in the body through the action of intestinal bacteria.

RDA 6mg (EU). Safe dosage up to 1,000mg. No known toxicity.

Healing qualities Fights infections and aids healing of wounds. Helps reduce side-effects of antibiotics. Can alleviate arthritic pain. An antidote to stress. If combined with vitamin C can cure some allergies.

Sample food sources (in mg per 100g) Brewer's yeast (9.50), organic lamb's liver (7.60), lamb's kidney (4.20), free-range egg yolk (4.60), wheat bran (2.40), peanut butter (2.10), raw mushrooms (2.00), salmon (1.80), lobster (1.63), soya flour (1.80), watermelon (1.55), hazelnuts (1.50), lentils (1.40), chicken (1.20), avocado (1.07), Stilton cheese (0.71).

Enemies Up to 40 per cent lost above boiling point. Leaches into cooking water. Destroyed by freezing. Harmed in food processing and canning. Caffeine, sulpha drugs, sleeping pills, the contraceptive pill and alcohol all have detrimental effects.

Vitamin B$_6$ or pyridoxine. Closely concerned with the metabolism of protein, so you will need extra if you are a heavy meat eater (but let's hope you are not!). Needed to produce effective antibodies and red blood cells. Works in cooperation with zinc.

RDA 2mg (USA and EU). **SONA** 10mg. Safe dosage up to 100mg. May be toxic at 500mg.

Caution Do not take if you suffer from Parkinson's disease and are being treated with L-Dopa.

Healing qualities Quells nausea including morning sickness. Reduces night cramps and numbness or tingling in the limbs, also premenstrual tension. A natural diuretic. Has anti-ageing properties. Helpful with skin and nervous disorders. Boosts the immune system.

Sample food sources (in mg per 100g) Brewer's yeast (4.20), wheatgerm (3.30), mackerel (0.84), haddock (0.35), organic beefsteak (0.33), free-range chicken (0.26), avocado

(0.50), bananas (0.50), dried fruits, especially currants, sultanas and prunes (0.26–0.30), tempeh (0.29), raw Brussels sprouts (0.28), raw leeks (0.25), raw red cabbage (0.21), raw broccoli (0.21).

Enemies Up to 50 per cent lost in juices through boiling, roasting or stewing unless reclaimed. Also lost through food processing, canning and long storage. Alcohol and the contraceptive pill have adverse effects.

Vitamin B$_{12}$ or cobalamin. This vitamin is needed to make red blood cells and the fatty myelin sheath around nerves. Together with folic acid it takes part in the synthesis of DNA (deoxy-ribo-nucleic acid) which governs the activities of each cell. Vegans can be deficient in this vitamin since its main sources are animal products, although it is present in yeast extracts; B-complex supplementation which includes this vitamin may therefore be advisable, otherwise there is a danger of pernicious anaemia and damage to the nervous system. Only very small amounts are needed and it is stored in the liver. Calcium aids absorption.

RDA 2mcg (UK and USA). 2.2mcg during pregnancy and 2.6mcg during lactation (USA). **SONA** 2 mcg. Extra needed if very large doses of vitamin C are being consumed. Safe dosage up to 1,000mcg. No known toxicity.

Healing qualities Along with folic acid prevents megaloblastic anaemia and is used to treat pernicious anaemia. Keeps the nervous system healthy. Good for the memory and sense of balance. Combined with folic acid promotes vitality and a feeling of well-being, thus relieving bad temper. Important for growth and appetite in children. Together with other B vitamins can ease menstrual flow.

Sample food sources (in mcg per 100g) Lamb's liver (81.00), lamb's kidney (79.00), mackerel (12.00), yeast extract (8.8), soya cheese (2.50), free-range eggs (2.40), lean beef (2.00), Mozzarella cheese (2.10), skimmed milk (0.40), tempeh (0.84), miso (0.21).

Enemies Stable to heat, but destroyed by acids and alkalis. Damaged by sunlight, the contraceptive pill, sleeping pills and alcohol.

Biotin. Occasionally referred to as vitamin H or coenzyme R, biotin is really a member of the B complex. It helps the body to change fats into fatty acids, which in turn aids energy production. Important for growth and for the maintenance of the nervous system, also for keeping the hair, skin, reproductive organs and bone marrow healthy. Another vitamin that is made in the intestines.

RDA 150mcg (EU). Safe dosage up to 3,000mcg. No known toxicity.

Healing qualities Slows down greying of the hair. Can prevent and heal eczema and dermatitis.

Sample food sources (in mcg per 100g) Free-range chicken liver (170.00), brewer's yeast (80.00), free-range egg yolk (50.00), wheatgerm (25.00), oatmeal (20.00), herring (10.00), mackerel (8.00), Camembert cheese (7.60), avocado (3.20), blackcurrants (2.40), raw leek (1.40).

Enemies Raw egg white prevents its absorption. Antibiotics and sulpha drugs, the contraceptive pill, alcohol and food processing are biotin destroyers. Up to 30 per cent is lost in cooking through discarded juices, unless reclaimed.

Folic acid or folacin. Another member of the vitamin B complex, although without its own number. Required to make certain components of DNA and RNA, it is therefore involved in passing on hereditary characteristics. Needed to make red blood cells and significant for growth and healthy nervous and digestive systems. It is stored in the liver until required.

RDA 300mcg (UK); 400mcg for pregnant women (USA).

SONA 800mcg. Safe dosage up to 3,000mcg. May be toxic at 15,000mcg.

Caution Megadoses may not be suitable for people who suffer from convulsions or cancer with a hormonal basis.

Healing qualities Prevents spina bifida and megaloblastic anaemia. Improves lactation. Protects against food poisoning. Good for the skin and an antidote to stress.

Sample food sources (in mcg per 100g) Organic chicken liver (500), soya flour (345), wheatgerm (331), raw endive (330), dark-green leafy vegetables (90–140), dry butter beans

(110), peanuts (110), Camembert cheese (102), almonds (96), cucumber (96), free-range eggs (51), kidney beans (50), beetroot (50).

Enemies Serious losses result from food processing, canning, leaching into cooking water, reheating, sunlight and long-term storage. Sulpha drugs and the contraceptive pill have damaging effects.

Vitamin C or ascorbic acid. Many animals make their own, but humans cannot, so frequent intake in the diet is vital. It is best absorbed in conjunction with bioflavonoids. It plays a part in the creation of collagen, a protein that holds tissues together and so is essential for the health of bones, cartilage, blood vessels, teeth and gums. Also needed for the synthesis of certain hormones and the effective absorption of iron from vegetables. Supplements should be taken in divided doses.

RDA 60mg (EU and USA). **SONA** 400mg. Safe dosage up to 5,000mg daily.

Caution Do not suddenly cease megadoses as 'rebound scurvy' can occur; gradually reduce amounts. Very high doses at around 20,000mg for extended periods may create kidney stones.

Healing qualities Prevents scurvy. Aids healing of wounds and bleeding gums. Boosts the immune system and prevents infections. Controls cholesterol levels. Promotes longevity. Protective against cancer.

Sample food sources (in mg per 100g) Acerola cherries (1,000–2,330), rosehips (1,250), blackcurrants (200), parsley (150), raw broccoli (110), raw green peppers (100), kiwi fruits (98), raw Brussels sprouts (90), lemons (80), oranges (71), strawberries (60), watercress (60), raw red cabbage (55).

Enemies Very unstable to all cooking, food processing and canning, particularly if copper, iron or nickel are employed. At least 60 per cent destroyed by heat, oxygen, baking soda and through leaching. Therefore, eat vegetables raw in salads. Smokers beware: each cigarette kills off 25mg of vitamin C. City dwellers also need extra as carbon monoxide impairs this vitamin.

Vitamin D. Calciferol or ergocalciferol (vitamin D_2) is produced in plants when exposed to UV light, while cholecalciferol (D_3) is formed in the skin of humans and animals in the same manner, hence the term 'sunshine vitamin'. The right amount is essential for healthy bones as it stimulates calcium and phosphorus absorption.

RDA 5mcg/200IU (EU and USA); more for dark-skinned people in northern latitudes and double for housebound adults and children. Safe dosage up to 1,000IU. Toxic at 2,000IU.

Caution Stored in the liver, therefore toxic with prolonged intake. Best obtained naturally rather than through supplementation.

Healing qualities Helps prevents rickets, osteoporosis, osteomalacia and severe tooth decay.

Sample food sources (in mcg per 100g) Cod-liver oil (210.00), herring (22.50), mackerel (17.50), salmon (12.50), tuna (5.80), free-range egg yolk (5.00), dried skimmed milk (2.10).

Enemies Smog. Destroyed in foods by light, oxygen and acids.

Vitamin E. Prevents polyunsaturated fatty acids in membranes and other body structures from harmful oxidation (i.e. combining with oxygen). Neutralizes the effect of free radicals (cancer-causing agents). Keeps the red blood cells healthy and prolongs their life. Selenium increases its potency. Best taken as d-alpha tocopherol with oily foods.

RDA 10mg/15IU (EU and USA); **SONA** 400IU. More for pregnant or lactating women or those going through the menopause. Safe dosage up to 800IU. May be toxic at 1,500IU.

Caution High-dose supplements are not advised for patients with rheumatic heart condition. Diabetics or those with an overactive thyroid or high blood pressure should build up amounts gradually and should not exceed 400mg daily.

Healing qualities A natural anticoagulant. Can be applied externally to reduce scar formation. Contributes to youthfulness of tissues. Alleviates fatigue through efficient use of oxygen. Increases fertility and helps prevent miscarriages.

Sample food sources (in mg d-alpha tocopherol per 100g) Wheatgerm oil (133.00), wheatgerm (22.00), hazelnuts (21.00), cold-pressed sunflower-seed oil (49.00), maize oil (11.00), soya-bean oil (10.00), olive oil (5.00), margarine (8.00–25.00), peanut butter (4.70), grapes (4.00), blackberries (3.50), avocado (3.20), free-range egg yolk (3.11), butter (2.00), spinach (2.00), parsley (1.80).

Enemies Freezing, so do not freeze bread. Food processing, commercial cooking and deep frying. Chlorine in drinking water. Ferrous sulphate, inorganic iron, employed in some vitamin pills destroys vitamin E (check the labels and choose an organic iron, e.g. ferrous citrate).

Vitamin K. K_1 (phylloquinone, phytylmenaquinone or phytonadione) is obtained from foods, while K_2 is formed in the intestines through the action of bacteria. K_3 (menadione or menaphthone) is a synthetic. This vitamin is concerned with the proper clotting of the blood.

RDA 70–140mcg (USA estimated). Safe dosage up to 600mcg. Toxic at 1,000mcg.

Healing qualities Can prevent coeliac disease and colitis. Protects against internal bleeding and haemorrhages. Helps control menstrual flow. Aids in the healing of nose bleeds.

Sample food sources Available in fresh leafy green vegetables, especially broccoli, spinach, cabbage and lettuce, also alfalfa and kelp. Yoghurt is another source.

Enemies Antibiotics prevent its formation in the intestines. Decomposed by baking soda and other alkalis, also aspirin. Radiation, freezing and food processing destroy it, as does light.

Minerals and trace elements

Like vitamins, these have particular physiological functions and are therefore vital to health. Those that are required in significant amounts are: calcium, chloride, magnesium, phosphorus, potassium and sodium; others are used in only tiny amounts of less than 100mg and are often referred to as trace elements. These include chromium, cobalt (as vitamin B_{12}), copper, iodine, iron, manganese, molybdenum, selenium and zinc.

Much has still to be discovered about the precise biochemical activities of minerals. Apart from sodium, potassium and chloride, which are easily absorbed by the body, most minerals can only be utilized with the assistance of carrier proteins. When you buy them in the form of supplements, therefore, check that the word 'chelated' appears on the label. This means that the mineral is attached to something that aids absorption, such as an amino acid. Gluconates, aspartates and citrates work in a similar way. Be especially careful when buying minerals in the form of compounds. For example a 100mg tablet of zinc orotate may contain only 15mg of elemental zinc, and it is this lower figure which you need to know.

Calcium. Humans contain a large amount of this mineral in their bodies, more than any other, some 2 to 3lb (1 to 1.4kg), most of it in the bones and teeth. It is constantly being lost and replaced, at the rate of about 700mg a day. It is obvious, therefore, that good dietary sources are vital. The small amount in the soft tissues and fluids helps to regulate nerves, muscles and hormones, and the clotting of blood. Best absorption is achieved if there is twice as much calcium as magnesium, and when vitamin D is available. Take chelated or as dolomite, with protein food.

RDA 800mg, including children 1–10yrs; 1,200mg 11–24yrs (EU and USA); 1,200mg during pregnancy and lactation and 1,000–1,500mg during menopause. Safe dosage up to 1,500mg. Toxic at 4,000mg.

Healing qualities When well absorbed, prevents rickets, osteomalacia and osteoporosis; also tetany (muscular twitching). Keeps bones and teeth strong. In conjunction with magnesium ensures a regular heartbeat. Alleviates insomnia in some people. Good for the nerves. Helps women who suffer from menstrual cramps.

Sample food sources (in mg per 100g) Whitebait (860),

cheese (720), spinach (600), whole sardines (550), nori and kelp seaweed (357), parsley (330), dried figs (280), almonds (250), watercress (220), salmon (196), spring onions (140), free-range egg yolk (130), skimmed milk (120), raw broccoli (100), tempeh (93).

Enemies Oxalic acid (in chocolate and rhubarb) and phytic acid (in unleavened bread) prevent absorption, as do too much fat and phosphate food additives. Excess salt increases its loss in the urine.

Chloride.
It forms the hydrochloric acid used to digest food. Helps regulate the acid/alkaline balance in the blood plasma.

RDA 750mg (USA estimated). Supplements unnecessary since the average intake from salt is too high.

Healing qualities Aids digestion. Checks loss of hair and teeth. Preventive against renal disease.

Sample food sources (in g per 100g) Salt (60.7), Marmite (6.60), shrimps (5.8), olives (3.75), Danish blue cheese (2.39), kippers (1.52), dried hijiki seaweed (1.40), wholemeal bread (0.86).

Enemies Sweating and vomiting.

Chromium.
Works with insulin to metabolize sugar. May also assist in the metabolism of fats. Chelated supplements are available. A good form to take is chromium gluconate, especially with protein food.

RDA 50–200mcg (USA estimated). Safe dosage up to 2,000mcg. Excess intake harmful.

Healing qualities Helps prevent diabetes and arteriosclerosis. Useful to hypoglycaemics. Aids growth. Regulates high blood pressure and blood fats.

Sample food sources Shellfish, lean meat, free-range chicken, fruit, brewer's yeast. Cooking in stainless-steel pans contributes to uptake.

Enemies Tea, coffee and smoking hinder absorption.

Cobalt.
This mineral is contained in vitamin B_{12} and is important for the health of red blood cells. Vegans may be deficient in it.

RDA 8mcg (estimated). Safe dosage up to 1,000mcg. Toxic in prolonged high doses, which may cause enlargement of the thyroid gland.

Healing qualities Helps prevent anaemia.

Sample food sources Lean organic meat and liver, shellfish, free-range eggs.

Enemies Same as B_{12}.

Copper. Approximately 100mg are stored in the human body, mainly in the liver, kidneys and brain. After being converted into enzymes in the liver, it is used to help the body absorb iron and to produce red blood cells. Works in cooperation with zinc. Supplements are rarely necessary, but if they are take ten times the amount of zinc simultaneously.

RDA 1.5–3mg suggested (USA). Safe dosage up to 20mg. Toxic at 50mg.

Caution Supplements are not recommended for anyone with Wilson's disease.

Healing qualities Protects against anaemia. Can relieve arthritis in some cases.

Sample food sources (in mg per 100g) Oysters (7.6), organic lamb's liver (8.70), crab (4.80), soya flour (3.12), cashew nuts (2.20), tofu (1.70), butter beans (1.22), lentils (0.58), parsley (0.52), walnuts (0.31), peanuts (0.27), wholemeal bread (0.27), mackerel (0.19).

Enemies Excessive intakes of zinc can reduce copper absorption.

Iodide/Iodine. An essential non-metallic mineral, of which about half is stored in the thyroid gland, which in turn controls the metabolism. If the soil is low in this mineral, local populations may suffer from goitre, an enlargement of the thyroid gland. Long-term deficiency can result in mentally retarded, underdeveloped children.

RDA 150mcg (from 11 yrs); pregnant women 175mcg rising to 200mcg during lactation (USA). Safe dosage up to 1,000mcg (WHO). No known toxicity.

Healing qualities Helps to control weight and keeps energy levels up. Improves mental capacities. Cures simple goitre and certain cases of hypothyroidism. Protects against radiation.

Sample food sources (in mcg per 100g) Iodized salt (3,100), seaweeds and haddock (120), yoghurt (63), free-range eggs (53), cheese (20–58).

Enemies Depleted soil. (The cabbage family contains substances that are goitrogenic in animals: excessive raw cabbage may inhibit iodine absorption.)

Iron. More than half the body's iron helps to constitute the haemoglobin of red blood cells, and a much smaller amount the myoglobin in muscles, both transporters of oxygen to the body's tissues. Some is involved in the creation of enzymes that assist in the release of energy from food. About one-quarter is stored as ferritin for future use. Red blood cells live for only about 120 days, after which they are remade using ferritin from the bone marrow. Iron is necessary for the proper assimilation of B vitamins. Women can often be iron deficient due to menstrual loss. Take the ferrous forms of supplements, with food.

RDA 12mg; 15 mg for menstruating and lactating women; 30mg during pregnancy (USA). Safe dosage up to 60mg. Toxic at 100mg.

Caution High doses are poisonous to children. Just 3g ferrous sulphate could be fatal.

Healing qualities Prevents and cures iron-deficient anaemia. Protects against disease via healthy blood cells. Good for the skin. Enhances energy and stimulates the appetite.

Sample food sources (in mg per 100g) Dried hijiki seaweed (29.00), organic liver (7.00–21.00), pumpkin seeds (15.00), cocoa (10.50), soya flour (9.10), black molasses (9.20), wheatgerm (8.50), parsley (8.00), lentils (7.60), minced beef (7.00), millet (6.80), haricot beans (6.70), free-range egg yolk (6.10), cashew nuts (6.00), peaches, apricots and dried figs (4.06–4.20), oatmeal (4.10), spinach (4.00).

Enemies Coffee and tea depress its absorption (tannins form insoluble salts with iron), as do phytates in unleavened bread and phosphates in eggs. Excess manganese.

Magnesium. Present in all living cells and necessary for the synthesis of proteins, nucleic acids, fats and carbohydrates. Especially important for muscle contraction and the health of the nervous system. Chelated supplements are available, or take as dolomite with protein food.

RDA 350mg; 600mg for pregnant women; 355mg for lactating women; 400mg for adolescent males (USA). Safe dosage up to 1,000mg. Toxic at 2,000mg.

Healing qualities Keeps the muscles in good trim. Promotes a healthy cardiovascular system. Relieves indigestion (a natural antacid). Counteracts depression. Helps prevent kidney stones and gallstones.

Sample food sources (in mg per 100g) Sage (428), brazil nuts (410), fennel seeds (385), soya flour (290), wheatgerm (270), cashew nuts (260), peanut butter (180), Marmite (180), oatmeal (110), shrimps (110), wakame seaweed (107), dried figs (92), tempeh (70), broccoli (60), Parmesan cheese (45).

Enemies Alcohol. Diuretics. High intakes of protein, calcium and phosphate can inhibit absorption.

Manganese. Up to 20mg of this essential mineral is stored in the bones, liver and kidneys. It helps to produce enzymes that are involved in the creation of cartilage components. It also activates other enzymes that ensure the utilization of biotin and vitamins B_1 and C. Assists in the production of thyroxine and is important for the proper function of the central nervous system. Take supplements as gluconate or orotate with protein food.

RDA 2–5mg estimated (USA). Safe dosage up to 15mg. May be toxic at 30mg.

Healing qualities Helps prevent ataxia (lack of coordination). Good for the memory. Keeps exhaustion at bay. Alleviates dizziness. Contributes to the health of the skeleton.

Sample food sources (in mg per 100g) Wheatgerm (12.30), split peas (8.00), oatmeal (3.70), soya flour (2.90), pineapple (1.60), tempeh (1.43), wakame seaweed (1.40). Present in tea.

Enemies Large amounts of phosphorus (including phosphate preservatives) and calcium can prevent absorption.

Molybdenum. Functions as part of several enzymes concerned with the metabolism of carbohydrates and fats, also the utilization of iron.

RDA 150–500mcg estimated (USA). Safe dosage up to 1,000mcg. Toxic at 1,500mcg (associated with gout).

Healing qualities Improves health of teeth. Helps prevent anaemia.

Best food sources Whole cereals, dark-green leafy vegetables.

Enemy Depleted soil.

Phosphorus. Present in all living cells and all natural food. In the human body the bones contain the most, up to 900g. It needs twice as much calcium to operate effectively. It is involved with many metabolic processes and biochemical reactions, as well as the transference of nerve impulses. Necessary for the absorption of niacin.

RDA 800mg adults and 1–10yrs; 1,200mg 11–25 yrs and for pregnant or lactating women (USA).

Healing qualities Keeps the heart and kidneys functioning well. Important for strong bones, teeth and healthy gums. Helps prevent rickets. Assists in growth and tissue repair. Promotes vitality. Cuts down arthritic pain.

Sample food sources (in mg per 100g) Brewer's yeast (1,750), yeast extract (1,700), pumpkin seeds (1,189), wheatgerm (1,050), whitebait (860), Parmesan cheese (810), soya flour (640), brazil nuts (607), basil (490), rolled oats (405), lamb's liver (400), prawns (350), goose (270), sirloin beef (244), sweetcorn (130), dried apricots (120), peas (83).

Enemies Antacids. Too much iron, magnesium or aluminium.

Potassium. Works inside the cells to balance water content and to regulate nerve and muscle functions. Activates various enzymes.

RDA 2,000mg estimated (USA). Safe dosage up to 5,000mg. May be toxic at 10,000mg.

Caution Potassium supplements are inadvisable for people with poor kidney function.

Healing qualities Keeps the brain clear and muscles and reflexes working well. Helps to lower blood pressure. Prevents excess fluid retention and useful for treating hypoglycaemia (low blood sugar).

Sample food sources (in mg per 100g) Brewer's yeast (1,900), dried figs (1,010), kelp (978), wheatgerm (950), almonds (860), raisins and sultanas (860), pumpkin seeds (817), dates (750), jacket potatoes (550), halibut (518), spinach (490), raw mushrooms (470), chick peas and butter beans (400), tempeh (367), bananas (350).

Enemies Coffee, too much salt, alcohol, diuretics.

Selenium. This essential trace element works in collaboration with vitamin E. They are both antioxidants; in other words they prevent damage to cells and premature ageing due to oxidation. Any supplements are best taken on an empty stomach. Just how much is available in the diet is dependent upon the soil in which the food is grown. For example, there is usually more in crops grown in America than in Britain.

RDA 70mcg (USA). Safe dosage up to 1,000mcg. Toxic at 3,000mcg.

Healing qualities Helps maintain youthful skin and trim muscles. Useful for treating dandruff. Protective against heart disease and cancer. May relieve menopausal symptoms. Important for the immune response.

Sample food sources (in mcg per 100g) Wholemeal bread (35.00), mackerel (35.00), Cheddar cheese (12.00), soya flour (11.00), free-range eggs (11.00), almonds (4.00), oatmeal (3.00), garlic (2.00), skimmed milk (1.00).

Enemies Depleted soil. Food processing.

Sodium. Essential as this mineral is, people in the West are dying from too much of it. It is a major cause of high blood pressure and heart disease. There is no need to have salt on the table or to add it to cooking, as sodium is widely available in many natural foods. There is also far too much of it in processed fare, especially meats and condiments, which should be avoided.

Of the 92g or so found in the human body, most is divided between the bones and the body fluids. It regulates the fluid balance, preventing excessive loss, and it also governs various functions of the nerves and muscles.

RDA 500mg estimated (USA). Supplements are not recommended since intake is already too high, causing serious potassium loss.

Healing qualities Prevents heat exhaustion. Helps to keep the muscles and nerves in good order. Usually stops cramp.

Sample food sources (in mg per 100g) Baking powder (11,800), Tamari soya sauce (5,160), gherkins (4,633), salt (3,876), miso (3,647), yeast extract (900–4,500), olives in brine (2,250), dried seaweed (872–2,500), bacon rashers (2,140), Feta cheese (1,440), kippers (990), canned salmon (509–570), wholemeal bread (550), peanut butter (350), lobster (330), raw celery (140), carrots (95), skimmed milk (50).

Enemy Heavy sweating.

Zinc. This is an important trace element, part of or closely involved with more than 70 enzymes, some of which are required for the production of DNA, RNA and also for the synthesis of protein. Among its many activities it is essential for healthy reproductive organs and for a balanced brain. It takes part in the formation of insulin and helps maintain the acid–alkaline balance in the body. It also affects the way muscles contract and is involved in immunity. Supplements are available as gluconate, orotate or sulphate and are best taken on an empty stomach.

RDA 15mg from 11yrs (EU and USA). More for lactating women. Safe dosage up to 60mg. Toxic at 400mg.

Caution If you have a risk of cardiovascular disease, do not take high doses of zinc (100mg or more) for prolonged periods, as the beneficial blood fats (i.e. the HDLs) may be reduced.

Healing qualities Its presence in saliva enhances taste.

Useful for the treatment of infertility. Controls cholesterol deposits. Can prevent diabetes by contributing to the formation of insulin. Maintains the health of the prostate gland. Eases menstrual flow. Can be used in the treatment of schizophrenia. Helps keep the brain alert. Speeds up healing of wounds. Boosts immunity. Eliminates white spots on the nails.

Sample food sources (in mg per 100g) Oysters (45.00), other shellfish (5.30–7.20), wheatgerm (17.00), organic lean beef and lamb (5.30), soya flour (3.90), miso (3.32), oatmeal (3.00), cheese (1.60–2.30), tempeh (1.81), free-range eggs (1.30), lentils (1.00), butter beans (1.00), peas (1.00), parsley (0.90), brown rice (0.70), raw broccoli (0.60).

Enemies Food processing, depleted soil, excessive perspiring (up to 3mg per day can be lost), phytate in unleavened bread.

Water

Those of us who live in countries where water is plentiful often take it for granted. The turn of a tap brings it gushing forth and we can put the kettle on and make as many cups of tea as we like. In fact we have to remind ourselves that we cannot live without it.

In hot countries dehydration, often through excessive loss of water in diarrhoea, especially among children, causes countless deaths. Most of our cells contain about 75 per cent water and they will quickly die if this level falls. Indeed water plays an important part in a host of their chemical reactions. Being a good solvent many nutrients can be carried about the body in the watery fluid of the blood. Waste substances can also be excreted in water via the kidneys.

As we all know, water regulates our temperature by cooling our bodies in the form of perspiration. We also lose it when we breathe out and of course when we urinate. We must therefore replenish this loss in our diet. Make sure you drink plenty (ideally at least 3 pints/1.5 litres daily and preferably filtered) so that your body can function efficiently.

Chapter 4

Poisons

During the months spent researching this book, I have been building a library of cuttings from quality newspapers relating to the subject. Most noticeable has been the number of headline stories concerning environmental pollution and ill health. Subjects covered include the connection between certain active ingredients of household insecticides and childhood brain cancer, the link between low sperm count in men and chemical pollutants, and the damage caused to human health and the world's life-support systems through relentless ozone erosion.

This makes depressing reading. Not only is human activity destroying our atmosphere and our earth, it is inevitably threatening our own species. In attempting to make our lives more comfortable and 'civilized', we have upset the very delicate balance of nature on which all life depends. To correct this now will take enormous political will, as yet hardly discernible, despite the constant campaigning of environmental groups. Meanwhile we have to cope with the situation as best we can, either by avoidance of polluting factors or, where this is impossible, by using nutrients to help expel toxins from our bodies.

Household chemicals

Perhaps the areas where we have greatest control of household chemicals are our own homes and gardens, yet we may not be fully aware how many hazardous substances are occupying our cupboards and sheds. Anything which is designed to kill small creatures, or other living organisms such as fungi, is also likely to be harmful to you and your family. The children mentioned in the newspaper article who have died from brain cancer were exposed to commonly used household pesticide sprays, flea collars on pets, garden and orchard insecticides and herbicides for the control of weeds. As we know, such chemicals are freely available in shops and stores. The death of a child is truly a terrible price to pay for the convenience of not having to brush cats and dogs daily or to pull up weeds by hand.

Some 70,000 chemicals are currently used in the home or in industry. A proportion of these is relatively benign, some are beneficial, but huge numbers are harmful, even if used correctly, and many are extremely hazardous. Take a look in your cleaning cupboard and ask yourself just how many of the bottles, aerosol cans and tins of substances there are truly necessary. No doubt magazine and television advertising combined with attractive packaging have encouraged you to buy them, but wouldn't a mild detergent and warm water work just as well in most cases? Apart from the money saved, you will be greatly reducing your risk of exposure to damaging chemicals, which can cause health problems ranging from skin irritation to cancer, or even, in some cases, death from inhalation of toxic fumes. For example if an acidic type of toilet cleaner (often based on sodium hydrogen sulphate) is mixed with bleach, a powerful reaction takes place, releasing dangerous chlorine gas into the air which, if breathed in, can be fatal.

On the subject of toilets, never use the freshener blocks designed to be inserted into the bowl or cistern. These frequently contain paradichlorobenzene, a chlorinated hydrocarbon which, apart from being a persistent environmental pollutant, is linked with liver disorders in humans and is known to be carcinogenic to animals. A bowl of potpourri or a sweet-smelling plant are natural alternatives that are both attractive and harmless. The same applies to air fresheners and fabric conditioners and other chemicals which have synthetic perfumes added, such as limonene which has a lemony smell. These all contain hydrocarbons, some of which cause cancer in animals. Several air freshener blocks work by inhibiting your ability to smell, which may leave you feeling spaced-out or hazy. It is far safer to open the window!

Stain removers are generally based on solvents, which give off fumes. When breathed in, chemical vapours quickly enter the bloodstream, via the lungs, and can place a large strain on the body's natural detoxification processes in an attempt to expel them. Most cause extreme irritation to the skin and eyes. Speedy immersion of stained articles in cold water followed by washing with warm water and detergent is a risk-free method – even so, wear rubber gloves. Baking soda is an alternative. Salt can also be a helpful cleaner.

There has been a high incidence of breast cancer among women who work in the dry-cleaning industry. Whenever possible buy clothes and furnishing fabrics that can be washed to avoid bringing hazardous fumes into your own home.

All oven-cleaners are dangerous. They are based on sodium hydroxide, or caustic soda, which is extremely toxic and corrosive. The aerosol type is particularly nasty because of increased risk to the eyes. Washing soda is much gentler, but even this can remove a layer of skin, so don't forget those gloves. Salt sprinkled on spills on the floor of the oven aids their removal.

At last some manufacturers, such as Ecover, are marketing safe cleaning products which are also environmentally friendly, so always choose these.

It is also wise to be careful in your selection of cosmetics. Talcum powder, which can be absorbed through the skin,

71

is thought to be responsible for some ovarian cancers and hair dyes are linked with breast cancer; go for natural henna or vegetable dyes that are harmless. Even shampoos may contain formaldehyde, an allergen, irritant and most probably a carcinogen. As for deodorants, many are based on aluminium chlorohydrate which can irritate the skin especially if grazed. Although the link between aluminium and Alzheimer's disease is currently disputed, this metal can depress your immune system. The best way to get rid of body odour is to have a good wash with a natural vegetable soap!

*

How about the contents of your garden shed? The range of toxic chemicals here can be ferocious yet none is really necessary. Moreover, pesticides will kill off many predators also, which you really need to encourage as your allies. For example the larvae of hoverflies are reliable aphid eaters, so attract these with the nectar that they most like, that of the poached egg plant, *Limnanthes douglasii*. Thrushes will demolish snails, while frogs and hedgehogs will eat unwanted slugs.

There are innumerable alternatives to outdoor chemicals, including ways of controlling diseases and weeds, which any good book on organic gardening will explain to you. While you are at it, make space for some vitamin-rich organic vegetables, such as carrots, spinach and broccoli, which will build up good health and protect against serious disease.

*

With the increase of DIY activities at home, people are now being exposed to yet more noxious chemicals. While painting our house, the glands in my neck began to swell alarmingly. It was a full two months before they had subsided to their normal size. I now seek out non-toxic paints from small companies, discovered through advertisements in Green magazines.

It is far better to cure the source of any dampness rather than cover it up with a damp-proofing fluid. This is likely to release hydrocarbon vapours which can cause coughing, irritation of the membranes and headaches.

Timber treatment uses chemicals that are among the most hazardous for the average DIY person. Some neighbours in our village had the beams of their fine fifteenth-century farmhouse injected with a kind of gel, which later oozed from the wood and had to be cleaned off by hand. The farmer's wife took on this job herself. Shortly afterwards she began to have trouble with her legs; each time she tried to take a step, her knees appeared to give way, resulting in an uncontrolled lurch. The doctors were mystified, but a neurologist eventually diagnosed damage to her central nervous system and identified the timber treatment as the cause. It is all too easy to become the unwitting victim of poisoning such as this. Do not take the risk.

Protective nutrients

Your susceptibility to the ill effects of pollutants and poisons will depend considerably on your nutritional status. People who are well supplied with vitamins and minerals on a regular basis in their diet are less likely to be harmed. The trace element selenium is particularly important in this respect. Animal studies show that it has a protective effect against most toxins. Even the herbicide paraquat, which has been responsible for wiping out thousands of hares, is less deadly to an animal which has been given selenium supplements. Wholemeal bread is a reliable source, as long as the wheat has not been grown in a soil-eroded area. If in doubt take a supplement of around 200mcg daily. Wholewheat also contains vitamin E which works in cooperation with selenium and enhances its effectiveness.

Zinc is another protective mineral because it is used by the body in the repair of DNA and RNA, which are often attacked by pollutants. If you are likely to be exposed to chemicals, a supplement of 15 to 20mg daily should be helpful. Eggs are a good natural source, as is wheatgerm. Include pumpkin seeds in your muesli or eat them as a snack with raisins; they are rich in minerals. Increase your vitamin A intake also by eating yellow fruit and green or yellow vegetables. This will augment the efficacy of the zinc.

Poisons described so far are mostly avoidable, so this is the obvious route to take. But what of environmental pollutants that we cannot so easily evade?

Clean water?

The water that runs from our taps looks clear enough, but aluminium has probably been used to clean it. Not long ago, some children on holiday in the south-west of England were affected by the accidental release of excessive amounts of aluminium into the local water supply. Resulting disorders included eczema, bowel complaints, listlessness and even speech problems. Filtration would be far safer, but of course this costs more. So people in Britain drink water that frequently exceeds aluminium levels permitted by EU regulations. If you suspect that this is happening, then increase your intake of calcium, iron and zinc (see chapter 3 for best foods); deficiency in these will allow greater absorption of aluminium. Recent research at Keele University shows that silicon prevents its uptake. This is available as a supplement. Use of a good home filter will also help to get rid of it.

Because of sewage contamination, water authorities have to use chlorine to kill off bacteria in supplies. Such treatment has been common for many years, but we now know that chloroform can be produced in peat districts or when chlorine reacts with other organic matter. This is linked to cancers of the colon, rectum and bladder.

Areas of arable farming are particularly vulnerable to high levels of nitrates in the water, which have leached into supplies from artificial fertilizers and from intensive

74

livestock units, as well as from the ploughing itself. Levels frequently exceed World Health Organization limits. After entering the body, nitrates change into nitrites which then combine with amines from our food. The compounds thus formed, nitrosamines, are carcinogenic and known to cause stomach cancer.

If the vegetables and other food plants have not fully utilized the nitrates to make protein, then we will also consume them this way – another good reason to eat organic produce, which is not saturated with artificial fertilizers. Other sources of nitrates are sausages, bacon, ham and pies containing cured meats. These are definitely not good for you, so stay off them and select your proteins from healthier sources, especially organic and vegetarian.

If you live in a region of intensive farming where your water supply is likely to be contaminated, then increase your intake of vitamin C from a good natural source such as an orange a day, and fresh tomatoes, green pepper and watercress in your salad. Give yourself extra protection with a supplement of at least 500mg. Vitamin C prevents the formation of those harmful compounds, the nitrosamines. Also select a water filter that removes nitrates; some do not. Of course the best thing of all that you can do is to campaign for a return to organic farming. This way we will all benefit from healthier food and water.

Many people have been concerned about the addition of fluoride to tap water to prevent tooth decay. Though now less popular, this is still practised in some regions and there is currently a renewed call for more widespread treatment in the UK from the Minister for Health. Any food processed in such places is also likely to contain fluoride. If the water is soft, then it is much more likely to be absorbed along with other unwanted minerals such as aluminium. The problem with fluoride is that it interferes with the chemistry of the body, in particular upsetting the action of enzymes. Research papers have been published linking it with cancer and in poorer countries with infant deaths. It is sad indeed, and unethical, that because some people are unable to give up sweets to prevent caries, others are forced to drink fluoridated water and endanger their health.

If you live in a fluoridated area, use a good water filter and make sure your intake of healthy minerals is adequate, especially calcium: whole sardines, cheese, skimmed milk, yoghurt, spinach and almonds are all excellent sources. Check that consumption of magnesium, zinc and iron is also sufficient (see chapter 3 for best foods). These will inhibit your absorption of unwanted minerals such as fluoride.

An alternative to filtering your water is of course to buy natural spring water in bottles, but this is expensive. Choose varieties that come from deep underground or from pure glacial regions, which are less likely to be contaminated. Reliable brands will give full descriptions on their labels.

Extreme measures had to be taken by an inhabitant of a village near ours. He had been suffering from severe headaches and nausea over a period of some three years. He noticed that the symptoms vanished during a trip to Sweden and therefore suspected an allergen, but patch testing at a specialist London hospital produced negative results. Finally he made the link with the tap water and had a well dug in his garden, since when he has been free from the distressing symptoms.

Fresh air?

Not far from where we live there is a tiny hamlet called Sibton. It is quaintly rural in character, with a handful of old cottages standing by a stream, each with a somewhat rickety bridge across it to reach the road. The inn is a favourite with local farmers, who gather round the roaring log fire on cold winter evenings exchanging news and jokes, various somnolent dogs and cats at their feet. Indeed, the place is a picture of English tranquillity, with green fields on all sides. It is some 10 miles (16 km) from the nearest small town and a good 35 miles (56km) from a large one. Yet even here air pollution levels have exceeded WHO safety guidelines on a regular basis, especially on hot summer days when low-level ozone increases, putting asthmatic children at great risk.

Without question the motor vehicle is largely responsible for our poor air quality. The average car spews out more than its own weight of air pollutants every year. Despite encouragement through lower prices to run cars on lead-free petrol, lead poisoning, especially among city children, is still rife. This damages the nervous system and blood and cell development, resulting in poor intelligence and other disorders. Additional poisonous substances from car exhausts include carbon monoxide that causes exhaustion and irritability and, in large doses, death; nitrogen dioxide impairs the function of lungs and increases susceptibility to viral infections; hydrocarbons irritate the eyes and throat, causing coughing; benzene is a carcinogen; aldehyde results in breathing difficulties; and acid aerosols induce asthma and bronchitis. Considering these appalling effects on our health, combined with deaths and deformities from thousands of accidents, the seductive advertisments which we regularly witness on our TV screens for these killers can only be described as repulsive. Yes, cars give us increased freedom of mobility, but can such a severe price ever be justified? Catalytic converters will help a little, but the continuing demand for yet more vehicles will quickly outstrip their benefits. In Mexico City the air is so vile that they sell oxygen from roadside booths at two dollars a shot. Is this how we want to live?

Well-nourished children and adults are more able to fend off the toxic effects of a heavy metal such as lead because certain nutrients will attach themselves to it and help expel

77

it from the body. Vitamin C and calcium work in this way, as do the amino acids methionine and cysteine. Zinc is also antagonistic to lead because it prevents its absorption in the intestine. If lead poisoning is suspected, therefore, increase the intake of oranges, grapefruit, peaches, grapes and bananas, eat lots of fresh salad with tomatoes and peppers and drink skimmed milk. Eat wholemeal bread and add wheatgerm to your breakfast dish. Have fish or poultry with your main meal. Additionally take at least 1g of vitamin C daily as a supplement together with 30mg zinc gluconate. Consider including 500mg L-methionine together with lesser amounts of vitamin B_6 and magnesium for two to three weeks.

Remember that there are other sources of lead poisoning, for example through food grown or displayed by a busy road. Some older houses may also still have lead piping to carry drinking water.

As far as smoking is concerned, only one rule applies if you value your health: don't. As we all know (but will rarely admit), cigarettes are lethal: they cause death by lung cancer, stroke, chronic bronchitis and emphysema, and coronary heart disease. They also contribute to many other diseases by lowering the body's resistance and depriving it of essential nutrients. Other directly related cancers are of the mouth, larynx, oesophagus, pancreas, kidney, bladder and cervix. Richard Peto of the Imperial Cancer Research Fund reckons that out of 1,000 young male smokers, one will be murdered, six killed in traffic accidents and 250 will die of smoking. This does not include peripheral vascular disease, which will most likely result in amputation of the legs, nor does it include birth defects in babies of smoking mothers. Despite dire warnings, smokers seem unable to grasp how appallingly destructive their habit is, not just to themselves but to others also.

Unfortunately it is impossible to avoid passive smoking on certain occasions. The immediate effect of a smoke-filled room, which contains too much carbon monoxide and insufficient oxygen, is the slowing down of brain activity. Long-term exposure greatly increases the risk of lung cancer and respiratory diseases as well as heart disease.

It is possible to help protect yourself with the antioxidant nutrients, especially vitamin C. Eat plenty of citrus fruits, kiwi fruit and fresh salads and take a vitamin C supplement of at least 1g daily (depending on the degree of exposure). The other antioxidant vitamins are A and E, so include a raw carrot in your salad and add a dressing containing cold-pressed sunflower or olive oil. If you sprinkle wheat-germ on your muesli then you will increase your vitamin E intake and at the same time obtain valuable amounts of the antioxidant minerals selenium and zinc.

You may not realize that your air at home or at work may be polluted by formaldehyde, a toxic gas released by some types of cavity wall insulation, also by chipboards and plywood, and by carpet backings. Low levels can cause headaches and irritation to the eyes and throat, and pro-longed exposure leads to cancer in animals. If this gas is likely to be present, make sure you have good ventilation and that chipboards are sealed. Spider plants are reputedly able to neutralize the gas. An ioniser may be helpful, too.

Radiation

In March 1986 operators at the Chernobyl nuclear power station in the former Soviet Union unwittingly allowed the water pressure to fall during a safety test. This resulted in a violent burst of reactivity and, within a second, power had increased almost five-hundredfold, blowing the lid right off the reactor. Millions of curies of dangerous radioactive material blasted into the atmosphere, contaminating vast areas of land as far away as Corsica. Shortly afterwards heavy rain spread the contamination to Western Europe.

Four years later a physicist from Newcastle University was measuring Chernobyl fallout levels in humans in Britain and his unit came to our local town for a week. I went along as a volunteer. After assuring me that no harm would result from the scanning equipment, I was asked to lie on the hard couch beneath it. Its movement was almost imperceptible as it took a full twenty minutes to scan my entire body. Although I had to keep my position, I was allowed to talk, so took the opportunity of asking questions that had been bothering me for some time. I explained that in 1986 I had encountered a personal disaster of my own, having found myself with breast cancer. Knowing how damaging radiation could be I had accepted the standard treatment of 5,000 rads of radiotherapy with considerable trepidation. Many Japanese had died from doses of only one-tenth this amount after the atomic bomb was dropped on Hiroshima. As a result of the Chernobyl accident, thousands of people have perished or will die prematurely from cancer and leukaemia. Currently more than 40,000 children in one nearby town alone have serious maladies ranging from thyroid cancers to birth defects. How was it that I was still walking around? He explained that certain areas of the body, especially the gastrointestinal tract, are more vulnerable to ionising radiation than others. If only a fraction of the 5,000 rads had been delivered in one go over my whole body, it would have killed me outright. But because it was given over six weeks on a small area in a controlled way, my body was able to cope with it. It was a relief to be able to talk so frankly; no one at the hospital would answer such searching questions truthfully, although one doctor did at least tell me how it worked: cancer cells are weaker than healthy ones and divide more rapidly, so they are most likely to be killed by the X-rays.

As a child I was brought up near the nuclear power station Windscale (now Sellafield), in Cumbria, and almost certainly drank milk contaminated in 1957 by an accidental release of radionuclides which fell on to the grass that was subsequently eaten by the cows. Could that have contributed in part to my later susceptibility to cancer? Some of the problem in assessing the risk of radiation doses is that it can be many years before mutated cells can be detected in the form of a tumour. Sometimes it is the following generation that suffers due to defective genes; childhood leukaemia around Sellafield is ten times the national average.

Radiation is both mysterious and frightening because you can neither see, smell nor taste it. Moreover, governments have an atrocious record of covering up the true facts of accidental releases and therefore cannot be trusted. Most of our knowledge comes from committed pressure groups and university researchers such as the one who had turned up in our locality. He explained that the Chernobyl fallout had a particular 'fingerprint' of caesium-137 which could be distinguished from any other. Yes, indeed, it was present in my body at the expected amount – too low, happily, to cause any damage. How had it arrived there? Almost certainly through the food I had eaten, even if it had been produced in Britain. Pollution in the form of radioactive fallout has total disregard for national boundaries.

Nutritionally, the best protection from ionising radiation is potassium iodide, which is distributed to people at risk in the case of a nuclear accident. By saturating the tissues of the thyroid gland with healthy iodine, it is possible to guard it against damage from radioactive iodine. Its best source is kelp, so if you live near a nuclear power plant or are likely to be suffering from unwanted radiation, then sprinkle some regularly on your soup. Another delicious seaweed is nori, which can be bought in flakes. Remember that nuclear power stations emit radioactive contaminants on a regular basis into the air and sea, which can be breathed in or consumed in food. Also take the antioxidant vitamins A, C and E and the minerals zinc and selenium which help to defend against injury to cells caused by free radicals, likely to occur if you are exposed to radiation. See the previous chapter for food sources. An additional dosage, for short periods only, of the amino acids cysteine and glutathione of 1g daily in divided doses, taken with orange juice, will give special protection to cells at times of need. Russian scientists advocate Siberian ginseng.

Not all radiation is artificially produced: 10 per cent comes from cosmic rays and 47 per cent from radon gas that emanates from uranium in the ground, especially present in granite areas. In other words we are exposed to it throughout our lives. Small doses of sunshine are of course good for us, but the thinning of the protective ozone layer in our atmosphere, mainly due to reckless release of chloro-fluorocarbons (CFCs) from aerosols, with an even bigger threat from halon in fire extinguishers, is becoming increasingly problematic. The extra ultraviolet radiation causes skin cancer and eye cataracts, it weakens the immune system, spoils crops and kills plankton. In most countries rates of skin cancer are increasing at 3 to 7 per cent per annum and in Australia death rates from this disease have risen by a factor of five in the past 50 years. Make sure you apply an effective suncream to block out UV radiation if you spend prolonged periods out of doors, and wear dark polaroid glasses to shield your eyes.

If you live in a granite area, keep your house well ventilated and have it tested for radon. Remedial work may be necessary to keep it out. As radon decays it forms short-lived radioactive particles which remain suspended in the air. If these are inhaled they irradiate the lungs, leaving them prone to cancer.

Despite much resistance from the public and a few of the more enlightened supermarkets, even some food is irradiated now in Europe to kill off bacteria. Unfortunately it also kills off up to 70 per cent of some vitamins. Always select food that is truly fresh.

Our modern way of life also subjects us to non-ionising, low-level radiation, notably from TV screens and microwave ovens that leak. Sit well back from the television, since there is evidence to suggest that long-term exposure to low-level radiation may cause blood disorders and genetic damage.

TVs, computers, overhead power lines and many other twentieth-century gadgets are surrounded by electro-magnetic fields, creating an electrical 'smog'. Biologists think that this could be interfering with the delicate electrical activity inside our cells, increasing the likelihood of mutation. Mobile phones are also under suspicion. One man is suing a particular production company, claiming that his wife died of a brain tumour that developed near the spot where her phone antenna was located. If you honestly cannot avoid this kind of pollution, then do take the antioxidant nutrients mentioned above.

Food contamination

Approximately one gallon (4.5 litres) of pesticides is sprayed on the fruit and vegetables consumed by the average person in one year. Although we have a marvellous natural detoxification system in our bodies, we are not biologically adapted to deal with such an array of poisons, traces of which inevitably end up inside us. Our own species, *Homo sapiens*, has been evolving for around 500,000 years, but poisonous chemicals have been used to control pests for only the last few decades. Because our livers do not know what to do with certain artificial chemical residues, they store them in our body fat. Here they can accumulate to produce health problems later.

In the Third World, where pesticides are often used indiscriminately, there are more than 10,000 deaths every year from poisoning, according to a recent calculation from Oxfam. In the developed world there are occasional deaths and a great many health problems attributed to pesticide poisoning, ranging from allergies and headaches to breast cancer and low sperm count.

It is hardly practicable to examine the body fat of humans for stored poisons, but fish can easily be analysed. In October 1991 Friends of the Earth published results of a survey of the contamination of freshwater fish with toxic chemicals from agriculture and industry. In 238 fish at 62 locations in the UK, 19 different toxic compounds were found at levels above government health guidelines or expected levels. Some fish contained a cocktail of poisons: for example an eel taken from the River Severn contained lindane (a wood preservative), dieldrin and cyfluthrin (both pesticides), and an eel from the River Frome contained DDT, TDE and dieldrin (all pesticides) and mercury, each over the respective standard. This is particularly worrying because DDT and dieldrin are officially banned, but obviously still used illicitly. Wildlife that depends on fish, such as otters and herons, will eventually die due to a build-up of toxins. This is known as bioaccumulation. If we eat the fish, then the poisons will also accumulate inside us. Thus, creatures (including humans) at the head of the food chain will suffer most.

Sadly, freshwater fish caught in the wild is generally no longer safe to eat in this respect. Nor are inshore fish, especially flat ones, because they are frequently polluted by heavy metals and industrial chemicals discharged into the sea. It is safest, therefore, to buy deep-sea fish, such as cod and haddock. Meat is also not free from this sort of contamination as pesticide residues find their way into animal feed. Antibiotics are added, too, in an attempt to prevent disease in their unhealthily crowded conditions. If you eat meat, choose organic or free-range produce only. It is worth the higher price.

Fruit and vegetables that come from abroad are more likely to be sprayed with extra chemicals, for example to delay ripening or to prevent potatoes from sprouting. Pesti-

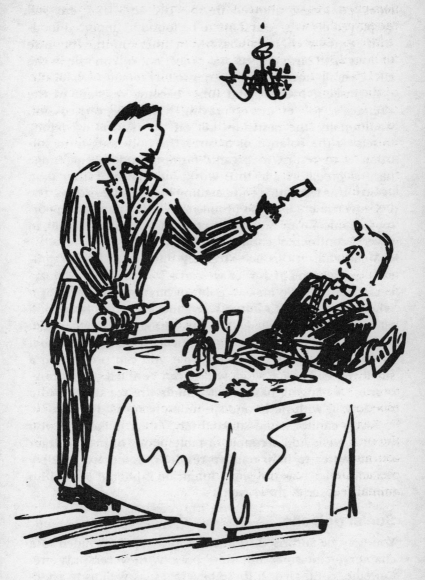

'A very wise choice, sir – it complements the pesticide perfectly!'

cides no longer allowed in the UK and USA are still employed elsewhere and are to be found in imported food-stuffs. Equally, chemicals banned in other countries because of links with birth defects and cancer are still on sale in the UK. Overall, however, it is better to buy food grown locally.

As insects, bacteria and fungi become resistant to the chemicals, so yet more spraying has to be carried out. Additionally, the pesticides kill off the natural predators, upsetting the balance of nature. The only long-term solution is to return to organic farming and to encourage natural predators and thus work with nature rather than against it. After much campaigning by pressure groups, the UK government is at last promising a little financial support for organic farmers, support that has been available in several continental countries for some time.

Meanwhile it can be extremely difficult to find organically grown food at a price we can afford. Some supermarkets stock it, so do make a point of buying it and ask for it when unavailable. Alternatively, make friends with local allotment-holders or, better still, grow your own fresh vegetables and fruit. This way you can be sure of food that is wholesome. It is surprising what you can produce in a small space. Even a window box can be filled with strawberries, a hanging basket with miniature tomatoes and a windowsill with herbs and sprouting beans and grains.

If you cannot avoid sprayed food, then make sure you wash it well. Add a couple of tablespoons of malt vinegar to the water to help remove residues. Some are horribly tenacious, such as the waxy fungicide 2-phenyl phenol on lemons, so scrub them well.

Social poisons

You may be surprised to find tea and coffee included in a chapter on poisons, but slow poisons they certainly are. Caffeine, contained in these beverages, as well as in chocolate and cola drinks, is an addictive stimulant. One cup of coffee can contain as much as 100mg of caffeine, while tea will give you approximately half that amount. Excessive intake may cause psychiatric symptoms, including insomnia, anxiety and nervousness. Physical problems can be wide-ranging, such as diarrhoea, tremors, migraine, palpitations, higher blood pressure and cholesterol, jumpy legs at night, and lumpy or painful breasts, plus crippling osteoporosis in later years. High coffee intake is associated with cancer of the pancreas. Drinking tea and coffee with meals can have an adverse effect on nutrient absorption: iron uptake can be reduced by two-thirds (very significant for women of childbearing age who may become anaemic); zinc absorption will also be inhibited.

Set against these problems is the fact that tea is a useful provider of manganese, so limited consumption could be beneficial in this respect. However, there are several other more nourishing sources, such as fresh vegetables and whole cereals. It is far better to drink herb teas and, as a coffee substitute, beverages made from chicory or dandelion roots, many of which have beneficial properties.

The other socially acceptable poison is, of course, alcohol, which depletes the body of nearly every vitamin, particularly the B vitamins, also E and many minerals. Such deficiencies will undermine the health, both physical and mental. Alcoholism, as we all know, will eventually damage the liver irreversibly, but there may also be severe injury to the brain, nervous system and heart. High doses of B vitamins (brewer's yeast is an excellent source), combined with nourishing food that includes plenty of protein, will help to heal the liver from the worst effects of cirrhosis as long as deterioration is not too far advanced. Vitamin E supplements may protect the cells from their increased susceptibility to oxidative injury and the cancers likely to result. Needless to say, it is essential to stop drinking. This could include skilled assistance in the form of counselling and support from a group (see Addresses). A healthy diet, as described under 'Food for lasting health' in chapter 2 and outlined in chapter 20, reinforced with multivitamin tablets will also greatly ease withdrawal symptoms. According to a Scottish study, evening primrose oil is useful in this respect. Take at least 2g daily.

Recent newspaper reports suggest that a regular glass of red wine may be protective against heart disease. Weighed against this are the results of a Norwegian study which show conclusively that people who include alcohol in their lifestyles, even in 'normal' amounts, run a 27 per cent higher risk of developing cancer than complete teetotallers. Clearly, it is not worth adopting for 'therapeutic' purposes.

Natural toxins

Just because vegetables, spices and herbs are 'natural', one should not conclude that they are all entirely safe. For example, cinnamon can bring on contractions in pregnant women, which could be dangerous in the early months. Some herbs can be very powerful and should therefore only be taken therapeutically on the advice of a qualified herbalist.

There are certain chemicals found in commonly used foods that, if taken in excess, could be carcinogenic. Compounds called psoralens are found in parsley, parsnips and celery; isothyocyanate is present in mustard seeds and horseradish; and alkaloids exist in the flowers (not leaves) of some herbs. Their negative effect is neutralized by the anti-oxidants, vitamins A, C and E and the minerals zinc and selenium, some of which are already naturally present in these foods. However, it is wise to limit your intake of such items. Certain raw beans can be toxic as well, but are quite safe if correctly cooked (see chapter 20).

Tyramine, present in some cheeses and meats and also yeast extract, pickled herrings and wine, can interfere with the action of neurotransmitters, the chemical messengers that direct nerve function, and precipitate headaches and migraines.

Another 'amine', phenylethylamine, which is found in chocolate, may also bring on headaches and even cause raised blood pressure. Chocolate is not good for you, tempting though it may be!

Cleaning up your system

Fortunately, our bodies have some marvellously efficient detoxification systems that cope well with unwanted substances and the particular demands of our modern lifestyles. Many poisons are broken down by the liver and rendered harmless before being excreted by the kidneys. Carbon dioxide left over from the chemical activities of cells is exhaled from the lungs into the atmosphere, later used by plants and converted back into oxygen – all part of the delicate way in which nature is balanced. Some wastes are sweated out through the skin, and of course much unwanted debris is excreted via the bowels after the goodness has been extracted.

The lymphatic system provides us with a cleaning and drainage network, which also removes waste products from cells along with the rubbish accumulated by the fighting forces of our immune system, such as dead bacteria. Unlike the blood circulation, the lymph has no pump to keep it on the move, but relies mainly on gravity and the action of our muscles. It is therefore vital to take some form of exercise to encourage the lymph to do its cleaning-up duties regularly. Brisk walking is beneficial, as are most sports. Any activity that involves small jumping movements is ideal, such as skipping or jogging, or bouncing on a mini-trampoline.

Exercise that gives good aerobic effect (that is making your heart beat faster and your face go pink) also increases the efficiency of your lungs in taking in oxygen and expelling carbon dioxide, while the perspiration will help to get rid of any extraneous urea not excreted by the kidneys;

this is the nitrogenous waste produced when the liver transforms amino acids into glycogen.

If for some reason you are unable to take part in energetic activities, then whole-body deep breathing, raising your arms to the side as you breathe in, will be advantageous.

Foods that detoxify

Certain foods and drinks have the reputation of being good cleansers, so it is worth setting aside a few days for a thorough spring-clean. Choose a time when demands are not too great, so that you can relax and rest when you feel the need, as you will be concentrating on foods devoid of saturated fat that are generally low in calories.

The average Western diet, which is high in fat and consists of lifeless processed foods and sugary, low-fibre confections, leaves the system distinctly bunged up. Constipation is common and faeces start to putrify in the gut, eventually causing very serious problems, some life-threatening, such as cancer of the colon. If elimination is not sufficiently frequent, faecal backflow can occur, whereby toxins are reabsorbed into the system – very unhealthy indeed. A good clean-out, therefore, must include fibre from natural sources.

High-fat, high-protein diets can also cause clogging up of the villi. These are tiny projections that line the small intestine in their thousands, giving it a huge surface area for the absorption of digested food. Clearly, our bodies cannot make the most of nutrients unless the villi are able to perform their function effectively. Low-fat foods, with protein from plant sources only, are therefore recommended as part of the detoxification plan.

Plenty of liquid, in the form of filtered or spring water, herb teas, or watered-down fruit juices, is essential for flushing out the kidneys. It is necessary to give up coffee, tea and alcohol entirely during your detoxification period. Healthy fluid balance can be established in the body by banning added salt and increasing your potassium intake.

There are two important ingredients that act as chelators: in other words they latch on to unwanted heavy metals and remove them from the system. These are pectin, found in fruits such as apples, and vitamin C.

The sulphur-bearing amino acids methionine and cystine are natural detoxifiers. During metabolism they yield sulphuric acid which interacts with other substances in a helpful way. Cystine can also bind harmful metals and thus protect the body. Some food sources are given in chapter 3.

Chlorophyll has the reputation of being a good cleanser, present especially in those dark outer leaves of vegetables such as cabbage, broccoli and spinach. It is best to eat these fresh and raw in salads, and of course always organically grown.

It is very important to re-establish beneficial bacteria in the gut, and yoghurt made from live culture, *Lactobacillus acidophilus* or *L. bulgaricus*, will do this if assimilated on a regular basis.

Four-day detox

A couple of days before commencing this programme, you will need to sprout seeds for the 'Raw day'. Recipes and advice about eating can be found in chapter 20.

Day 1 (Friday) Elimination menu
On waking: Peppermint tea
Breakfast: High-fibre Muesli with soya or skimmed milk
Mid-morning snack: Slice of wholemeal bread with whole peanut butter (salt- and sugar-free); nettle tea
Lunch: Freshly squeezed orange juice, topped up with spring water and a dash of lime juice; Avocado and Pistachio Salad with oatcakes; whole fresh grapes
Tea: Banana; nettle tea
Dinner: Slice of fresh melon; Three Beans Feast; cup of Caro or dandelion coffee
Before bed: Camomile tea

Day 2 (Saturday) Rest day

Grapes and mineral water as required. Take the liquid half an hour before the fruit.

Day 3 (Sunday) Raw day

On waking: Glass of freshly squeezed orange juice with a slice of lemon, topped up with spring water

Breakfast: High-fibre Muesli with fresh fruit in season

Mid-morning snack: Fresh-pressed apple juice topped up with spring water; banana

Lunch: Cabbage and Grape Juice; Sprout Salad with Yoghurt Dressing

Tea: 1 whole apple, including skin; cup of nettle tea

Dinner: Beetroot and Cucumber Juice; Walnut Coleslaw; rice cake; fresh pineapple; peppermint tea

Before bed: Cup of camomile and spearmint tea

Day 4 Renewal day

On waking: Blackcurrant tea

Breakfast: Spiced Compôte with goat's milk yoghurt and wheatgerm

Mid-morning snack: Handful of nuts mixed with pumpkin seeds and sultanas; nettle tea

Lunch: Grapefruit; Vitamin C Salad; Hummus; slice of wholemeal bread with non-hydrogenated margarine

Tea: Date Square; fennel tea

Dinner: Avocado vinaigrette; Baked Stuffed Onions; fresh mango; peppermint tea

Before bed: Cup of camomile tea

This programme can be adjusted to suit your own needs. The number of elimination days can be increased if you are especially bunged up. Equally, the rebuilding time can be extended, keeping to raw food for longer and introducing cooked foods more gradually. The rest day is best kept to no more than one and is not recommended for anyone with metabolic problems such as diabetes or hypoglycaemia, nor for pregnant women.

Chapter 5

The Healthy Kitchen

As knowledge about transmission of diseases has progressed, so cleanliness and personal hygiene among Western people has improved, to the point where we now take our plentiful supply of running water and our sewerage system for granted. Indeed, the fitted kitchen with its sweeping work-top and gleaming sink is currently the aspiration of most young couples, as is the bathroom with coloured suite and shower – each a mark of affluence. Competition to sell new kitchens is fierce and advertisements are persuasive. Names such as 'Monte Carlo' or 'Princess' or 'Whisper' are dreamed up to entice the purchasers, hoping to convince them that the melamine-faced chipboard is something exotic, priceless or mysterious. Be that as it may, fitted kitchens are certainly hygienic, providing few corners for bacteria to breed. The result is that food preparation and ablutions can be performed in considerable comfort. Yet it has taken us many centuries to reach this civilized state.

In Roman times public health and sanitation were well advanced and the first aquaduct brought fresh water into the city as long ago as 312 BC. Public baths were huge edifices, those of Diocletian having 3,000 rooms! The remains of closets linked by waterways have also been discovered among the ruins of Pompeii, dating from before AD 79. Yet it took more than 1,700 years for the first water closet to be built in London. Romans seemed to understand intuitively that it is not possible for people to live in crowded conditions and remain healthy without fresh water, proper sewers and clean streets.

In the European cities of the seventeenth century, a few brick-lined sewers existed, but an open gutter down the street was more common, which regularly received the contents of chamber pots emptied from windows. 'Modern' houses had cesspits in the basement with a small hut built on top and a wooden board with a hole in it. These were called 'houses of easement' – but they were far from comfortable and the stench was indescribable, especially on those rare occasions when they were cleaned out. Pepys tells us that one day, while carrying on a conversation with a certain lady, she made use of his chamber pot. These were generally kept in a cupboard in the dining room and, as the Duc de la Rochefoucauld related, it was 'common practice to relieve oneself while the rest are drinking . . . without concealment'.

Thankfully, our attitudes concerning waste disposal have altered considerably since then and we now know how important it is to wash hands after visiting the lavatory, otherwise bacteria from the gut can be passed on via comestibles to others and cause food poisoning or even more serious disease such as typhoid. Equally, if water supplies become contaminated, then a great many people will become ill after drinking that water. Literally millions of bacteria can infest the intestine of one diseased person; if the faeces end up in a stream or river, the bacteria may eventually infect a reservoir. This is how dangerous diseases of the alimentary canal, such as cholera, are passed on.

Avoiding food poisoning

Clearly, it is pointless preparing delicious, health-giving food unless basic rules of hygiene are followed. Patients may end up worse rather than better. Unfortunately some health food restaurants and shops are run on a somewhat amateur basis and cleanliness is not always up to standard. I have twice had food poisoning from a macrobiotic restaurant in London, even after making rigorous complaints the first time.

One of the most common forms of food poisoning in western countries is caused by the bacterium *Clostridium perfringens*. Luckily it is rarely fatal, but after being ingested along with infected food the bacteria produce spores and a toxin that irritates the intestines, resulting in diarrhoea.

The following story demonstrates how easily infection from *Cl. perfringens* can occur if simple precautions are not followed. Jenny is a busy mother with three children. Her husband, Len, runs his own garage and motor repair business and Jenny works there part-time looking after the accounts and general correspondence. Preparing evening meals for everyone can sometimes be a rushed affair. The weather is cold, so she decides to make a filling hotpot. She peels and chops the carrots, onions and potatoes on a board; then, being in a hurry, she scrapes the peelings off and without washing it proceeds to chop up the meat. She cooks the hotpot and she and the children eat as soon as it is ready at 6pm. Len, however, has meanwhile telephoned to say he has an urgent job to finish and will be back late, so Jenny leaves his food in the oven, but switches it off. It is 9 o'clock before he finally returns home and Jenny warms up his dinner. He wakes up in the early hours of the morning with abdominal pains and diarrhoea, but the rest of the family is unaffected.

The fault here lay in the preparation of the meal. The soil from the vegetables contaminated the meat and *Cl. perfringens* ended up in the hotpot. The spores can withstand normal cooking and reheating and they particularly like warm, moist conditions that lack oxygen such as the bottom of Len's portion of the dinner. Here they germinated and produced vegetative bacteria which then quickly reproduced themselves. The quantity of bacteria in Len's hotpot by the time he ate it was enough to make him ill. Jenny and the children, however, consumed their portions piping hot, straight from the oven.

This case of food poisoning could easily have been avoided either by washing the chopping board after preparing the vegetables, or by having a separate board for cutting up the meat. Equally, the bacteria could have been brought into the kitchen on the meat itself and for this reason raw meat must always be stored apart from cooked food. They can also arrive via dirty hands or on the legs of flies. These, together with soil, pets and vermin, are the most common sources of infection with various food-poisoning bacteria.

Bacillus cereus is slightly different in that it is carried into the kitchen on cereals, especially rice. It too produces spores that survive cooking and will then germinate if the rice is kept warm for a while. The resulting vegetative bacteria multiply and produce a nasty toxin, often not destroyed by reheating. Prevention is simple: wash cereals before cooking and always put leftovers in the fridge. Any reheating needs to be rapid and thorough, followed by immediate serving. Never reheat more than once.

Salmonella is reckoned to be present in 80 per cent of chicken carcases. Luckily it is destroyed by heat and does not form spores. It is essential, however, to defrost frozen poultry thoroughly, otherwise the temperature at the centre of the bird may not be sufficient to kill the bacteria. A 3-lb (1.5-kg) bird will take 10 hours at room temperature. It is also best to cook any stuffing separately to avoid possible contamination. Salmonella is also present in eggs and on their shells. Always wash your hands after breaking eggs. Make sure you cook them thoroughly and never risk eating them raw.

Humans are the main carriers of *Staphylococcus aureus*, passing it to food through sneezing or coughing over it and from uncovered septic cuts or spots. The bacteria are killed by cooking, but they produce a toxin in favourable conditions which can resist half an hour's boiling. Food is often contaminated after cooking or with gentle reheating. Meats and milk products are especially susceptible. Testing a trifle for sweetness and then putting the licked spoon back into the custard for a further taste could easily affect this dessert if the cook is a carrier and if it is then left in a warm place before being consumed. It makes good sense not to put unwashed utensils into food, nor to sneeze over it, to cover all cuts with waterproof dressing and not to touch spots while cooking.

In recent years Listeriosis has become a problem, being widely present in soil, water and sewage. This bacterium can not only survive refrigeration temperatures, it actually reproduces in cold conditions, and can cause very serious illness, including loss of an unborn child. Coleslaw, soft cheese and chicken have been past trouble-makers, and of course any cook-chill meals are potential hiding places for this bacterium. If you keep to fresh, home-made food you are unlikely to encounter this type of poisoning.

Perhaps the most frightening of all is botulism, which is highly toxic and damages the central nervous system, causing complete muscular collapse and almost certain death from inability to breathe, unless an antitoxin can be administered in time. Fortunately the bacteria are easily destroyed in oxygen and by heat, but there have been occasional instances of poisoning from canned food. Always make sure that tins you buy are not 'blown', which may indicate incomplete sterilization, nor damaged in any other way.

Needless to say, rats and mice must be kept well away from homes as they carry bacteria such as salmonella in their intestines and on their fur and feet. If you keep your kitchen clean, avoid leaving food out, and ensure that rubbish is well wrapped, then you will not encourage them. Remember that one pair of mice can produce up to 2,000 offspring in one year! Cockroaches also like a ready supply of food, especially at night, and warm, dark corners in which to hide. If you remember to put food away before going to bed they are unlikely to set up home in your kitchen.

Perhaps the copy from this Health Education poster will convince you that houseflies and bluebottles are unwelcome guests: 'Flies can't eat solid food, so to soften it up they vomit on it. Then they stamp the vomit in until it's liquid, usually stamping in a few germs for good measure. Then when it's good and runny they suck it all back again, probably dropping some excrement at the same time. And then when they've finished eating, it's your turn.' Ugh! Don't use chemical sprays to get rid of them, which may poison you, too. Shoo them out of the window or put up a sticky fly paper.

If you observe basic rules of personal hygiene, keep food preparation and storage areas and utensils clean, defrost thoroughly and avoid keeping food warm for extended periods before serving it, then you are unlikely to poison anyone. You cannot totally prevent bacteria from coming into your kitchen, but you can prevent them from getting into meals and multiplying and thus causing illness. People are unaffected by small numbers because the body's defences, such as the acid in the stomach, can easily deal with them.

Natural remedies

Mild cases of food poisoning can be treated naturally by replacing lost fluid with regular cups of camomile tea, which is very soothing, and by avoiding food while the upset lasts. As soon as the patient feels able to, take live bio-yoghurt mixed with wheatgerm and a little honey. This will reintroduce healthy bacteria into the intestine and re-supply the body with B vitamins, which will almost certainly have been excreted. Thin vegetable soups will also help to replace lost liquid and vitamins. A good remedy for diarrhoea is blackberry leaf tea (see chapter 20). Small children will require only a few teaspoons daily while adults may need up to three cups.

It is important to have plenty of rest to speed recovery. Any serious cases of food poisoning will need a doctor's help, which should be sought immediately. Rehydration powders, available at chemists, may be necessary.

Pots, pans and packaging

My mother always used to say that the best way to clean an aluminium pan was to cook rhubarb in it. Nor was this entirely a joke. I remember looking into the pan afterwards as a child and realizing that I could almost see my face in it. What I failed to understand was that in this 'cleaning' process the acid had actually caused traces of aluminium to leach into the rhubarb, which we then ate.

Our bodies contain very small quantities of aluminium from natural sources, but there is good evidence that higher levels can damage us in the long term. The link with Alzheimer's disease is currently disputed, although one recent survey in southern Norway, where lakes are high in aluminium due to the action of acid rain on rocks, shows that the disease is particularly prevalent there. We have already seen in the last chapter how children suffered after the accidental contamination of water in Cornwall with this metal. So the best advice is to play safe and substitute stainless steel for aluminium pans. They are expensive, but if you shop around you will find good-value cookware in certain chain stores. While you are at it, buy a vegetable steamer to sit inside one of the pans. It is also best to avoid non-stick pans, since the Teflon can eventually flake off and end up in the food. It is a suspected carcinogen.

As for casserole dishes, glass is cleanest, and pottery is all right so long as the glaze contains no lead. Do not buy red or orange enamelled cookware as cadmium may have been used as a colouring pigment and this could migrate

99

into food, especially if the pot is chipped. Cadmium is extremely toxic and low levels over prolonged periods can harm the vital organs.

A certain amount of packaging is obviously necessary to keep food fresh and free from dirt, but aluminium in the form of foil containers or as a lining for cartons can contaminate its contents especially if acidic. However, if you are switching from convenience meals to fresh produce – and hopefully this book is rapidly convincing you that you must! – then you are less likely to be encountering this problem. Old-fashioned grease-proof paper is handy for wrapping sandwiches and so on. As far as your own storage is concerned, small stainless-steel containers are very useful for left-overs in the fridge and polythene bags are fine for the freezer.

Make sure that any clingfilm you buy is free from plasticizers or vinyl chloride monomer – that is, not made from PVC. These chemicals are toxic and they are soluble especially in fat, so never wrap cheese or cooked meats in film. Also do not use in the microwave, nor to wrap or cover food that is still warm. Fortunately clingfilm is now more commonly made of polyethylene which does not need plasticizers.

In America the Environmental Protection Agency did some tests on milk delivered to schools in cartons and found that levels of dioxin were 1,000 times higher than limits thought to be safe. It had migrated into the milk from the chlorine bleach used to whiten the cartons. We have always been led to believe, especially by advertisements, that 'whiter than white' is also the healthiest. Not so: dioxin is a poison that produces a nasty skin rash in humans after only mild exposure and it causes cancers and birth defects in animals. Britain may be considered old-fashioned or sentimental by other European countries for wanting to retain its tradition of having milk delivered to doorsteps in glass bottles, but at least we know it is dioxin-free. As a bonus to the environment, the glass is automatically recycled. Dioxin may also be present in tea bags – make sure it is not by writing to the manufacturers, or by buying all teas loose, including herb teas.

Storage without spoilage

As you will have seen from chapter 3, many vitamins are unstable and easily destroyed under certain conditions, especially vitamin C. While plants are growing they use enzymes and oxygen to produce the vitamins, but after maturity or picking, this action is reversed. Since light and warmth are favourable to enzyme activity it is important to slow this process down by storing vegetables in a cool, dark place, such as the bottom drawers of the refrigerator. This way vitamins will last longer. Enzyme activity is also speeded up after chopping, so salads need to be consumed very fresh and vegetables cooked straight after preparation. Even if you have little or no garden space for your own produce, seeds and beans can be sprouted on your windowsill in a large glass jar. These are full of goodness and ideal for salads. Just keep them moist and rinse three times a day until ready.

Vitamins B_2 and B_6 are unstable in light, so any foods containing these must be kept in a dark, cool place, including milk, cheese, fish, eggs and bread.

Vegetable oils can easily go rancid in warmth, producing those dangerous free radicals. Oily nuts, especially walnuts and brazils without shells, need to be put in the fridge, too, as does wheatgerm.

Some foods can be safely frozen, but not those containing vitamin E which will be destroyed, and to a lesser extent vitamin B_6. Do not therefore freeze wholemeal bread or cakes, nor indeed any dishes that include other grains, eggs, soya beans, green vegetables or beef.

Chapter 6

Digesting Your Food

In order to digest an average dinner, an amazingly complex chemical process takes place inside our bodies which results in solid chunks of food being broken down and dissolved to make a solution. Molecules thus formed are so small that they can pass through the wall of the alimentary canal and right into the bloodstream.

Let us imagine an accountant called Philip who lives on his own. He loathes cooking so eats a substantial midday meal at the pub round the corner from his office. At one o'clock on Thursday he examines the menu: steak-and-kidney pie, chips and peas, followed by apple crumble and custard. Just the smells emanating from the kitchen have already provoked Philip's stomach to generate an acidic juice and his mouth to produce saliva. Once the meal arrives and he starts to chew, the salivary glands are stimulated still further and the food becomes slippery enough to swallow. Meanwhile an enzyme in the saliva called amylase has been working on the starch in the potatoes, breaking it down into dextrins and maltose.

One mouthful of chewed chips slides down Philip's oesophagus into his stomach, followed by a mashed ball of steak-and-kidney pie. The arrival of the food stimulates the glands lining the stomach walls to produce more juices, consisting of hydrochloric acid, mucus (to protect the stomach's lining), salts, enzymes and another protein called intrinsic factor. The enzyme pepsin sets to work on the steak and kidney, splitting the long chains of amino acids (which make up the protein) into smaller chains called polypeptides. Intrinsic factor attaches itself to the vitamin B_{12} in the meat, and later in the milk from the custard, allowing absorption and ultimately the formation of fresh red blood cells. The muscles in Philip's stomach walls churn up the food with the gastric juice.

He downs a pint of beer and that afternoon works away at a client's tax return, unaware that his lunch is gradually leaving his stomach for his duodenum (or upper part of the small intestine), where most digestion and absorption takes place. Here the chyme has prompted a hormone called secretin to be produced and it travels via the blood to the pancreas, telling it to release salts (which help to neutralize the acid) and more digestive enzymes into the small intestine. The gall bladder has also been triggered to secrete bile, which breaks down the fat from the meat, milk and pastry into droplets, and yet more enzymes are released from the wall of the small intestine. The fat droplets can now be digested by an enzyme made in the pancreas called lipase.

Starches from the chips, pastry, crumble and custard will be acted upon by amylase to form maltose, which in turn is broken down by maltase into the single sugar molecules (monosaccharides) of glucose. Similarly, the sugars from the peas and apples will be broken down into fructose. The polypeptides from the part-digested steak-and-kidney protein are further broken down in the duodenum by the protease and peptidase enzymes. Meanwhile the alcohol from his pint of beer has passed straight through the walls of Philip's stomach into his bloodstream, giving him a pleasantly euphoric feeling.

The lower part of the small intestine, the ileum, is where most absorption takes place. Its internal surface is formed into rounded folds, each of which bears thousands of

THE DIGESTIVE SYSTEM

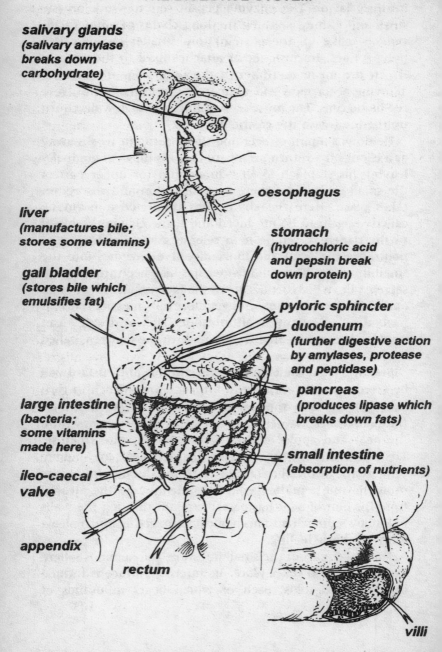

salivary glands
(salivary amylase
breaks down
carbohydrate)

oesophagus

liver
(manufactures bile;
stores some vitamins)

stomach
(hydrochloric acid
and pepsin break
down protein)

gall bladder
(stores bile which
emulsifies fat)

pyloric sphincter

duodenum
(further digestive action
by amylases, protease
and peptidase)

pancreas
(produces lipase which
breaks down fats)

large intestine
(bacteria;
some vitamins
made here)

small intestine
(absorption of nutrients)

**ileo-caecal
valve**

appendix

rectum

villi

minute projections called villi. If laid out flat, it is reckoned that they would produce an area about the size of a tennis court! All of these are supplied with a dense network of blood capillaries. The molecules of Philip's digested lunch, such as the glucose from the starches and amino acids from the proteins, are now minute enough to pass through the walls of the villi right into the bloodstream, along with vitamins and mineral salts. These are the essential ingredients that Philip needs to keep his body going and his brain ticking over, providing him with energy as well as nutrients for repair and maintenance work.

By about 10pm, Philip is thinking about going to bed, and his lunch has travelled some 23 feet (7m) to his large intestine (or colon), pushed along by muscular waves called peristalsis. Here more absorption takes place, especially of water and salt, leaving semi-solid faeces. This consists mainly of plant fibre, nitrogenous remains, dead cells and bacteria and water. It could be another two days before the remains of Philip's lunch arrive in his rectum for storage and final expulsion.

It is remarkable that such a complex system functions so well every day, despite the many ways in which we mistreat it, through gobbling food, taking in too little fibre and so putting a strain on the colon, or too much fat that clogs up the delicate villi, or through stress that causes the stomach to generate too much acid. Yet many disorders can result, most of which are entirely preventable. What a pity it is that we give our digestive tracts so little consideration. The following are some of the things that can go wrong, together with the ways in which nutritional therapy can help correct such disorders.

Teeth and gums

I have my parents to thank for my good teeth. As children we were never allowed sweets except after meals, and then only if teeth were subsequently brushed. In any case the rationing of sweets for a considerable period after the Second World War meant that they were not easily obtainable. The result is that, in half a century, I have only ever had one filling – just a small white one behind a front tooth. Both my parents kept most of their teeth until they died and I hope to retain all of mine.

The number of dental cavities is directly related to sugar intake. One Harvard researcher has shown that this problem increased one-thousandfold after sugar became a significant part of the Western diet. The reason for this is that bacteria thrive on the sweet plaque that forms on and between teeth after sugar or refined carbohydrates have been eaten. The bacteria cause it to ferment and an acid is produced which dissolves the enamel. Acid from fruit can also damage the teeth directly. At the same time, there is evidence that a lack of vitamin B_6 will hasten any decay.

Care of the teeth with regular brushing and flossing, combined with the cutting out of sticky, sugary snacks and refined carbohydrates, and an adequate intake of vitamin B_6 will ensure healthy teeth and gums. Whole foods will not encourage rot: for example brown rice will cause no damage, whereas Rice Crispies, especially if sugar-coated, will.

Jamie was a happy kid, but whenever he smiled the erosion of his milk teeth was noticeable. His mother blamed his poor dental health on constant sucking of his baby feeder, which invariably contained Ribena. The acid from the blackcurrants combined with the sweetener had given his teeth no chance, damaging the enamel irreparably. Jamie's parents, like many others, also complained about the prevalence of confectionery in machines in public places and at check-out points of shops, always within a child's reach. Forbidding the treat invariably produced cries and wails, while giving him what he wanted resulted in instant quiet. No wonder parents often succumb to this form of gentle blackmail. But the result all too often is dentures as a young adult.

Periodontal disease

Jack was an actor in his thirties who worked in repertory companies, often with long hours of rehearsal followed by evening performances and little time to eat properly or take much care of himself. He began to notice his gums bleeding when he brushed his teeth, but put off going to the dentist until some months later when he finally returned home.

Meanwhile the condition worsened, his gums became inflamed and an actress in the company hinted that his breath was not as sweet as it might be. Having some knowledge of vitamin therapy, she suggested that each day he take 3g of vitamin C complex that included the bioflavonoids rutin and hesperidin. He also cut sugar from his coffee and tea. After some weeks the bleeding and inflammation had subsided.

Jack's dentist warned him that if the gum disease returned, he would be running the risk of losing his teeth altogether. He stressed the importance of flossing and using a toothpick to prevent build-up of plaque, good advice that Jack thereafter followed.

The munching of tough whole foodstuffs has a massaging and cleansing action on the gums, which helps to keep them healthy. Conversely, a diet high in refined carbohydrates will encourage the growth of bacteria in the pockets formed as the gums fall away from the teeth in periodontal disease. A switch to a wholefood diet that is low in sugar will keep your gums healthy and guarantee longer-lasting teeth.

If you cannot bear the thought of life without cakes, then pick out some sugar-free recipes from chapter 20. You will be surprised how delicious they are!

Scurvy

Bleeding, weakened gums can often denote the early stages of scurvy, caused by a lack of vitamin C, now making a come-back owing to reliance on nutrient-deficient convenience and junk foods. Regular intake of fresh fruit and vegetables will ensure the avoidance of this disease.

Mouth ulcers

These are common and can be due to a shortage of B vitamins, especially B_6, B_{12} and folic acid, also iron or vitamin A. Add dried peaches to your muesli and pick out some recipes using molasses from chapter 20, both good sources of iron. Do not eat unleavened bread which prevents its absorption. Take wheatgerm for other B vitamins, along with green, orange and yellow fruit and vegetables for the folic acid and beta carotene, also avocados and beans.

If you are a vegan, you are most likely to be short of vitamin B_{12}, available mainly in meat, so add spirulina seaweed or yeast extract to your diet and include plenty of soya protein. Alternatively take a B complex supplement of at least 500mg daily.

If the ulcers are very persistent they could be due to a food intolerance, so try cutting out wheat and dairy products for a while.

Oesophagus and stomach

The oesophagus is the narrow tube that connects the throat with the stomach. Often we treat it unkindly by bolting food or not chewing it thoroughly and forcing down a bolus that is too large and rough. In our haste, we then send down another ball of food that has not benefited from complete predigestion in the mouth. A few years of this, and uncomfortable pockets of distension in the oesophagus will become permanent.

Hiatus hernia

This is a protrusion through the diaphragm around the place where the oesophagus joins the stomach, causing the symptom of heartburn, especially when lying down. This indicates a backflow of gastric juices. Overweight, middle-aged people are the usual sufferers.

Thorough chewing and unhurried eating in relaxed surroundings will avoid this problem. If it should occur, the patient needs to be propped up at night and must avoid stooping and tight clothes. Have a light supper early and do not eat before going to bed. Since losing weight is crucial, read the notes on obesity in chapter 16. It is best to exclude meat, not only because of its high-fat, calorific content, but also because it requires an acid environment in the stomach for digestion. Alcohol also increases the secretion of gastric juices, so cut this out, too. Smoking has to be banned because it encourages leakiness of the sphincter (the value that prevents blackflow of gastric juices). In a study at St Stephen's Hospital in London, Professor John Yudkin showed that eight out of nine patients with hiatus hernias improved substantially if they gave up refined carbohydrates, especially sugar, which is known to contribute to gastritis.

Since surgery is not always successful and carries a risk of post-operative mortality, do consider your stomach when you eat. Many hernias are entirely avoidable.

Stomach ulcers

Ulcers can occur in both the stomach (gastric ulcers) and duodenum (duodenal ulcers) and are caused by damage to these areas from the hydrochloric acid needed to digest food. Both types seem to be connected with stress and turbulent emotions which are then repressed.

Jeremy was a clergyman. He had grown up in a poverty-stricken area of Leeds in northern England, one of seven

109

children. He was a highly sensitive youngster and suffered much bullying, especially as he had an angelic voice and sang in the local church choir. At the age of 14 he suffered from severe pains under his right ribs, especially during the night or a couple of hours after eating, and his doctor diagnosed a duodenal ulcer. Indeed, he had recurring trouble with his digestive system most of his adult life. He was aware that the symptoms worsened when he was under stress and tried to plan an unhurried existence. However, being highly conscientious, he worked extremely hard for long hours caring for his parishioners. Invariably he took everyone else's problems too much to heart.

From bitter experience he knew that hot spicy foods had disastrous consequences, and the nutritional solution in those days was to prescribe a sloppy, milky diet. We know now, however, that the result of that can be heart disease at an early age from the excess saturated fat. Milk, in any case, is not a good idea, nor is any animal protein, for these require an increase in acid to digest them. Small, frequent meals are best, since these will keep the hydrochloric acid busy and therefore less likely to attack the stomach itself. Eat slowly and chew well. If necessary seek the support of a counsellor to help cut down on stress, which can often be self-inflicted, stimulating the release of extra acid.

Important healing factors are vitamin A along with B_6 and zinc, while vitamin E helps to prevent ulcers in the first place. Vitamin A is involved in the formation of the glycoprotein that protects the stomach from its own acid. Eat plenty of carrots, therefore, along with pumpkin when available, also apricots, cantaloup melon, sweet potatoes and dark-green leafy vegetables. If you have been used to refined carbohydrates you will be low on vitamin E, so make a gradual change to wholemeal bread and have wheatgerm with your breakfast cereal or porridge (make this from finely ground oatmeal for a gentle start to the day); you can also add wheatgerm to cooking (see chapter

20). Never eat bread that has been frozen. Cut out sugar, which can irritate the stomach, also coffee and strong tea because these stimulate gastric acid secretion. Lentils, avocados, dried fruits and a little fish will increase your B_6 intake. Zinc is widely available in food (see chapter 3), but a supplement of 20mg three times a day will speed up healing. Balance this with a supplement of beta carotene of around 25,000IU daily and 500mg of vitamin B complex. Reduce dosage with improvement.

Raw cabbage juice is not just a folk remedy for healing peptic ulcers; studies in America and Russia have proved that it is often more efficacious than modern drugs and this special quality has been termed vitamin U or anti-ulcer factor. Sip the fresh juice after eating and pain should diminish in five days; within a fortnight healing should be well advanced.

Indigestion and dyspepsia

We have all suffered the niggly discomfort of indigestion at some time or other, perhaps after a fried breakfast, or fish and chips cooked in old fat, or simply by eating too quickly or too much. Dyspepsia is the term given when the discomfort is experienced just below the breastbone. Antacids are sometimes useful for temporary relief, but do not rely on these as many contain aluminium which is toxic, and they also interfere with absorption of essential minerals. Magnesium is very alkaline and can be safely used instead.

Make a note of any offending foods and avoid those in future. Check out whether you are intolerant of wheat, milk, sugar and indeed anything sweet, since these can often cause stomach problems. Also cut back on smoking, alcohol and stimulants including coffee and tea, all of which can exacerbate dyspepsia. Instead of ordinary tea, use camomile or fennel, which are very soothing. Peppermint tea also assists digestion. The pawpaw, fruit of the papaya tree, has some outstanding properties. When not yet ripe

111

it produces a latex named papain which contains enzymes similar in action to pepsin, mentioned at the start of this chapter. This is a remarkable aid to digestion and is available at health food shops. (See also 'Poor digestion' in chapter 19.)

The gall bladder

This organ stores the greenish liquid known as bile which is produced in the liver, then released into the duodenum when needed. It acts rather like washing-up liquid by breaking down fats into droplets.

Gallstones

If the bile becomes too high in cholesterol, this can precipitate out as crystals which can then block the duct leading to the duodenum. Symptoms are acute pain and perhaps vomiting, especially after a high-fat meal.

Gallstones are generally uncommon among vegetarians because of their low intake of fat and the amount of fibre consumed. Slender people are also unlikely to suffer from this condition.

Geoffrey enjoyed good living. Recently he and his wife had retired to a delightful house in the country, but they were wealthy enough to have everything done for them in the way of improvements and decorations and to hire a regular gardener. This left Geoffrey with little to do apart from browsing through *The Times* each day and patronizing the local golf club, where he was more regularly seen in the bar than on the green. Gastronomy had become an abiding interest, especially when travelling abroad, where all the specialities were indulged in to excess. As a result, his girth had expanded considerably.

His wife made a few attempts to introduce some healthier fare into his diet, but these were generally dismissed with scorn. After all, he reasoned, he had worked hard all his life and now he deserved to enjoy himself.

It was after a trip to the south of France that the pains started. He had rarely been ill and their intensity frightened him. The doctor diagnosed gallstones and warned that a low-fat diet was now essential, otherwise surgery might be the result. He prescribed medication to dissolve the stones.

Nutritional therapists know that lecithin, largely a product of the soya bean but also found in eggs, nuts, liver and wheat, has the ability to dissolve gallstones. Patients should take an initial 4 to 6 tablespoons daily, cutting back to 1 to 2 after recovery to keep the blood fats normal. Since vitamin C is needed for the production of bile salts, deficiency of this vitamin can result in bile which is too concentrated and hence the formation of stones. Any gallstone patient should therefore be given 2g of vitamin C daily in small amounts, preferably combined with about 400mg of magnesium which will aid its metabolism. A deficiency in vitamin E can bring about stone formation; equally, if foods containing this vitamin are supplied, stones will dissolve of their own accord. A supplement of 200IU daily is therefore recommended combined with regular intakes of wheatgerm, nuts, soya beans and cold-pressed sunflower-seed and olive oils.

Herbalists often suggest chicory, which is good for the liver and assists in healthy bile production, so take one cup of chicory tea daily (see chapter 20) and include raw endive in salads. It is well known that people who exist on wholefoods rather than a refined diet are far less likely to suffer from this disease, so a switch to the Health-Giving Diet described towards the end of chapter 2 and outlined at the start of chapter 20 is essential. This is especially important for women on the contraceptive pill who have an increased risk of gallstones.

The small intestine

As we saw from the story of Philip's lunch at the start of this chapter, the lower part of the small intestine (the ileum) is where most absorption of digested food takes place. By now starch has been turned into glucose, proteins into amino acids and fats into fatty acids and glycerol, tiny molecules that can pass into the bloodstream. The fine capillaries that collect these nutrients join up to form larger veins, which in turn combine into one large one called the hepatic portal vein. This carries the nutrient-rich blood to the liver. What happens here will be described in the next chapter.

Appendicitis

At the bottom of the small intestine where it joins the colon, there is a pencil-like projection, the appendix, once thought to be useless but now known to play a part in the lymphatic system. The appendix of grass-eating animals is where digestion of the cellulose takes place. In 'civilized' humans, the appendix frequently becomes blocked and inflammation sets in, ultimately spreading to the surrounding area and causing abdominal pain and vomiting. A burst appendix (peritonitis) is extremely dangerous and can be fatal. A fellow student studying English in my year at university died this way. He was only 19. Highly intelligent and well liked, he had his whole life to look forward to. We were stunned by an appalling sense of waste yet, like many diseases of modern Western people, a refined diet lacking in roughage is to blame. Appendicitis is not a problem in undeveloped countries. The following case is typical.

Jane was 12 years old. She was an only child so most of her food fads were pandered to. For the past year she had been suffering from occasional tenderness in her lower right abdomen and recurring bouts of constipation. Her mother was extremely concerned but had little knowledge of nutrition and continued to supply her with her favourite Sugar Puffs for breakfast and white bread sandwiches for lunch. There were always treats for tea, such as fairy cakes and jellies, and trifle for puddings. The doctor prescribed a laxative. Jane's condition deteriorated.

One night she had severe pain and vomiting and started to run a temperature. This time the doctor diagnosed appendicitis and she was rushed to hospital and operated on shortly afterwards. The nurses tempted Jane back to food with ice cream and rice pudding, but of course the constipation continued and she was terrified of bursting the stitches with all the straining. Luckily her mother happened to read an article in a woman's magazine about the importance of fibre in the diet and gradually switched to wholemeal bread and flour and introduced Jane to more fresh fruit and vegetables. As a result she began to feel much stronger and was relieved to be free of the constipation.

If Jane's mother had introduced the fibre at a much earlier date, the appendicitis could probably have been avoided altogether, because the roughage prevents hardening of the stools and blockage. Additionally, by keeping the faeces moving, harmful bacteria are less likely to proliferate. It is astonishing that hospitals still disregard this most basic piece of information regarding nutrition and frequently feed patients on the very diet that made them ill in the first place!

The large intestine (colon and rectum)

The main purpose of the colon is to absorb water from the undigested matter. Healthy bacteria here are able to assimilate part of the remaining fibrous material, creating fatty acids and some vitamins which can then be absorbed by the colon. Diseases of the large intestine are unfortunately very common among Westerners.

Diverticulosis

Studies have shown conclusively that this disease is the result of a low-fibre diet. This produces hard, compacted faeces which, over time, distort the mucous membrane lining the large intestine, creating pouches that can become inflamed. It is a disorder frequently found among middle-aged and older people in the West, with almost one-third of retired Americans suffering from it. Symptoms are pain in the lower left abdomen, either constipation or diarrhoea and possibly internal bleeding. A ruptured diverticulum may be extremely serious and can result in major surgery with colostomy, so do not risk allowing this condition to worsen.

A high-fibre diet (see chapter 20 for recipes) can be very effective in healing disorders of the colon. Because the roughage is able to absorb water, this results in softer stools and easier movement through the intestines. This should be combined with generous daily doses of live yoghurt made with the acidophilus culture to restore healthy bacteria. Fluid intake needs to be increased.

To reduce inflammation and speed up healing, take 250mg of vitamin C six times a day combined with about 100mg of vitamin B complex. These can be taken with the Fortified Soya Drink described in chapter 20.

Constipation

Vegetarians rarely suffer from this irksome condition because their fibre intake is more than half as much again as that of omnivores, while vegans, whose diet is entirely plant-based, consume twice as much as meat eaters at around 47g daily.

So, if you suffer from constipation, switch to whole grains such as brown rice and eat wholemeal bread. Instead of meat, introduce beans and lentils and nuts, and eat more fresh fruit and vegetables (see chapter 20 for high-fibre recipes). Figs and prunes are naturally laxative, as are red currants and blackberries. Honey and olive oil are more gentle in their action. Muesli for breakfast, containing rolled oats and fresh apple, is particularly good for you as these ingredients contain water-soluble fibre which will soften the stools. The husks of the plantain seed (psyllium), available from health food stores or by mail order (see Addresses), act as a bulking agent and are excellent for intestinal health. You will need to increase your fluid intake in the form of herb teas and fruit juices: aim for 2 litres (3½ pints) daily. And don't forget that important daily dose of live yoghurt.

Piles (haemorrhoids)

These are basically varicose veins that form in the rectum or anus, often resulting in discomfort and itching. They are linked with obesity and generally caused by long-term constipation and straining. Laxatives, rather than easing the condition, seem to make it worse. As with constipation, this sort of medication is not the answer, but rather a high-fibre diet with emphasis on foods that absorb water and keep the faeces soft.

In addition to losing weight, which you will achieve by cutting down on fat and sugar (see 'Obesity' in chapter 16 and recipes in chapter 20), this condition can be eased by following the cure for constipation described above. Surgery should then not be necessary.

Irritable bowel syndrome

Rebecca is a violinist with a well-known symphony orchestra. About eight years ago her mother died unexpectedly from cancer and since then she has suffered persistent 'tummy troubles' with bouts of diarrhoea, abdominal pain and rumbling stomach. She has noticed that the symptoms are always worse prior to an important concert when she is feeling tense or if she spends long periods travelling away from home. She has also discovered from experience that certain foods can aggravate the condition, so tries to adjust her diet accordingly, but finds this difficult when away and reliant on restaurant fare. Most debilitating are the spells

117

of acute fatigue which overtake her, especially in the mornings, making getting up a real struggle.

Her general practitioner had suspected *Candida albicans* (see chapter 11), but she had not responded to the treatment. It was only after having herself tested for food allergies that she discovered that she was intolerant of wheat. After giving this up in all forms and taking daily doses of live yoghurt together with plenty of fresh fruit and vegetables and lots of fluid, she was able to keep the condition well under control. Furthermore, regular counselling for six months helped her to manage stress and she was finally able to banish the disease altogether.

IBS is not always triggered by a food intolerance, although this is frequently the cause. Sometimes the colon can be invaded by too many abnormal bacteria which can give rise to continual problems. The number of bacteria in the gut has been reckoned to be something in the region of 10 billion per gram! The balance between beneficial and harmful bacteria can easily be upset, particularly after taking antibiotics, or as the result of a poor diet. In addition to live yoghurt and vegetarian wholefoods, especially fruit and vegetables, supplements of lactobacillus will help speed up recovery.

If a food intolerance is suspected, try excluding the following in addition to wheat: corn, dairy products and citrus fruits, all of which have been found to worsen the syndrome. Tea, coffee, and alcohol can all produce IBS-like symptoms, so replace these with mineral or spring water, fruit juices and herb teas.

Anyone who has suffered from frequent bouts of diarrhoea is likely to be vitamin deficient and should take a multivitamin and -mineral supplement until better. The Fortified Soya Drink (see chapter 20) should also prove a useful addition. The best herb tea for diarrhoea is made from blackberry leaves (see chapter 20). Small children need only a few teaspoons daily, while adults will benefit from up to three cups.

It is worth noting that constipation (q.v.), rather than diarrhoea, can also be a symptom of IBS.

Chapter 7

Internal Regulators

You may have heard of the term 'homoeostasis', which means 'staying the same'. When applied to human beings, it describes the way in which body fluids are regulated to provide a constant internal environment, so that the chemical reactions vital for life can take place successfully. Two kinds of organs which have this important job are the liver and kidneys.

After eating, the nutrient-rich blood from the alimentary canal passes through the liver, which extracts surplus glucose, storing it in the form of glycogen, sometimes referred to as 'animal starch'. After a meal high in carbohydrates, this can form as much as 6 per cent of the weight of the liver. When the blood-sugar level starts to fall between meals, the liver allows some of the stored glycogen to re-enter the circulation as glucose. Thus, it keeps the sugar level within a steady range. If it falls too low, the result can be disastrous, causing damage to the brain cells and coma.

The blood also flows through the kidneys, which filter a staggering 7,000 pints (3,750 litres) daily or thereabouts. If it is too concentrated, more water will be reabsorbed back into the body, and therefore little urine will be formed. Conversely, if the blood is too dilute, less water is retained and plenty of urine will be passed. Thus the balance of fluid is kept stable. At the same time, the kidneys control the levels of salts and acids in the circulation, which in

HOMOEOSTASIS

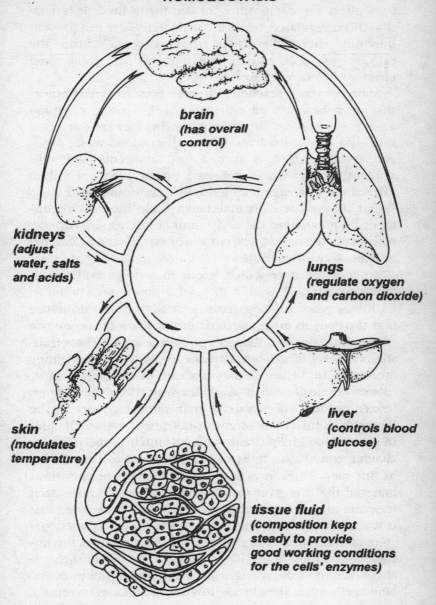

brain
*(has overall
control)*

kidneys
*(adjust
water, salts
and acids)*

lungs
*(regulate oxygen
and carbon dioxide)*

liver
*(controls blood
glucose)*

skin
*(modulates
temperature)*

tissue fluid
*(composition kept
steady to provide
good working conditions
for the cells' enzymes)*

**Homoeostatic processes keep the internal environment of the
body constant.**

turn affect the composition of the tissue fluid. It is vital that this is regulated, because fluctuations here can prevent important chemical reactions from taking place inside the cells. For example, a small change in acidity can stop some enzymes from working.

Many of these reactions produce poisonous substances that must be removed efficiently. If, for instance, amino acids are not needed for making protein, they are converted into glycogen by the liver. During this process waste nitrogen results, which is turned into ammonia and subsequently urea. This is collected by the blood and then filtered out and excreted by the kidneys in the urine.

Our kidneys therefore maintain a stable internal environment by preventing the body from becoming dehydrated, by keeping the correct acid/alkaline balance, and by helping to expel unwanted matter.

Yet it is the liver which is our most important detoxification organ. It is able to render poisonous chemicals harmless, whether they occur naturally or are introduced into the body as drugs. Bacteria in the colon produce toxic compounds by their action on amino acids. These substances travel in the bloodstream to the liver, where they are modified before being excreted in the urine. Hormones are dealt with in a similar way when they are no longer needed. Alcohol is detoxified by enzymes in the liver, which turn it into carbon dioxide and water. The pint of beer which Philip drank with his lunch in the previous chapter would take most of the afternoon to be oxidized in this way. There is a limit to the amount of poisonous material that the liver can cope with. We all know what happens to chronic alcoholics – cirrhosis of the liver, that is scarring and hardening, with eventual loss of function.

In addition to storing glycogen, the liver reserves the fat-soluble vitamins A and D until the body needs them. It also saves the iron released from the haemoglobin of red blood cells when they break down so that it can be reused.

These are only some of the many functions of the liver and kidneys, yet it can be seen from this brief description how important the health of these organs is, as the well-being of the whole body is heavily dependent upon them. As with any part of the body, if not treated with respect, they are vulnerable to disease.

Kidney stones

Henry's complexion was pallid in the extreme. Although he was quite plump, it was clear that he was a sick man. He had been suffering from excruciating pains in the loins and X-rays had revealed several stones in his kidneys, one almost as large as a bird's egg. Questions concerning his diet revealed that he was a heavy meat eater and somewhat addicted to coffee and tea, always with the addition of a heaped spoonful of sugar. As far as bread was concerned, his preference was for white rather than wholemeal and he had a definite liking for biscuits and cakes. Being quite afraid of the surgeon's knife he was hoping to be able to dissolve the stones with a change of diet. He agreed that it was going to be difficult, however the pain was so bad he was prepared to try anything.

Urine tests had shown that he was excreting excessive amounts of calcium and oxalic acid, the most common causes of stones. The nutritional therapist told him that he must cut down drastically on meat and preferably give it up altogether. The reason for this is that when meat is metabolized, both oxalic acid and uric acid are formed, which inevitably end up in the urine and these can both lead to kidney stones. Vegetarians are 50 per cent less likely to suffer from such problems than omnivores. Furthermore Henry must reduce his intake of refined carbohydrates, especially sugar, as this can raise the level of calcium in the urine of certain people. Equally, Henry must not add salt to his food, nor indeed cook with it, because too much sodium also encourages loss of calcium via the urine, which over time can be deposited as stones in the kidneys.

Henry groaned when he heard that not only should he give up alcohol, but tea and coffee also. It is known that alcohol increases susceptibility to stones, probably by reducing the effectiveness of the protective nutrients magnesium and vitamin B_6, while tea and coffee are high in the problematic oxalic acid. Instead, herb teas were recommended, especially sage, which is rich in magnesium, and dandelion coffee, and of course plentiful amounts of filtered or spring water. He must aim to produce 4 to 6 pints (2 to 3 litres) of urine daily. Foods exceptionally high in oxalic acid are chocolate, rhubarb, beetroot, spinach and peanuts, and are best avoided.

It seemed easy enough to switch from white to wholemeal bread. Bran, being high in phytate, reduces the amount of calcium in the urine. Indeed, the therapist stressed the importance of fibre, saying that Henry should eat adequate amounts with every meal, concentrating on whole grains and fresh fruit and vegetables. These are doubly beneficial, since they contain magnesium, particularly brown rice, wheatgerm, broccoli and peas, and also apricots, bananas, figs and coconut. She encouraged him to sprout alfalfa seeds for their magnesium content. Rather than meat, which is directly associated with stone formation, beans should become a staple of his diet, especially butter beans, haricot, mung, red kidney and soya, as well as chickpeas, all of which have useful amounts of vitamin B_6 as well as magnesium, and of course they are a beneficial source of dietary fibre. Fish should also be included because of its B_6 content, especially mackerel, herring, salmon, tuna and sardines. The essential fatty acids from fish oils are known to be very healthy for the kidneys.

Additionally, the nutritionist told Henry to take 300–400mg of magnesium per day plus 20–40mg of vitamin B_6, balanced with a 500mg B-complex tablet. She explained that these nutrients together help to keep minerals in solution rather than crystallizing to form stones. They would also help to dissolve the existing ones, combined with the healthy diet.

He asked whether he should reduce his calcium intake. This is a controversial point, although the latest study (1993) concludes that dietary calcium is helpful. Since he drank only a small quantity of skimmed milk (no more than $1/2$ pint/275ml) daily, the therapist reckoned that for the sake of the health of his bones he should maintain this, but reduce his intake of high-fat cheese. The magnesium supplement would ensure proper metabolism of the calcium.

The therapist had further advice for him. His job as a teacher was both stressful and sedentary, a bad mixture. Chronic stress causes the release of hormones into the bloodstream, including cortisone, and this draws minerals from the bones, which can end up deposited in the kidneys. Equally it is well known that immobilization contributes to calcium loss, encouraging calcium-phosphate stone formation. So he had to find a way of managing strain. He took up deep relaxation and meditation and revived his former hobby of swimming.

Henry's progress was slow but steady and the stones gradually reduced in size until they could be passed. He is now free of the terrible pain and has incidentally lost some of the excess weight due to the high-fibre diet combined with the exercise, which pleases him greatly.

Urinary tract infections

Women's particular anatomical make-up seems to leave them more prone to infections of the urinary tract than men. These should be reported to a doctor, since they can lead to other more dangerous disorders.

As a guide to prevention, it is known that vegetarians who include garlic and ginger in their diet are less likely to suffer from them than omnivores. Indeed, garlic is toxic to many unwanted viruses, bacteria and fungi.

The best dietary cure is plenty of vitamin C taken several times a day, totally about 2–3g. This helps the immune system to clear up most minor infections. Cranberry juice is particularly recommended as an excellent remedy, while juniper oil has useful antiseptic and diuretic qualities (although this is not suitable for use during pregnancy).

A copious amount of fluid in the form of clean, filtered or spring water is essential. Rice Water is particularly soothing (see chapter 20).

Cystitis

Women's fashions have sometimes been blamed for the prevalence of this irritating condition. It was a real problem in the 60s when tight jeans and miniskirts were both the rage, combined with nylon underwear which prevents the skin from breathing freely. It is also regarded as the newly-wed wife's disease, being linked with unaccustomed sexual activity.

Betty was a classic case. She liked to show off her slim figure with skin-tight trousers, and to feel pretty underneath with slinky briefs. She had recently moved in with her boyfriend and was embarrassed by her frequent trips to the toilet and distressed by the burning sensation on passing urine. Her doctor explained that potassium citrate would alleviate her condition by making her urine alkaline. It was also important for her not to drink alcohol as this can cause irritation to the bladder.

Indeed, this cleared her cystitis up within about five days, but a later recurrence took her to a nutritional therapist who recommended that she replace all junk food with a wholesome diet low in sugar and saturated fats. It was important that she drink plenty of fluid to flush out the germs before they could take hold and make herself tea from blackcurrant leaves, a natural diuretic, but avoid ordinary tea and coffee, both of which can be irritating. Another traditional remedy for cystitis is a beverage made from juniper berries (see chapter 20); drink one cupful in the morning and evening for at least a week. Use of garlic in her cooking would help to vanquish unwanted bacteria. Additionally, live yoghurt would maintain the health of the gut, an important consideration bearing in mind that the infection generally travels to the bladder from the anus.

These recommendations, together with meticulous personal hygiene, certainly helped to keep the cystitis at bay and Betty rarely suffered from the problem again.

Enlarged prostate

The prostate is a small gland in males that adds fluids to sperm. It is also a storage place for zinc. Older men sometimes suffer from prostate enlargement that causes difficulty in passing urine due to strangulation of the urethra (the tube leading from the bladder). The most common treatment is surgery, which generally results in infertility.

Before resorting to the knife, it is well worth trying zinc supplementation, since there is evidence that the swelling can be due to a diet low in this mineral, often lost in food processing. It is also sweated out through the skin in perspiration. Take chelated zinc in a dosage of about 25–30mg daily until the swelling goes down. Thereafter reduce the amount to 15mg. This mineral needs to be balanced by extra vitamin A, so initially include a beta carotene supplement of around 15,000IU. It is important to avoid all refined and processed foods and keep to a nutritious diet rich in zinc (see chapter 3 for best food sources) and in essential fatty acids, also needed by the prostate. These can easily be supplied by 2 to 3 teaspoons of cold-pressed safflower-seed oil per day, perhaps as a salad dressing, or alternatively linseed oil.

A high intake of caffeine has been linked with prostate problems, so it makes sense to cut out coffee and tea.

Bill, a 60-year-old catering manager, had suffered from the discomfort of a swollen prostate for some months with the accompanying frequency of urination and the anxiety that this gave him. Having a special interest in nutrition he decided to do some research and luckily found a booklet in his local pharmacy which explained the importance of sufficient zinc. He bought a supplement of zinc gluconate at 15mg, which also incorporated 75mg calcium, 50mg vitamin C and 750IU vitamin A. At the same time he increased his consumption of oily fish. He took only one tablet daily, but within a month felt very much better and within three months was completely cured.

Infections of the prostate can be controlled with good doses of vitamin C. Take around 2g divided into small amounts during the course of each day.

Chapter 8

The Body's Pump

During the writing of this book, heart disease has been much in the news in Britain: James Hunt, having survived the hazards of Formula One car racing, collapsed and died recently of a heart attack at the early age of 46, while the Labour leader, John Smith, has just suffered the same fate at 55 years. Not long ago Cabinet Minister Michael Heseltine, close contender for the premiership of the Conservative Party, lay in a Venetian hospital in intensive care, one of the lucky 50 per cent who would recover. Having reached 60 years, he was in the high-risk age group.

British people have the unhealthiest hearts in the world, with the Scottish and Irish the top scorers in cardiac failure. It is the commonest cause of premature death in the UK, accounting for 31 per cent of men under 65 and 14 per cent of women. Contrary to popular opinion, it is three times more likely to strike down the manual labourer than the executive. The financial burden to the National Health Service is estimated at around £500 million, yet only one-fiftieth of this amount is spent in efforts to prevent it. The disease costs the UK about £2 billion per annum in lost earnings calculated on the staggering total of 40 million working days.

Before the Industrial Revolution, with its attendant changes in eating habits and lifestyles, heart disease was a rarity. Much of the blame, therefore, has to be attributed

129

to the appalling UK diet. A switch from high-fat, high-sodium, over-refined junk food to an intake of whole grains, plenty of fresh fruit and vegetables without added salt, makes a noticeable difference to premature death rates, as has been proved in recent years in America and Australia, where emphasis has been laid on these simple preventive measures, combined with regular exercise and no smoking.

Considering that there are some 60,000 miles (96,500 km) of blood vessels in each human being, it is quite astounding that the circulatory system keeps going as well as it does. Part of its work is to transport oxygen and nutrients to the cells and to remove their waste products. Indeed, the network of capillaries is so dense that all 60 trillion cells have access to nourishment. Some capillaries are exceedingly fine, measuring only 0.001mm in diameter.

After collecting the digested food from the tiny villi in the intestine, the blood carries the nutrients in solution to the liver, following which the glucose, salts, vitamins and some proteins are transported to every part of the body. Eventually they seep through the walls of the capillaries into the tissue fluid. The cells, being soaked in this fluid, can now absorb the nutrients and use them for the chemical reactions that maintain life.

Meanwhile, in the lungs, oxygen has combined with haemoglobin in the red blood cells. The newly oxygenated blood, now bright red, travels down the arteries, through the smaller arterioles and finally to the capillaries. Here, the oxyhaemoglobin breaks down and so the oxygen becomes available for use by the tissues. Equally, the blood carries away the carbon dioxide from the respiring cells, through the venules and then the veins and back to the lungs, from which it is breathed out.

The blood also transports hormones, made in the body by various glands, to the parts that need them. Additionally, it is important for the maintenance of correct temperature, keeping the extremities warm.

In the previous chapter, a description was given of how the liver and kidneys ensure that the cells are bathed in a liquid that stays the same in its composition (homoeostasis). All the tissue fluid is derived from blood plasma and it is the job of the circulation system to replenish this fluid.

The organ that keeps the blood on the move is of course the heart. It is amazingly efficient, sending a red cell round the entire circulation in as little as 45 seconds. The pumping action, caused by the contraction and relaxation of the heart muscles, creates blood pressure, which you can feel at particular points, for example on the wrist below the thumb joint. The number of beats per minute varies from individual to individual: this can be between 50 and 110 when resting, and as much as 200 during excessive exertion. Special muscle cells at the top right of the heart initiate the beat, which is regulated by two sets of nerves from the brain, according to the needs of the body. Yet if these nerves are severed, the heart will still continue to beat.

Basically three main things can go wrong with the circulatory system: the pressure can increase unhealthily (hypertension) or become weak or irregular; the vessels can become hardened and liable to burst (arteriosclerosis); fatty deposits or clots can block the vessels up (atherosclerosis and thrombosis).

Hypertension

When taking blood pressure, doctors note two measurements in the arteries: the one caused by the heart contracting and the other when it relaxes, producing a reading such as 120/80. If you show a reading above 140/95 you are suffering from high blood pressure or hypertension and could be heading for trouble.

Several factors can contribute to this disorder including smoking, chronic stress, some oral contraceptives, certain anti-inflammatory drugs, lead poisoning, obesity and a fatty diet. Hardening of the arteries will raise blood pressure, as will an imbalance among the chemicals that regulate the circulation, the hormone-like prostaglandins and steroids. Too much salt leads to fluid retention which can result in hypertension, as can other mineral imbalances.

The main problem with this condition is that a blood vessel may burst due to the extra pressure. If this happens in the brain, a stroke will occur, damaging the nervous tissue, with death the possible outcome.

*

Margery had a history of hypertension and circulatory disorders in her family. She herself was overweight and chocolate biscuits and alcohol were her consolations whenever she felt a bit depressed or lonely. She had recently retired and was missing the companionship of her work colleagues. Perhaps she should go to her doctor for a checkup. After taking her blood pressure he warned her that she was a possible stroke candidate and that she must lose weight. He also recommended that she reduce her salt intake by not having it on the table and that she give up alcohol. However, Margery found these therapeutic measures extremely difficult to follow. She disliked preparing food, especially just for herself; snacking seemed so much easier. After a month of struggling with the new regime, she finally gave in again to her craving for chocolate biscuits, and the glass of wine soon became supplemented with a few straight Scotches. She was vaguely aware of tingling sensations in her right arm, but thought nothing of it.

The inevitable happened. She was pottering about in her back garden when she collapsed. Luckily her neighbour happened to look over the fence and, seeing her crumpled up on the lawn, quickly rushed to her aid and called an ambulance. When she finally came out of the coma in hospital she felt very disorientated, especially on discovering that her right arm and leg refused to move and that she had trouble in coordinating her speech.

Margery needed almost two months of regular physiotherapy before she was mobile enough to leave the hospital. Having come into a small inheritance she was able to afford further rehabilitation at a private centre in the country, where the care was of a high standard. The dietary regime was strict, but this time she took it seriously; the effects of the stroke had been so frightening that she was now well motivated to look after herself properly. She lost some weight and her staggered lurches gradually began to resemble proper steps. She learnt from the excellent resident nutritionist that by following some simple measures her high blood pressure could be substantially reduced, which in turn would greatly lessen the risk of another stroke. At the same time she could take particular nutrients to increase the flexibility of the blood vessels, making them less prone to bursting.

She was astonished to learn that her intake of sodium was probably as much as 40 times the amount her body needed, bearing in mind her sedentary lifestyle, and that not only must she cut out added table salt, she must also avoid all processed and convenience foods (all high in sodium), canned foods preserved in brine and all obviously salty fare such as bacon and cheese. She was also fascinated to hear that humans have evolved from hunter-gatherer African tribes, who naturally sweated out considerable amounts of sodium as they looked for their daily supplies under the hot sun. They instinctively searched for salty flavours to replenish those losses. Our liking for sodium has been ruthlessly exploited by food companies to the detriment of our health. It also has useful preservative qualities that contribute to shelf life and therefore profits. This mineral is widely present in virtually all natural

133

foodstuffs in sufficient quantities to maintain health and there is no need to add more. It took Margery a while to adjust to meals prepared without salt, but after a few weeks her taste buds began to appreciate the subtleties of natural flavours. In August 1982 a study by T. C. Beard et al. was reported in *The Lancet* showing that 80 per cent of hypertensive patients put on a low-sodium diet were able to reduce or stop their drugs within three months. This knowledge encouraged Margery.

However, it is not just a question of low sodium, but of the crucial balance between this mineral and potassium. Potassium deficiency greatly increases the risk of hypertension and the more salt you take, the less your body can use the available potassium. Primitive hunter-gatherer humans consumed about 16 times more potassium than sodium, whereas modern Westerners eat four times more sodium than potassium. This imbalance creates serious health problems and needs to be reversed if we are to avoid premature deterioration of cell function. Although potassium is widely available in foods, especially in green leafy vegetables, about half is lost by boiling; a switch to light steaming means that all but 6 per cent of this mineral is retained.

Vegetarians have lower blood pressure on average than omnivores and this may have something to do with their higher intake of potassium from fresh vegetables. At any rate, Margery was strongly advised to boost her consumption of plant foods and cut down on meat. Anyone who has great difficulty in cooking without salt can switch to a substitute such as Biosalt or Ruthmol which have the correct potassium content. It is a disgrace that doctors often put hypertensive patients on diuretics which cause potassium loss without also giving supplements of this mineral; such drugs are probably doing more harm than good.

Potassium has a direct benefit on the circulatory system by dilating blood vessels and relaxing the muscles that surround them. It also counteracts the effects of stress hormones that push up blood pressure. Margery was given a daily supplement of 2.5g.

Magnesium is another mineral that relaxes muscles, including those around blood vessels. A study by T. Dyckner et al. reported in volume 286 of the *British Medical Journal* in 1983 proved that this mineral helps to reduce blood pressure in hypertensive patients. Excessive alcohol causes a deficiency by acting as a diuretic and thereby promoting its loss in the urine – another incentive for Margery to give up those double Scotches.

Calcium also helps to lower blood pressure in about half of patients, although it is not fully understood why. It makes good sense, however, to take a combined calcium and magnesium supplement in the form of dolomite; Margery was prescribed 2g daily. Zinc has a similar effect at about 30mg daily balanced with 3mg of copper.

Another protective food is fish oil which contains EPA (eicosapentaenoic acid) and DHA (docosahexaenoic acid) from the omega 3 family of polyunsaturated fatty acids. Patients who take regular doses of cod-liver oil (3 to 4 tablespoons daily) note a significant lowering of blood pressure within a month, after which the amount needs to be reduced in case of vitamin A toxicity. Fish became an important part of Margery's diet. Anyone who cannot tolerate the fish oil will benefit from 3g daily of evening primrose oil, which contains another important fatty acid, GLA (gammalinolenic acid), of the omega 6 family. While raising the level of polyunsaturated fats in the diet, saturated fats and hydrogenated oils must be reduced for maximum benefit.

Of the vitamins, C helps to build strong walls to blood vessels, and the bioflavonoids, especially rutin, toughen up the fragile capillaries. Clearly these are vital nutrients for stroke candidates. The recommended supplement here is 2g per day of ascorbic acid with 200mg of rutin.

Luckily Margery was fond of garlic, a truly magical

ingredient for a healthy circulation, reducing blood pressure and lowering cholesterol and triglyceride levels. Garlic pearls are perhaps a more sociable alternative, although the chlorophyll in green vegetables and parsley help to freshen the breath. Another age-old remedy, ginseng, is know to improve the flexibility of blood vessels as well as counteracting hypertension.

The switch to a wholefood diet meant that Margery's intake of dietary fibre had increased significantly. Hair analysis had shown that her lead levels were too high – another source of hypertension. This could be remedied by the phytate in the wheat fibre, which attaches itself to body lead and helps to extract it from the system.

By the time Margery returned home, she was almost back to normal and her blood pressure was on the way down. Understanding fully how nutritional therapy would keep her well, involved her in preparing healing foods for herself (see recipes in chapter 20). She was even able to give up the chocolate biscuits, knowing that sugar can increase hypertension.

At the same time she bought herself a dog and the regular walking provided much-needed exercise. To reduce tension she joined a relaxation class. Here she learnt how deep breathing can slow the heart rate. As an added bonus she made some good friends there which kept her loneliness at bay. When Margery went for her check-up a few weeks later, her doctor was astonished at her improvement.

Coronary heart disease

Colin is a self-employed builder, physically strong, but a life-long forty-fags-a-day man and overweight with a 'beer belly'. Despite the smoking, he had always considered himself to be reasonably fit until at the age of 53 he began to suffer from chest pains. He was repairing a roof early one morning when he experienced the first symptoms: a gripping pain behind his breastbone, which spread up into his neck, causing a feeling of suffocation, and then down his left arm and over the upper part of his abdomen. He climbed down his ladder with great difficulty and lay on the ground until the pain gradually subsided.

His doctor suspected angina pectoris and this was later confirmed by an electrocardiogram and blood tests. The pain was the result of the heart muscle being deprived of the blood supply needed to keep it working properly, due to clogged-up arteries. He was instructed to give up smoking which was damaging his blood vessels, and to avoid fatty foods and lose weight. Yet Colin was nicotine-addicted and, try as he might, he just could not cut out cigarettes. His angina attacks became more frequent, although somewhat alleviated by the drugs prescribed, which helped to dilate the blood vessels.

Finally, as feared, Colin suffered a heart attack. Fortunately he was at home at the time. The pain in the left side of his chest was intense and he turned deathly pale, cold and sweaty. His pulse became so weak and his breath so gasping that his wife thought he would die, but the ambulance managed to rush him into intensive care in time to save his life.

If only Colin had been able to quit smoking and follow proper nutritional advice in the early stages of angina, the heart attack would most probably not have occurred. In this disease the arteries become increasingly blocked by fatty deposits consisting mainly of cholesterol and triglycerides. Yet there are nutrients that can actually reverse this process and thin the blood out. Another factor is the stickiness of the little pieces of blood cells called platelets, normally available to aid the healing of wounds through causing the blood to congeal. Here again, nutrients can correct stickiness so that clots do not form in the wrong places.

EPA (eicosapentaenoic acid), an active ingredient of omega 3, found in fish oil, is especially beneficial to heart disease patients. This both thins the blood out and reduces its stickiness. Studies have shown that it lessens by more than half the manufacture of TXA_2, a thromboxane produced by blood platelets that promotes clotting. Equally, EPA stimulates the blood vessel walls to put out more PGI (prostacylins) that discourage the clotting action. If patients eat plenty of oily fish, especially herring, mackerel and salmon, then blood cholesterol levels will drop to a healthy level – even if eggs are consumed (although this is not recommended) – as will the triglycerides. Salmon oil in particular reduces the VLDLs (very low-density lipoproteins), forerunners of LDLs (low-density lipoproteins), which are high in the 'bad' cholesterol that gets deposited in blood vessel walls.

If Colin had taken fish oils, he would have noticed his angina pains lessen considerably. Not all cholesterol is bad by any means. Indeed, the body generally makes more than twice as much as we consume in food because it is needed for making steroid hormones, the manufacture of bile and for the structure of cell membranes. High-density lipoproteins (HDLs) pick up cholesterol from the tissues for transportation to the liver and then excretion. This sort of cholesterol is popularly referred to as 'good' because it is being removed from the body.

A couple of portions of fish per week is very protective against heart disease. If EPA is taken in capsules, then the antioxidant vitamins C and E should also be included to counteract potential ill effects of any rancidity. Patients with heart disease will profit from doses of EPA ranging from 300 to 3,000mg daily, depending on severity. An alternative is a teaspoon each day of cod-liver oil; this can be bought with a pleasant mint or orange flavour. A word of caution, though: it is easy to overdo a good thing. Do not exceed recommended doses or you may bleed more than usual if you cut yourself. In any case all heart disease patients should consult their doctors before taking supplements.

Vegetarians are not likely to suffer from heart disease, especially if they do not smoke, but protective factors similar to those in fish oils are found in linseed oil and the herb purslane. Linseed oil actually encourages the cells to make EPA. Evening primrose oil at 2 to 3g per day can also reduce blood cholesterol.

Calcium has cholesterol-lowering effects too, especially if combined with a low-fat diet. Patients improved in only six weeks with 400mg of elemental calcium taken three times daily. This is particularly beneficial if combined with 200mg of magnesium.

Vitamin C is not only a useful antioxidant, it can actually break up clots at a dosage of at least 2g daily, it lowers the amount of fats in the blood and increases the ratio of the 'good' HDLs. It is even more effective if taken with bioflavonoids, especially rutin.

Multiple benefits are also provided by vitamin E at between 200 and 800IUs daily, especially if taken along with selenium at a dosage of 70mcg up to 1,000mcg. Do check with your doctor first, however, as such supplementation can conflict with anticoagulants. A natural way to take selenium is in the form of wholemeal bread or brazil nuts – just two will provide you with your daily needs – or soya beans are another good source. It is well known that the lower the level of selenium in the blood the greater the risk of heart disease. Studies have shown that selenium and vitamin E have natural anticoagulant properties by promoting prostacyclin levels, the prostaglandin that discourages clotting. These nutrients offer marked relief from the pain of angina and vitamin E is better at thinning blood than aspirin.

Angina sufferers will gain from another nutrient, vitamin B_6, which at about 40mg per day diminishes the stickiness of platelets and hinders the formation of an enzyme in the blood called thrombin; this converts the plasma protein fibrinogen into fibrin, insoluble strands of fibres in which red cells become trapped, thus making a clot. Remember to take B complex also, as this group of vitamins needs to be balanced.

Another magic ingredient is the amino acid L-carnitine. Research in Italy showed that patients who had died of heart attacks had a deficiency of this substance in the heart muscles. In a different study chronic angina sufferers were prescribed 1g twice a day. After only four weeks they were able to exert themselves much more without incurring pain. Carnitine helps to keep the blood clear of fats by ensuring their efficient burning for energy. It is found only in animal products, but humans also manufacture their own. However, vitamins B_6 and C, together with iron and the amino acid lysine, are essential for the production of carnitine, so that a deficiency in any of these nutrients could result in low levels of this important substance. Best sources of lysine are lean lamb and fish, another good reason to go in for seafood. In addition to lowering blood fats, carnitine raises those 'good' HDLs that help to keep the blood clear of cholesterol. Dosage can range from 500 to 3,000mg daily depending on need. Muscular weakness can be a sign of deficiency.

Coenzyme Q is also concerned with the release of energy from food, working in cooperation with vitamin E. It is the 'spark' that initiates the conversion of carbohydrates to energy in the presence of oxygen. More than 90 per cent of patients given this quasi vitamin showed improvement in the pumping action of the heart within a month. Angina patients were also significantly helped. It could be that some people are not able to make enough of this substance in their bodies to ward off heart disease, maybe due to a deficiency of the necessary complementary B vitamins, and a supplement of 30–60mg could be helpful. This coenzyme is also depleted by stress and ageing.

Wonder foods are garlic and ginger, both of which have passed with flying colours in scientific studies. When eaten daily, blood cholesterol decreases. Walnuts and avocado pears have a similar effect. Garlic also significantly lowers triglyceride levels while at the same time promoting those 'good' HDLs. In one experiment patients ate up to ten cloves per day, with outstanding results . . . even if they did become unpopular with other members of the family! Perhaps it is well worth being unsociable for the sake of a sound heart.

Apart from smoking, Colin was also a coffee addict. It is now known that drinking more than two cups per day is connected with high blood cholesterol and low HDLs. On the other hand, chicory has the reverse effect and can be used as a coffee substitute. As for sugar, a high intake brings about a loss of chromium, another nutrient that helps to keep the blood clear of fatty blockages. Heart disease patients must therefore cut out sugar and increase their consumption of wholewheat bread and pasta. Refining flour removes nearly all of this vital mineral.

Frightened by the appalling experience of the heart attack and relieved to be alive, Colin this time was sufficiently motivated to adopt a wholefood diet. While too weak to cook for himself, his wife was glad to support him in this by learning to select ingredients that would do him good. She substituted soya products for much of his meat, thereby providing him with a useful source of lecithin. This substance is a natural emulsifying agent, since it is partly soluble in water as well as in fat, and for this reason has been adopted by the food industry as an additive. In the body it can prevent and reverse atherosclerosis by causing blood fats to be broken down into such small particles that they can pass right through the walls of the arteries and then be used by the tissues. It can be bought in granules and sprinkled onto food.

Colin's new wholefood diet had the advantage of

increased dietary fibre which binds to blood fats and escorts them out of the body. At the same time it effectively raises the 'good' HDLs and lowers the 'bad' LDLs. Oats and legumes were more or less new to him, but they were particularly recommended. Pectin from fruits such as apples and oranges is a healthy type of water-soluble fibre. Colin rarely ate fresh fruit prior to his heart attack, but it now features every day on his menu along with fresh vegetables. As he has lowered his intake of saturated fat by eating less meat and switching to skimmed milk, so his weight has dropped.

The hospital helped him with a gently graduated exercise programme by handing him a card every so often with a new goal written on it. At first he could scarcely climb the stairs when he arrived home, but his strength returned as his vascular health improved, until he could walk several miles in a day.

Giving up smoking was hardest of all, but he finally achieved this by joining a self-help group. The support of others in similar predicaments encouraged him to stay the course. As for the garlic, this has become a joke in the family. Recently Colin and his wife have learnt to introduce main courses made from beans and lentils, such as those described in chapter 20, and sandwiches are now spread with non-hydrogenated margarine rather than butter.

Varicose veins

This is another problem that lifelong vegetarians are unlikely to develop, on account of their higher intake of dietary fibre; generally speaking they acquire at least half as much again from their diet as omnivores. This means that they rarely, if ever, suffer from constipation, thought to be one cause of varicose veins due to the frequent straining at an overloaded, clogged-up bowel.

Women appear to be more prone to varicose veins than men, often the result of pregnancy. The growing foetus has high requirements for vitamins, especially C and E, and grabs these from the mother's bloodstream, leaving her depleted of these nutrients which are essential for the health of her circulation. Replacing those lost vitamins will certainly help, especially if the vitamin C is taken with the bioflavonoid rutin (about 200mg daily), known to be useful in the treatment of varicose veins.

People who have to stand for lengthy periods at work, such as hairdressers, are other candidates for this disorder, as continuous pressure is put on the valves in the blood vessels; these are designed to prevent the circulation from running the wrong way. It is wise, therefore, to sit down from time to time, with feet raised, to relieve the strain.

Although surgery is frequently used for varicose veins, this unfortunately does not solve the basic problems, as the condition can easily recur. The only lasting remedy is to switch to a wholefood diet which is high in fibre (see recipes in chapter 20) and rich in nutrients. Wholemeal bread and plenty of fruit and vegetables are especially important. If you are overweight then cut down on saturated fats.

Surprisingly, varicose veins can often prove to be an emotionally based disorder. Stress or repressed negative feelings such as anger provoke a rush of blood to the legs to supply the large muscles for action, either fighting or running away. If this happens often enough, but no action results, pressure will inevitably build up in the veins. The solution is to express your feelings safely by saying what you need to say to the person concerned and then having a good kick at a large cushion. Additionally exercise such as running or a sport like squash helps to disperse aggression that has built up physically in the body.

Chilblains

I clearly remember the agonies we endured as children every winter from chilblains. My sister's ankles were purple and swollen, while my little toes were the worst affected, sometimes almost doubling in size and itching mercilessly. Trying to cram bulging feet into shoes first thing in the morning was a painful process. It was such a common problem at our spartan boarding school in the north of England that there was little or no sympathy from the house matron, and the creams we rubbed on hopefully were useless. Exercise was certainly good for us, but running around the hockey field in perishingly cold conditions in knee socks and shorts was frequently torturous as the blood rushed into our feet, causing even more intense irritation.

Since chilblains are often the result of poor circulation, any nutrients that improve it will help to keep this uncomfortable disorder at bay. The wonder ingredient for the blood is EPA (eicosapentaenoic acid) found mainly in fish oils. Children will therefore benefit from a regular spoonful of malt with cod-liver oil, especially in winter – take care not to exceed doses stated on the jar as this is rich in oily vitamin A which can be toxic in large amounts – plus at least two portions of oily fish per week, especially herring, mackerel or salmon. Additionally it is advisable to take an antioxidant vitamin, either C or E, to counteract any harmful rancidity in the fish oil (check the bottle as it may already be included) at about 250mg or 200IU respectively.

It is obviously prudent to ensure that the child wraps up very warm in winter when going out in cold weather, with really thick socks and gloves and a woolly hat that covers the ears, since it is the extremities that are most prone to chilblains.

Food for healthy blood vessels

If you follow the Health-Giving Diet outlined in chapter 20, you will already be well on the way to protecting yourself from cardiovascular disease, since it is low in saturated fat and salt, excludes refined carbohydrates and is high in fibre and all essential nutrients.

While cutting back on red meat, cheese and full-fat milk, increase your intake of fish, especially the oily sort, including salmon, mackerel and herring. Other important sources of protein are soya beans along with tofu and tempeh, also lentils and nuts. Be wary of eating too many eggs, at most three or four per week.

Emphasize fresh vegetables, just lightly steamed or eaten raw in salads, and make sure you have these every day. Make your own French dressings from cold-pressed plant oils and include plenty of garlic. Have this also on avocado pears. Eat at least two pieces of fresh fruit daily, especially citrus, kiwi and berry fruits.

Do not use added salt at all; switch to Biosalt, LoSalt or similar to flavour cooking, which contain good levels of potassium. Better still, use sea seasonings and plenty of garlic and ginger.

Start each day well with home-made muesli, using rolled oats and adding apple or pear complete with well-washed skin, along with dried fruits and nuts and a liberal sprinkling of wheatgerm. Always eat wholemeal bread and pasta and choose non-hydrogenated margarine. Replace refined cakes and biscuits with wholemeal goodies low in sugar.

Instead of coffee have a chicory substitute and reserve alcohol for special occasions only. At the same time maintain a regular exercise programme and, of course, do not sabotage your excellent healthy eating habits by smoking.

Chapter 9

The Breath of Life

Every single one of our 60 trillion cells needs oxygen in constant supply. Without it we can last little more than three minutes. The brain in particular has a heavy requirement for it, using as much as one-quarter of the intake.

So how does the oxygen reach all the cells? The air we breathe in contains approximately 21 per cent of this element. After passing down the windpipe, or trachea, it enters the two bronchi, which subdivide into a mass of tiny bronchioles, only about 0.2mm in diameter. These lead into minute air sacs called alveoli – some 350 million of them! Because the number is so huge, the total surface area from which oxygen can be absorbed is very large indeed, even though the lungs are crammed into a comparatively small space within the ribs. It is the movement of the ribs and diaphragm that forces the lungs to contract and expand – and so we breathe in and out.

The alveoli are surrounded by abundant capillaries carrying blood that has had its oxygen removed by the activities of the cells. It is only through the presence of oxygen that the body's cells are able to release the energy from food and make use of it. Carbon dioxide is produced as a waste and this is carried away in the blood back to the lungs, where it is exchanged for fresh oxygen. The walls of the alveoli are so thin that oxygen can pass through by diffusion and is thus absorbed by the blood. The CO_2 is surrendered similarly.

Our breathing apparatus is kept clean by the action of minute cilia that line the inside of the nose and windpipe. By a continual flicking action, they drive the fluid called mucus, which has trapped specks of dust and germs, upwards to the top of the trachea. This is then swallowed and the unwanted matter is dealt with by the stomach acid.

Unfortunately our respiratory system is vulnerable to infection, despite this clever defence mechanism, since the viruses and bacteria can so easily be breathed in, attacking the nose, throat or lungs, where the dark, moist, warm conditions provide an ideal breeding ground. If your immune system is working effectively due to good nutrition and healthy lifestyle, then you are far less likely to submit to infection. Even the TB bacterium can be conquered in this natural way without the afflicted person ever being aware of having caught the disease; a scar showing up on an X-ray of the lungs is the only tell-tale sign.

Cigarette smoke, as most of us are aware, can do irreparable damage to the intricate mechanisms of the respiratory system, with approximately 100,000 people per annum dying prematurely in the UK alone from smoking-related diseases. The tiny cilia cease their cleansing flicking motion, the bronchioles constrict and the mucus builds up. The air sacs in the lungs become so fragile that they finally burst and the blood can no longer be effectively oxygenated. Studies with animals show that a minimum of seventeen different substances in tobacco smoke cause lung cancer. This disease has increased by 4,000 per cent over the last hundred years, almost entirely as the result of widespread nicotine addiction. One nasty by-product is acetaldehyde, but its toxicity can be lessened by the vitamins C and B_1, combined with the amino acid cysteine. Generous amounts of vitamin C will replace the loss due to smoking and a

147

supplement in addition to food sources is important for anyone exposed to tobacco fumes.

Atmospheric pollution can also seriously harm the human breathing apparatus. A report published in July 1993 by the highly regarded Environment and Forecasting Institute in Heidelberg, Germany, makes alarming reading. This assesses the environmental damage attributed to the motor car alone. Assuming that the average life of a car is 10 years and that it is driven for 8,000 miles (13,000km) per annum, it will pollute more than 2 billion cubic metres of air – a staggering amount – even supposing that it is fitted with a three-way catalytic converter and runs economically on unleaded petrol. This takes into account extractions of raw materials and their transportation, the actual production of the car, its usage and its ultimate disposal. Low-level ozone pollution and nitrogen dioxide are particularly hazardous for asthma sufferers, a disorder which has increased thirteenfold among infants in the last 30 years. In Britain, one-third of the population breathes air which is contaminated beyond EU safety regulations. Over in Los Angeles the situation is appalling: children have already lost 15 per cent of their lung capacity by the age of 11 years due to damage from atmospheric pollution.

At least certain nutrients can help to offset some of the worst effects of our foul air. The antioxidants can prevent the 'rusting' of the lungs from pollutants such as low-level ozone and nitrous oxide. Vitamin E together with selenium work in this way. They also contribute to the mending of any injured DNA inside cells.

Asthma

During an attack the airways of the bronchi become uncomfortably narrow due to contraction of the muscles that encircle them. This produces wheezing and trouble with breathing, especially when expelling the air from the lungs. Swelling in the bronchi may also occur, with the extra generation of mucus, which is then hard to cough up. Such attacks can be very alarming, especially if they last for several hours; they may even be fatal in some cases. There seems to be a positive epidemic of asthma at present, with one child in seven in the UK affected; indeed the number of cases has doubled since the 1970s. Every four-and-a-half hours someone in Britain dies from an attack.

Some people seem to be especially sensitive to environmental irritants, in particular dust, smoke, animal dandruff and pollen. Certain foods can also trigger an attack and patients should therefore test for intolerances (see chapter 11 under 'Allergies'). Problem fare frequently includes wheat, cow's milk, eggs, hazelnuts or celery. As many asthma sufferers will confirm, psychological factors can play an important part and stress and anxiety can make the condition worse.

Most patients discover from experience what the allergens are that provoke attacks and make every effort to avoid such substances. However, certain social situations can make this awkward. Some irritants such as ozone or nitrogen dioxide are not even visible and, with such widespread pollution of the atmosphere, it is impossible to avoid them, even in the countryside.

Since asthma is potentially very serious, ventilators and drugs that dilate the bronchi need to be available for quick relief. However, it is worth knowing that vitamin C is a natural antihistamine. If 250mg is taken every ten minutes during an attack, its severity can be significantly lessened. As a preventive measure, 1 to 2g daily has proved helpful. This amount builds resistance to the effects of harmful airborne substances. Additionally, if exercise provokes wheezing, this can be alleviated with a 500mg dose of vitamin C taken about an hour beforehand.

The mineral magnesium is implicated in muscle relaxation and supplements can therefore ease symptoms: try

400mg daily. This can also be taken in the form of Epsom salts (magnesium sulphate).

Experience has shown that if 100mg of vitamin B_6 is given daily to children who are asthmatic, the number of attacks as well as their severity is diminished. It is thought that some symptoms may arise from an inability to metabolize this vitamin correctly.

Avoid all food preservatives, flavour enhancers and colouring agents: monosodium glutamate (E621–3), if eaten regularly, can induce spasms of the breathing muscles, while metabisulphite (E223) is known to aggravate asthma attacks. This is used as a preservative, particularly in wines and squashes. Here again, vitamin B_6 can counteract the worst consequences if such substances are consumed unwittingly. Painkillers such as aspirin can also induce wheezing.

A friend of mine, also a writer, has struggled with asthma most of her life. Whenever she comes to stay the entire house has to be carefully vacuumed and the cat is banished to the outhouse, amidst indignant mewing. Since Angela is allergic to feathers as well as animal fur, she arrives complete with her own pillow and duvet that contain non-irritating stuffing. She also has to avoid various foods, especially eggs and nuts – quite a problem as she is a vegetarian. She is aware that stress aggravates her condition, so she has taken up meditation and has attended a time-management course, both of which assist in keeping her breathing easy. She keeps up her intake of vitamin C with a daily supplement and by eating plenty of fruit, vegetables and salads. She has also cut out sugar and all other refined carbohydrates, which can aggravate symptoms, and reduced saturated fats. Luckily she is not wheat-sensitive, so obtains her B vitamins from wholemeal bread and wheatgerm. Both ginseng and garlic are traditional remedies which she finds useful. By adjusting her diet and lifestyle she has learnt how to avoid asthma attacks almost completely and rarely has to resort to an inhaler.

Another tip from Angela: after learning that an ionizer encourages dust to settle by emitting negatively charged ions, making it less likely to be breathed in, she bought one for the bedroom.

Hay fever

Along with other allergic diseases, this is very much a modern malady, being virtually unknown in the early part of the last century. Some researchers have pointed out that it started among the wealthier classes who could afford the luxury of sucrose. It is interesting that grass, sugar and wheat belong to the same botanical family, so is it just chance that grass pollen is the most frequent irritant in hay fever and that wheat is the main culprit as far as food intolerances are concerned? At any rate, if you do suffer from hay fever, then you would do well to cut out sugar and other refined carbohydrates. Also check out whether you are intolerant of wheat or any other foodstuff, especially eggs, cow's milk and yeast, including alcohol (see the end of chapter 11 for more details on food allergies). By cutting out any possible allergens, you will lower your overall sensitivity and are less likely to find yourself with streaming nose and eyes in the spring. Pollen counts tend to be worst when the weather is warm and sunny, so you may be better off inside on those days.

It is important to boost your consumption of vitamin C, so eat plenty of fruit, especially oranges, strawberries and kiwi fruit, and salads with green peppers, tomatoes, red cabbage, raw broccoli florets and watercress. And don't forget those other green vegetables. These also contain magnesium, a mineral which will help counteract the allegeric symptoms. You will find more of this in brazil nuts, whole cereals and soya beans. Include delicious nut roasts in your diet, therefore, and some original tofu dishes

151

(see chapter 20 for recipes). During the spring and early summer take supplements as well: at least 1g of vitamin C daily and 250mg magnesium. If you suffer from stress, then include a B-complex tablet of at least 500mg.

As with asthma, emotional upheavals can greatly worsen hayfever, so try to find ways of staying calm. Meditation and yoga are of proven value.

Chronic hay-fever sufferers may find relief from the amino acid methionine in combination with calcium, which have an antihistamine effect. Take 500mg of L-methionine with 400mg of calcium twice daily for up to three weeks. Additionally, boost your immunity with 15mg of zinc and 100mg of vitamin B_6.

Coughs and colds

As far as the medical profession is concerned, the problem with colds is that there is a minimum of 80 varying strains of the virus. One of these infects the mucous membranes of the nose and pharynx, causing the familiar runny nose and watery eyes with sneezes. Each of these propels millions of infectious droplets into the air only to be picked up by some unwitting passer-by – and so the virus is passed on.

It is well known that some 'colds' are psychosomatic in origin, expressing an unconscious need to cry. These are best treated with counselling or at least a heart-to-heart with a close friend.

As with all infectious diseases, healthy nutrition that keeps the immune system in top working order will prevent them from taking hold. A diet that is rich in fresh fruit, vegetables and salads, with a good percentage of it eaten raw, and low in saturated fats and refined carbohydrates, will ensure that the cold virus will be an unwelcome visitor.

If you are unlucky enough to develop a sore throat or catch a cold, then as soon as you feel it coming on, take at least 500mg of vitamin C four times a day until the symptoms ease, after which you can gradually reduce the amount. This, together with 5mg of chelated zinc three times daily or zinc lozenges, will curtail its duration. You can also make yourself a herbal gargle which will relieve a sore throat (see chapter 20). Cold germs dislike warmth, so wrap your head up in a woollen scarf at night and put on plenty of clothes during the day.

If you are troubled by catarrh, avoid dairy produce and take one garlic oil capsule three times a day. These will also alleviate coughs, as will the soothing herbal remedy called the Vegetable Cough Remover available at health food shops. My mother used to make us a delicious hot lemon and honey drink and blackcurrant tea, both classic remedies that will aid recovery (see chapter 20 for information on healing beverages).

Bronchitis and emphysema

An ordinary cold can sometimes turn nasty and spread into the windpipe and bronchi. This secondary infection may be generated by bacteria and is generally accompanied by a sore throat and cough with raised temperature. There may also be chest pain. Smokers are especially susceptible to bronchitis, as are the elderly, mostly during the winter months.

While antibiotics may have to be taken to control serious bacterial infections, high doses of vitamin C (3g daily divided into frequent small amounts), together with chelated zinc (30mg), will help to fight off the invaders. Vitamin A is particularly important for the health of the mucous membranes and for the production of the white cells of the immune system, so take 10,000IU daily as beta carotene. Make sure your intake of B vitamins is adequate by adding wheatgerm to your diet. This will also supply you with vitamin E, another nutrient involved in the production of antibodies. If you have to take antibiotics, then eat plenty of live yoghurt to correct any damage to your intestinal flora.

Avoid all refined carbohydrates, which deplete you of essential nutrients, and, as with all infections, have plenty of fresh fruit, salads and vegetables, preferably raw – or juiced if you have little appetite. Keep away from saturated fats. Drink lots of fluid, especially rose hip and blackcurrant teas (see chapter 20 under 'Beverages and Herbal Remedies').

There is another sort of bronchitis which is not instigated by infection but rather by cigarettes or polluted air which irritate and ultimately damage the bronchi and lungs. Before the Clean Air Act in the UK, the London 'smogs' used to be notorious, with 4,000 people per week dying from chronic bronchitis in 1952. It is very common among cigarette smokers. The fragile cilia cease to beat, so that they cannot clean the airways of mucus and unwanted particles. If the pollution continues to enter the lungs, the delicate walls of the alveoli (the tiny air spaces) will burst and the overall surface area will be greatly reduced. This means that the exchange of oxygen and carbon dioxide to and from the blood can no longer operate efficiently and the patient will become constantly breathless, even when inactive.

Owen is a typical case. Now in his late 50s, he has been an addicted smoker since the age of 15 when he first took it up in a misguided effort to prove to his schoolmates how 'grown-up' he was. Even the horrible discomfort of recurring bronchitis each winter, with fever and hacking cough, did not put him off cigarettes. At a time in his life when he should still be full of energy, he has been forced to retire early from his job as a painter and decorator and can now barely stagger out into the garden to mow the lawn. He wheezes constantly and frequently has to stop to catch his breath.

After the doctor's gloomy prognosis, his wife took him to a nutritional therapist to see if anything could be done at this late stage. The therapist explained that the damage to his lungs was permanent and that nothing could reverse that, but certain nutrients could assist him in metabolizing oxygen so that he would be less short of breath. Giving up smoking was, of course, vital. She prescribed vitamin E and iron supplements (400IU and 20mg daily respectively). The diet sheet she gave him was high in complex carbohydrates, which require less oxygen than fatty foods to be metabolized, with the emphasis on whole grains, peas, beans and lentils, vegetables and fruit. The B vitamins, especially niacin, are needed for the burning of these, so she also recommended 500mg daily of a B-complex supplement. Since the remaining connective tissue needed to be strengthened, the vitamins C and A would sustain this process, so she also included 1g daily of the first and 10,000IU of beta-carotene.

Owen managed to stick to this programme and experienced gradual improvement with less exhaustion. The therapist also encouraged him to take up singing to increase the efficiency of his injured lungs. Being Welsh, he took to this idea readily and joined a male-voice choir, thereby discovering an absorbing new hobby. While he could never be entirely cured, at least his decline was halted and it became possible to live a more normal life by making the most of the lungs he still had left.

Influenza and pneumonia

We are all familiar with the symptoms of 'flu: a temperature, but also feeling shivery, usually a headache and pains in the bones and muscles, together with a cough. It takes about 10 years to develop immunity to a particular strain of 'flu virus, by which time any epidemic has died out and a new variety is on the attack. It can be dangerous if secondary bacterial infection develops because it may turn into pneumonia. Antibiotics were able to limit mortality rates from the 1957 pandemic, which spread from China via Hong Kong, but in 1917–19, before their invention, an

155

equally extensive and vicious onslaught resulted in more deaths than those due to the fighting during the entire First World War.

As with colds, people seem to imagine that they should not give in to 'flu but rather stagger into work as long as it is possible to walk and thereby spread the infection. Naturally, the best way to limit it is through isolation. While that attitude remains, however, the only other way to avoid catching it – or at any rate markedly reduce its effects – is to boost your immunity with excellent nutrition. There is plenty of advice about this in chapter 11.

Meanwhile, if you have the misfortune to fall victim to a passing 'flu virus, there is much that you can do nutritionally to get rid of it soon. Any fever quickly depletes the body of vitamins, so these must be replaced as follows: 2g vitamin C, 200mg pantothenic acid and 10mg each of vitamins B_2 and B_6, all to be taken immediately, then half quantities every three hours for the first day, gradually reducing the amounts as the symptoms ease. You will also require plenty of fluid to prevent dehydration: Lemon Barley Water is excellent for calming a fever, Ginger Brew is based on a traditional folk remedy and Lime-Blossom Herb Tea is very soothing (see chapter 20 for recipes). If you do not feel like eating, then take the Fortified Soya Drink, which will supply you with protein and other important nutrients, and Miso and Onion Soup (also described in chapter 20). As you return to solids, keep to fresh fruit, vegetables and pulses, and avoid refined carbohydrates and saturated fats (including dairy products), both of which reduce your immunity. See also the section on colds and coughs for other helpful suggestions.

It is important to rest, especially if you are old, to give the body maximum chance to fight the infection, and to keep warm.

If you treat yourself nutritionally as described, then it is unlikely that the 'flu will progress to pneumonia. Should this type of bacterial infection occur, then your doctor will prescribe antibiotics to reduce the inflammation of the lungs. Take plenty of live yoghurt to reinstate healthy intestinal flora which the drugs will deplete and keep up the anti-fever nutrients.

Tuberculosis

This is a disease long thought to have been vanquished in the West by the effective use of antibiotics, yet a recent article in the *Guardian* warns against complacency. In New York drug-resistant strains have emerged among the poor and homeless and Tower Hamlets in east London has a much higher-than-average incidence of TB: 50 per 100,000. Among disadvantaged groups and ethnic minorities statistics are considerably worse at 160 per 100,000 in the UK, whereas overall national rates are just 5 in every 100,000. Worldwide there are up to 2 million deaths per annum. Overcrowding and poor hygiene are largely responsible for its spread as the bacterium can survive for many weeks in dirty, damp places.

Good diet and fresh air were the traditional remedies, and indeed this remains wise advice, for the bacterium dies in sunlight. It is also well known that people with sound immune systems conquer the disease without realizing they have been affected by it. Chapter 11 will tell you about maintaining a healthy immune system, which will prevent a disease such as TB, combined with clean, well-ventilated living conditions.

In case of any infection, the length and severity can be significantly reduced by taking 500mg of vitamin C, 50mg pantothenic acid (vitamin B_5) and 2mg each of vitamins B_2 and B_6 six times a day, together with regular cups of Fortified Soya Drink (see chapter 20), gradually easing amounts as the disease abates. To prevent scarring of the lungs, take 300IU vitamin E daily.

Cystic fibrosis

The prognosis for this sad condition is better now than previously, with many sufferers surviving into adulthood thanks to improved treatment with antibiotics for the severe chest infections to which the patients are highly vulnerable. Parents have to be trained in special care for children with this disease, which includes draining mucus from the respiratory tract.

Sometimes babies are also born with a poor ability to secrete digestive juices. This very often means difficulty in breaking down and absorbing foods along with many nutrients, especially the fat-soluble vitamins A, E, D and K, so supplements of these need to be given at above RDA levels. Children should also be tested for mineral deficiencies which ought to be rectified.

It is extremely important to adhere to a healthy diet (see chapter 20) and good intakes of vitamin C and zinc will help guard against the recurrent infections.

Chapter 10

Chemical Messengers

Although we are not generally aware of it, messages are constantly being passed around our bodies, either via nerve impulses from the brain telling different muscles and glands how to function, or else via special chemicals which are released into the bloodstream and aimed at particular organs – a somewhat slower method. These chemicals are collectively known as hormones. The blood picks them up from the endocrine glands, namely the pituitary situated at the base of the brain, the thyroid at the front of the neck, the two adrenal glands above the kidneys, the nearby pancreas and the ovaries or testes. Many important body functions are affected and controlled by hormones, including growth and reproduction, as well as chemical reactions connected with metabolism that keep us alive.

Some women are conscious of the ebb and flow of their sex hormones throughout their monthly cycle, while most people are familiar with the sudden rush of adrenalin in response to stress. When a part of the endocrine system goes wrong, however, the results can be dramatic with serious illness following; diabetes is one such disorder.

Diabetes mellitus

In chapter 6, in describing the journey of Philip's lunch through his digestive system, the pancreas was mentioned as secreting enzymes. This organ has another role, however, and that is the production of two hormones, called glucagon and insulin. When the amount of sugar in the blood declines, glucagon is released. On reaching the liver, it prompts cells located there to convert some of its stored-up glycogen into glucose and so the blood-sugar level is corrected. Insulin works in exactly the opposite way: after a meal, when the blood is rich with sugar, the pancreas secretes this hormone, which then also targets the liver. This time liver cells are provoked into extracting glucose from the blood and then keeping it in the form of glycogen, and so the blood-sugar level is again regulated, but downwards. The balancing act involved is another example of homoeostasis described in chapter 7, in which the internal environment is kept constant.

The disease known as diabetes occurs either when the pancreas produces insufficient insulin or when, having secreted the hormone, the body's cells are then unable to incorporate it into their metabolic processes. Either way, the patient does not have normal control over blood-sugar levels, which may swing wildly. If they rise too high, the person will become extremely thirsty and will have an overwhelming urge to urinate as the body tries to rid itself of the sugar. For this reason diabetes was bluntly referred to as 'the pissing sickness' by seventeenth-century English people. The Latin name, *diabetes mellitus*, accurately describes this symptom, meaning 'sweetness running through'. If they swing too low, the brain cells, which are heavily dependent on glucose, will be unable to function properly and the result may be coma. In advanced cases, coma may equally occur if blood sugar rises too high due to failure to administer insulin.

If the diabetes starts in childhood, then insulin will have to be injected to keep the blood sugar steady as there will be underproduction of the hormone, due possibly to genetic factors or maybe as the result of injury to the pancreas from a virus. If, however, the disease starts in the middle

160

years, as is often the case, then the chances are that insulin is being produced but the body's cells cannot absorb it. This type is generally described as 'non-insulin-dependent', and control with nutrition alone is usually very effective (although more serious conditions may have to be treated additionally with anti-diabetic drugs). It is therefore a programme for the adult-onset variety that we will concentrate on here; however, the dietary recommendations will also significantly assist any diabetic. All are prone to other serious illnesses as well, including blindness, kidney dysfunction, nerve defects, gangrene, strokes and heart disease, but such hazards can be largely prevented with healing nutrients.

Like many other maladies discussed in this book, the steep rise in the incidence of diabetes is a consequence of our modern way of life. Researchers who have studied peasant farmers in East Africa have noted that the occurrence of diabetes is well under 1 per cent. Yet when they examine the affluent *nouveau riche*, the 'Wabenzi' (that is those who own a Mercedes Benz!), 8 per cent of this over-fed, sedentary group has the disorder. It seems that the body's natural mechanism for dealing with sugars has become confused by overburdening it with an excessive amount of simple carbohydrates and so, in the end, the blood-sugar levels rise unchecked.

The two most important ways to avoid diabetes, and to control it if you have it, are to lose weight if you are too heavy and to take regular exercise. Permanent weight loss is discussed in chapter 16 and you will find low-fat, sugar-free recipes at the end of the book. As for exercise, this will help your body to make better use of the available insulin.

Your doctor will doubtless explain to you that the aim in working with nutrition is to keep your blood-sugar levels steady, thereby avoiding those highs and lows that will make you feel miserably ill.

Doreen is now in her late 60s and is almost blind, having suffered from diabetes for 25 years. This is especially sad for her as her garden was her greatest joy. Now she can no longer witness the spring flowers popping through the earth, nor see the delicate blossoms of her favourite roses.

She described the strange sensation as her sight deteriorated: like a spider's web being pulled across her eye. She knew then that internal bleeding was damaging the retina. Had she found out about nutritional therapy at an earlier stage, some of this deterioration could have been averted. Just 500mg of vitamin C daily would have strengthened those fragile capillaries, while bioflavonoids could have stopped the build-up of excess fluid in the eyes.

Diabetics also have problems with blood clots; the specialized red blood cells called platelets clump together too readily due to an abnormal fatty acid content. This can result in strokes as well as eye damage. Eating plenty of oily fish such as salmon, herring and mackerel, or taking linseed oil, will help to correct this, as will 500IU of vitamin E daily.

To begin with, Doreen found the diet recommended by her doctor hard to adhere to, but the experience of going into a coma alarmed her so much that she had to change her attitude. One Sunday she decided to visit her sister who lived in another town. She caught the country bus in the late morning, planning to take sandwiches with her to eat on the way. When she searched inside her bag she realized to her horror that she had left them in the kitchen by mistake. This meant she would be unable to eat for at least another one and a half hours. She crossed her fingers and prayed that her blood sugar would remain steady that long. Towards the end of the journey she started to feel faint. She broke out in a cold sweat and her heart began to palpitate. By the time the driver called out her destination she was in trouble. She staggered to her feet and managed to climb off the vehicle, only to reel about on the pavement as if she were drunk. A passer-by laughed at her, thinking she had had one too many. Her legs would no longer hold her up and she fell to the ground in a heap. Fortunately her sister, who had offered to meet her at the bus stop, arrived just at that moment and quickly summoned medical help. Doreen was soon revived with an injection of glucagon.

After this episode she joined the British Diabetic Association (see Addresses) and with their help maintained a dietary regime that kept her blood sugar steady. Since she had always had a sweet tooth, giving up sticky cakes – especially doughnuts – seemed like a real hardship, but she soon discovered the delights of sugar-free goodies (chapter 20 contains recipes); excluding simple sugars and artificial sweeteners was an essential part of the programme. More than half her intake of calories had to be from unrefined complex carbohydrates which were high in fibre. This meant she had to emphasize fresh fruit and vegetables, whole grain products and legumes (there are high-fibre recipes in chapter 20).

The results of a study published in May 1985 of Seventh Day Adventists, who are lifelong vegetarians, showed clearly that they were only half as likely to develop diabetes as other Americans. Further studies have demonstrated that a diet rich in fibre and complex carbohydrates reduces blood glucose and therefore insulin requirements by up to 50 per cent. Taking the soluble fibre in the form of around 10g of xanthum gum or guar gum is especially valuable in this respect, while pectin delays the rate at which food passes through the digestive system, so bringing about a gradual release of glucose into the bloodstream. Doreen made sure, therefore, that she ate plenty of oranges and apples. (On the subject of fibre, it is not advisable to take extra wheat bran as this can bind to valuable minerals and extract them from the body.)

She had to reduce her proportion of dietary fat to only

one-third or less of calories, especially cutting back on the saturated variety. This meant little or no meat and only low-fat dairy products in restricted amounts. She also had to restrain herself from reaching for the salt-shaker or from buying those much-appreciated bottles of wine. Her doctor had warned her that she must lose weight to improve her prognosis and she was delighted that after only two months on her diet she easily lost half a stone (3kg) and maintained her new weight without any extra effort.

Research during the last 15 years has shown chromium to be an essential trace element which works together with the amino acids cysteine, glycine and glutamic acid and vitamin B_3 (collectively called Glucose Tolerance Factor or GTF) that helps insulin to get the glucose into cells. Considering that the refining of flour removes nearly all the chromium from our bread, otherwise the main source for this mineral, it is hardly surprising that Westerners suffer from deficiency, with resulting late-onset diabetes. Do eat fresh wholemeal bread, therefore – organic if you can find it. Or better still, make it yourself. All older diabetics will benefit from chromium supplementation, found in brewer's yeast tablets, which will also contain GTF. Take at least three tablets three times a day; indeed you can safely take three times this amount. Brewer's yeast contains other B-complex vitamins; B_6 and B_{12} help in blood-sugar control and combat symptoms such as tingling and dizziness. It is worth experimenting to discover what dose suits you best.

If the glucose is unavailable to cells, then the body will invade fat and protein stores for urgently needed fuel. The unfortunate consequence of this is that fats build up in the bloodstream, leaving diabetics highly vulnerable to strokes and heart disease, a potentially lethal situation. All the more reason to prevent this happening by taking chromium and following the advice in chapter 8 concerning such problems that beset the circulatory system. Needless to say, it is vital that diabetics do not smoke, which will only exacerbate all these complications.

Not only will vitamin C strengthen capillary walls, it will help to heal leg ulcers and avoid bruising, both common in diabetics, as well as keeping the blood cholesterol down: 1g daily in small amounts is a useful dosage, together with plenty of oranges, kiwi fruit, green peppers and broccoli.

You may have been losing zinc in your urine, so include a daily supplement of 15mg. This mineral is important for healing and will also combat leg ulcers; check chapter 3 for food sources. Moreover, it is involved in the production of insulin so is especially valuable to diabetics. However, too much will not be better for you; more than 25mg daily may deplete the 'good' blood fats. Chromium, on the other hand, will raise the beneficial HDLs (see chapter 8).

Russian researchers have identified an anti-diabetic substance in ginseng called ginsnenin. It is worth the expense because it helps to keep blood sugar on an even keel. The powdered root can be bought in tablets and you will need to take about 400mg daily. The reason why the price is so high is because it is harvested only every six years, after which the land is left for a whole decade before replanting. Do you know you can grow it in your own garden? The root can then be boiled to extract the active ingredients. It might be worth experimenting.

As for fenugreek, this is reckoned by some experts to be more effective than many anti-diabetic drugs at lowering blood glucose. You can sprout the seeds in a jar on your windowsill and they are delicious eaten in salads.

Garlic, once again, is wonderfully medicinal. Tests in India have shown that it reduces the concentration of sugar in the blood of both healthy people and diabetics, so use it regularly in cooking. If you really cannot stand the taste, then garlic-oil capsules are a handy alternative, although they may not be so efficacious.

The best drink for diabetics is sage tea (see chapter 20,

under 'Infusions'). This will also assist in keeping blood sugar under control.

To prevent those swings in glucose eat a little often rather than gorging yourself every now and again; six small, well-balanced meals are far better than three big ones.

Hypoglycaemia

This condition of low blood sugar is surprisingly common, yet all too often – as in my own case – it is misdiagnosed, or even worse, sufferers are dismissed as neurotic hypochondriacs. Some of the symptoms can sound as if they are psychosomatic in origin: poor concentration, irritability, mood swings, tiredness, headaches, anxiety and insomnia, but when experienced subjectively the patient definitely knows there is something physically wrong. This becomes more obvious when other pointers are taken into account, such as blurred vision, trembling limbs, faintness, extreme hunger and/or nausea. However, the issue may be complex because stress can be associated with hypoglycaemia. Blood-sugar tests need to be carried out over a period of at least three hours, preferably five, to give a reliable indication of the drop in blood glucose. Ideally it should be measured while symptoms are occurring. Few hospitals will provide this service, though.

A hypoglycaemic attack can be extremely alarming. Even though I am now an expert at keeping my blood sugar steady and rarely travel far without an emergency packet of nuts and raisins and a banana in my bag, I have occasionally been caught out. One such time was when John, my husband, and I were first going out together. Some of his archaeological finds were being displayed in a local church and we arranged to meet first at his cottage at about noon. I assumed he would offer me lunch, or perhaps we would buy a meal at the local pub; little did I realize at that time that he was the sort of person who often skips meals without ill effect, especially when carried away by some enthusiasm.

Keen to show me his discoveries, we went straight to the church, where I was introduced to several members of the local history club. All were proud of their village, a quaint place indeed, boasting several half-timbered medieval houses along its winding main street. The most interesting of these had been researched in detail and I was shown dozens of photographs illustrating particular features. Absorbing as this was, my concentration began to deteriorate, and the subject of food became a matter of urgency. I wandered over to John's stand, where he was holding forth on the way of life of Roman soldiers with tremendous zest. How I envied his energy! His finds were fascinating: a baby's skeleton, dice, innumerable fragments of pottery, several Roman coins, an ancient ruler and so on. These items entered my consciousness only dimly as the pain behind my eyes increased and my vision started to blur. By now feelings of faintness were setting in and I started to panic. I muttered something to John about looking for something to eat and groped my way out of the church, keeping my head as low as possible, hoping that the blood supply might reach my brain somehow and that my behaviour did not appear too peculiar. The light outside was dazzling and I fumbled in my handbag for my sunglasses. If only I had brought my emergency nut supplies!

Realizing that the pub was only serving drinks, my search for food became desperate. Should I borrow John's car? No, better not; it could be dangerous to drive in this condition. Finally a tea tent on the village green came into view. What luck! Images of asparagus quiche and salad with fresh-pressed orange juice floated across my imagination, only to be dashed on entering the marquee: the fare being served was scones with butter and jam, sugary fairy cakes and tea. Most people would be glad of such offerings, but sugar has a disastrous effect on hypoglycaemics – a sudden rise in energy followed by a rapid drop, often accompanied by nausea and fainting. Another problem: there was a long queue. I propped myself up by holding on to the backs of chairs, smiling in a forced way at any vaguely familiar face, hoping no one would notice anything odd. At last my turn: two scones and butter, please, but no jam, with tea. Before passing out altogether I crammed them into my mouth, all thoughts of elegant eating thrown to the winds. At least they would keep me going for another half-hour or so and then perhaps I could raid John's cupboards for some protein.

He was photographing the Morris dancers when I emerged from the tent feeling temporarily revived. Once again I could enjoy myself, sing along with the music, appreciate the gaudy colours of the costumes and laugh at the high jumping and earnest expressions of the dancers. Before my blood sugar crashed again John, distinctly perplexed by my behaviour, nevertheless obligingly took me home and put some substantial food in me. It is hard indeed to describe to a person with normal metabolic processes the wild swings in well-being that hypoglycaemics have to endure, simply by not having the right food at the right time. Happily the condition is totally controllable with correct diet.

So what causes hypoglycaemia? Rather than having an insufficient supply of insulin, as in diabetes, the patient generally produces an excess of the hormone. This means that too much sugar is extracted from the blood and driven into the cells for burning, leaving the bloodstream depleted. The organs that have a very high requirement for glucose, such as the brain and the eyes, immediately feel the effects, hence the loss of concentration and coordination, the faintness, the blurred vision and so on. The same happens if a diabetic takes too much insulin.

It is advisable to test the activity of the thyroid gland, as a hormonal imbalance here can result in low blood sugar. Equally, stress can upset hormonal and therefore blood-sugar levels by stimulating the pancreas and adrenals. Very rarely the disorder occurs because of a tumour on the pancreas, so severe cases should be thoroughly investigated.

Remember that doctors know little or nothing about the chemistry of nutrition, since they do not study it in medical school. The advice you receive from your general practitioner on the subject of low blood sugar may therefore be erroneous: the classic reply is to drink a cup of sweet tea, or to eat starchy or sugary foods. Nothing could be worse! Most people with this condition have what is known as 'reactive' hypoglycaemia; in other words, the blood sugar falls low in reaction to simple sugars. Moreover the quicker it rises, the faster it falls and the more pronounced the symptoms. As with diabetes, therefore, the aim is to keep the blood-sugar curve as gentle as possible and the best way to do that is to eat foods that take a long time to digest. Since refined carbohydrates are absorbed instantly through the gut, avoid these absolutely and concentrate on the complex carbohydrates (whole grains, fresh fruit and vegetables and legumes), which are also high in fibre, and on protein, because it helps to control insulin.

If you suspect that you are suffering from hypoglycaemia, then keep a diary for a couple of weeks, noting down what you have eaten and when, and exactly what time the symptoms occur. After a while you will probably begin to notice a pattern. My worst time in the day is 11.30am and the best is after supper in the early evening. You need to arrange your programme so that you can eat something sustaining just when your blood-sugar level is dropping, which could be as often as every two hours. Forget society's rules about when meals should be served; you will have to re-invent your own! Like me, you may have to eat lunch

169

at 11.30am. Certainly you will be better off having a little, often.

Notice which foods aggravate your symptoms and avoid these. Packet breakfast cereals such as Frosties or Sugar Puffs, and any sweet biscuits or cakes, especially if made with white flour, will all be real trouble-makers, as will sugar (or artificial sweeteners) in coffee or tea, and any canned or alocholic drinks. Indeed, caffeine, alcohol and tobacco, like sugar, all provoke insulin production, which in turn lowers blood glucose. Also, test yourself for food intolerances, especially wheat and dairy products, which can exacerbate symptoms in some cases (see next chapter).

Fibre will be very helpful to you because it slows down the digestion of other foods in the intestine. The complex carbohydrates, that is whole grains, legumes, fruit and vegetables, all contain dietary fibre and will give you good glucose tolerance. Experiment with a variety of grains because some will provide more gradual sugar release than others, for example pumpernickel and wholemeal rye bread are better than whole wheat in this respect. Maintain your diary entries noting down which foods give you a feeling of well-being and for how long. Increase your protein intake, emphasizing nuts and fish especially, also free-range eggs and poultry, low-fat dairy products, and lean meat in moderation. Indeed, the Health-Giving Diet outlined in chapter 20 will be a good starting point for you.

The most important meal of your day will be breakfast. The standard fare of cornflakes with milk and sugar, or white toast and marmalade with cup of coffee, will play havoc with your blood glucose and by mid-morning you will feel terrible. Make sure you have some form of protein such as scrambled eggs on wholemeal toast or fish cakes accompanied by a herb tea or fruit juice, and your energy will be released gradually, keeping you going for several hours. Instead of biscuits and coffee mid-morning, eat a fruit-and-nut bar (without added sweetener) or a mixture of nuts, raisins and pumpkin seeds and/or a banana, with herb tea or dandelion or chicory coffee. Keep up the principles of high complex carbohydrates and high protein meals throughout the day. You may well be thought eccentric especially if, like me, you take to lentil cutlets for breakfast, but what does it matter if your new diet cures your erratic blood levels and you end up feeling great?

Various supplements will also help you. The B vitamins are crucial to energy metabolism, together with chromium and organic iron, and you will derive all you need from brewer's (not baker's) yeast tablets. Take three tablets of 250mg three times daily, supplying up to 200mcg chromium. Zinc is a part of, or necessary for, more than 70 enzymes, so you are likely to benefit from a supplement of 15mg daily, especially if you do not eat meat and dislike oysters. Other useful minerals are manganese, magnesium and potassium, but you will already be boosting your intake of these through your extra supply of whole cereals, fruit and vegetables. Cut down on salt, though, to make potassium more available to cells.

If you are under stress, do find a way of managing your time better and of relaxing, and take 250mg vitamin C four times daily (but not too late in the evening). You may also like to refer to 'Insomnia' in chapter 16 if you tend to wake in the night feeling hungry.

Regular exercise of just a few minutes each day, plus a good work-out of about 40 minutes three times a week, will greatly improve metabolism and regulation of blood glucose.

Goitre

As mentioned at the opening of this chapter, the thyroid is one of the endocrine glands producing hormones that carry messages to other parts of the body. In this case thyroxine is the chief hormone and its supply affects the rate of metabolism in many cells. If it is deficient, then the person

171

will quite literally slow down as the basal metabolism falls and the circulation becomes sluggish. Its main constituent is iodine and a diet lacking in this essential trace element results in goitre, with its main symptom an enlarged thyroid gland. In the past, when populations were dependent upon locally grown foods, if the soil was low in iodide, such as in Derbyshire in central England, then goitre was endemic. If depletion was severe, children would fail to develop properly, leading to cretinism or dim-wittedness. When researchers assessed the iodine status of 22 children aged two to three years in affluent Dortmund, Germany, in 1992, they were astonished to discover that half were deficient and at risk of goitre.

The correct intake of iodine will cure goitre, the daily amount recommended by the EU and USA being 150mcg. Most doctors will suggest adding iodized salt to food, but high sodium is bad for the cardiovascular system. Kelp is a much better option. Fish, including haddock and cod, eggs, dairy foods (especially yoghurt) and almonds are excellent sources.

Since thyroxine uses niacin (vitamin B_3) for proper synthesis, it is a good idea to ensure adequate intake of this nutrient. This is available in brewer's yeast and wheatgerm, lean meat and poultry, fish, eggs, dates and avocados.

Too much iodine can be toxic, the maximum safe intake recommended by WHO being 1,000mcg a day. It is worth mentioning that the red food-colouring erythrosine (E127), found in items such as glacé cherries, tinned strawberries and luncheon meat, is very high in iodine and may be restricted in future.

The characteristics of thyrotoxicosis, due to too much thyroid hormone in the body, include sweating, loss of weight and prominent eyes. However, it is generally due to an overactive thyroid rather than an unbalanced diet. Like goitre, it is more frequently diagnosed in women than in men. Hyperthyroidism can be significantly helped with

172

vitamin A, so eat plenty of carrots and apricots and consider taking a supplement of beta-carotene. Interestingly, some foods inhibit the activity of the thyroid gland in animals, including the Brassica (cabbage) family, peanuts and soya beans. Any such disturbance, though, needs specialist treatment.

Chapter 11

Your Defence Forces

The immune system is often likened to a nation's military defences which must be perpetually on the alert to beat off potential invaders. These are a constant threat to survival and include attack from viruses, bacteria and fungi as well as other parasites. Such defences also need to be capable of repairing wounds and dealing with any mutiny from within, such as errant cells that threaten to form a malignant tumour.

The external defence mechanisms are fairly obvious, such as hairs in our noses which trap unwanted particles, tears that remove specks from our eyes, or the oil on our skin that is naturally antiseptic. If the attackers defy these external defences and slip through on to home territory, then other forces are set in motion, which are of two kinds: general and specific.

Inflammation is one general defence method in which cells release particular chemicals, such as histamine, thereby encouraging the blood vessels to dilate. Plasma proteins arrive on the scene to assist in healing and repair work, while white 'scavenging' blood cells attack any invading bacteria by gobbling them up in a process known as phagocytosis. Some of these scavengers are able to dispose of as many as 100 bacteria before themselves expiring.

Yet the phagocytes may not be the victors, in which case another general defence mechanism will come into operation, namely the lymphatic system. Its main purpose is for drainage, but in addition to removing fluid from the tissue spaces, it collects foreign bodies and dead material, which are swept along the fine capillaries into the larger lymphatic vessels. Situated in clusters along these, especially in the neck, armpit and groin, are the lymph nodes which trap the debris in a fine network of fibrous tissue. The resident scavenger cells known as macrophages then devour the unwanted organisms, while other white cells may produce antibodies against them. At the same time new white cells develop here called lymphocytes, some of which are carried into the bloodstream to boost the immune defences.

Canny bacteria may outwit all of these defences, in which case having entered the bloodstream they face another hurdle: the spleen. This is a spongy organ near the stomach which filters the blood and, like the lymph nodes, it also contains resident macrophages which will attack any remaining invaders.

Despite these ingenious general defence processes, particularly vicious pathogens capable of causing nasty infections may outmanoeuvre the lot. Their presence will, however, trigger the body's specific immune responses, which are individually designed to deal with any particular invader. Even more astonishing, they have a memory, so that the body is unlikely to fall victim to, say, scarlet fever more than once. Vaccination, by which the person is injected with a treated form of the pathogen, relies on this natural process for its effect. Tiny molecules called antigens, on the surface of each pathogen, provoke the immune system to produce antibodies, which then lock into the antigens and weaken the bacterium so that it disintegrates or so that scavenger cells can then devour it more easily.

Lymphocytes that produce antibodies are known as B-cells because they mature in the bone marrow. These are different from the other sort of white cells, the T-cells, which develop in the thymus.

You might well wonder how it is that we become ill at all with such an effective barrage of defences. It really depends on whether the white cells can produce antibodies more quickly than the bacteria can multiply. The immune system may be impaired, due to factors such as poor nutrition, stress or, occasionally, damage to genes, in which case the invaders take hold and disease results. Certain viruses can change their antigens through mutation so that the immune system is unable to recognize them; epidemics of influenza have occurred in this way.

All the more reason to keep your defences healthy so that you are well equipped to fight off disease. Sound nutrition makes a very significant difference to the numbers and quality of the white cells. Clearly, a well-fed army is far more likely to be successful in battle than an under-nourished one!

Boosting your immune system

The first line of defence facing potential aggressors is the mucous membrane that lines the body's apertures. Here, resident white cells either gobble up invaders or else secrete antibodies. Vitamin A must be at hand for this to happen; indeed, if it is undersupplied, fewer antibodies will be available to fight off unwanted organisms and disease will more easily set in. Severe deficiency will actually cause the thymus and spleen to shrink so that only restricted numbers of white cells will be produced. Vitamin B_6 is also necessary for the health of mucous membranes and this cooperates with B_2 to assist in the manufacture of antibodies. Any deficiency in pyridoxine will seriously impair immunity.

In order to manufacture those defensive B- and T-cells, the body must have vitamin A present in good supply, preferably as beta-carotene. Vitamin C is essential for the production of a particular variety of white cells, called T-killer cells, which attack invading organisms directly with a cell poison and also raid tumour cells. Zinc is the most valuable mineral with regard to T-cell creation and iron must be available, too, because the haemoglobin which is derived from this mineral carries the oxygen to the developing white cells.

Antibodies require other nutrients also, especially pantothenic acid (B₅), vitamin E along with selenium, and zinc which cooperates with vitamin B₆. Folic acid plays a crucial role as it takes part in the formation of red and white blood cells. Moreover, healthy cell division cannot occur without it.

Once formed, white cells must remain active and need protection for their dangerous defensive work. Vitamins C, E and the trace element selenium assist both macrophages and phagocytes in these ways.

For wounds to heal, pantothenic acid and zinc need to be freely available. Zinc and selenium have a further use in that they assist in the excretion of heavy metals from the body, such as lead, cadmium and mercury, all of which suppress the immune system.

Whenever someone is under stress, hormones called corticosteroids are released into the bloodstream which, if they are allowed to circulate for too long, can damage immunity. Fortunately ascorbic acid can counteract this negative effect, so always take extra vitamin C if you are under any prolonged strain.

Immunity-boosting foods

The most basic requirements for healthy immunity are sufficient calories and protein. It is common knowledge that undernourished people are more susceptible to illness. On top of that certain nutrients, in particular those described above, make special contributions to a fully functioning system and many of these will be automatically supplied if you switch to the Health-Giving Diet (see chapter 2, towards the end, and the start of chapter 20). You need to accentuate yellow-orange vegetables and fruit, also dark-green vegetables for the beta-carotene. These are even more valuable if eaten raw, maximizing the available vitamin C and other nutrients including folic acid, for example by including grated carrots and broccoli florets in salads. Sprout alfalfa seeds and add these, together with green peppers and tomatoes, also rich in ascorbic acid. Sprinkle on a dressing made from cold-pressed plant oils to supply that protective antioxidant vitamin E, mixed with cider vinegar flavoured with garlic (see 'French Dressing' in chapter 20).

Citrus fruits, cantaloup melon, strawberries and black-currants when in season are all valuable for their vitamin C content. Eat seafood regularly for the minerals, especially salmon, tuna and herring, also oysters if you like them, being the best food for zinc. Seeds, including pumpkin, sesame and sunflower, are useful for the same reason and an excellent spread is dark tahini. Also include mushrooms and root vegetables like beetroot (again, these can be chopped or grated into salads raw). Other high-grade protein sources are eggs, legumes and nuts, while desiccated liver can be taken as a supplement by non-vegetarians.

Whole grains together with extra wheatgerm, yeast extract and black molasses are all wonder foods for the immune system, containing many nutrients that help create and maintain white cells, including selenium, zinc and iron as well as B complex and vitamin E. Here again, brewer's yeast is well worth taking as a food supplement for an extra ingestion of B vitamins. Additionally ginseng is reputed to be a natural immunity-booster, as is the herb echinacea. My herbalist also recommended three teas to me while recovering from cancer, made from an infusion of red clover, sweet violet or mistletoe.

178

Infectious diseases

During this century orthodox allopathic medicine has made enormous strides in prevention of infectious diseases through vaccination. By altering antigens in the laboratory and then injecting these into the person, antibodies and memory cells form against that particular disease, providing immunity to it. In 1939 about 2,500 people died of diphtheria in Britain alone, but today the disease is a rarity. Smallpox, which was once such a scourge, has now been wiped out. Unfortunately, as with all medical intervention, vaccination is not without risk and there has been the occasional case (about 1 in 330,000) of brain damage from the whooping cough vaccine.

The development of antibiotics has been another medical success story of the twentieth century; these are selective poisons effective against bacterial infections including syphilis, tuberculosis and tetanus. Here again, though, there have been drawbacks and their overuse for minor maladies has rendered them less potent as organisms have built up resistance to them. Antibiotics have various side-effects. They can, for example, depress the immune system and they are also likely to harm the natural flora of the intestine so that unwanted bacteria such as *Candida albicans* can more easily flourish. If you have to take antibiotics, eat plenty of live yoghurt because the *Lactobacillus acidophilus* will replenish the beneficial flora.

Any serious infection needs a doctor's attention without delay, but the patient can be helped with a natural boost to the immune system by following the recommendations in this chapter. Vitamin C in high doses can be particularly useful against viral infections including mumps and measles, shingles, viral hepatitis, viral encephalitis, viral pneumonia and possibly even poliomyelitis, but any such treatment must only be carried out by a specialist. In developing countries, courses of vitamin A reduce

179

mortality from infections by at least one-third. For infections of the respiratory tract, such as coughs and colds, see chapter 9.

Immune-deficiency diseases

Genetic defects, environmental or emotional factors, poor nutrition, stress, ageing and drugs such as steroids, as well as unknown reasons or a mixture of causes, can all lower immunity allowing illnesses to develop, the more common of which are discussed below.

Aids

Aids is an acronym for the condition called Acquired Immune Deficiency Syndrome, in which a virus known as HIV (human immunodeficiency virus) attacks the defensive white cells directly. As a result, the sufferer is unable to ward off diseases that the immune system would normally deal with routinely and ultimately the infected person is likely to die from one of these. Until the Aids epidemic, some such illnesses were almost unheard-of or were only known to affect animals, such as PCP (pneumocystitis carinii), a virulent type of pneumonia, or toxoplasmosis that destroys the brains of cats. People with compromised immunity, such as drug addicts, will probably succumb very quickly, but those who adopt a positive attitude combined with excellent nutrition designed to boost immunity increase their chances of living for many years. There is no medical cure, despite millions being spent on research, and the future still looks bleak. Like other viruses, it breeds right inside the cells, so how do you kill the virus without also killing the cells – in this case those of the immune system? Additionally, it has a nasty habit of changing both its genetic material and its antigens, becoming ever more elusive.

Infection is transmitted via sex or blood, so prevention is fairly straightforward. All donated blood for transfusions is now screened, needles for injections must be carefully sterilised, and people such as firemen who clean up after traffic accidents have strict instructions to wear gloves and other protective clothing. Those in long-term stable relationships are at low risk of infection, otherwise use of a condom is a fairly reliable and simple solution. Nevertheless the World Health Organization forecasts that there will be at least 40 million cases worldwide by the end of the century, which is a frightening prospect.

People who are HIV positive will benefit considerably from making a conscious choice to strengthen their immunity by following the nutritional guidelines above (see 'Boosting your immune system' and 'Immunity-boosting foods'), thereby helping to fend off dangerous diseases. Equally, Aids patients can give their bodies the best chance of replenishing a weakened immune system by supplying the nutrients that are necessary for the building of new white cells.

At the same time some may be suffering from diarrhoea and weight loss. Often high-fat diets are suggested, but this is bad advice because bodies under such strain cannot easily absorb so much cholesterol. Dr Monty Berman, who has a wealth of experience in treating Aids patients in London, suggests that a variety of complex carbohydrates in small amounts (for example brown rice and other cereals, pulses and potatoes) allows the body to regain its normal metabolic level most readily. He recommends bread made from corn rather than whole wheat. Most importantly, the patient needs to tune in to his or her own nutritional needs and follow those. Foods which are easy to assimilate include porridge with skimmed or soya milk, vegetable and lentil or chicken soups, scrambled eggs, low-fat cottage cheese, grilled fish, chicken breast, shrimps, well-cooked beans in modest amounts, couscous, pasta or rice noodles, lightly steamed vegetables, potato salad and other salads in small quantities, bananas, melon, grapes, mixed fruit salad (fresh), rice cakes and occasional corn bread. Fortified Soya Drink (see chapter 20), being packed with nutrients as well as protein, is always useful for maintaining energy when the body is fighting disease, while live yoghurt will help to restore the health of the gut.

Viral disturbance of essential fatty acid metabolism may contribute to weight loss and diarrhoea. Twelve Aids patients at the Muhimbili Medical Centre in Dar Es Salaam were given capsules containing evening primrose oil and fish oils. After three months they had put on weight and suffered less from fatigue, diarrhoea and skin rashes. Moreover their T-lymphocyte immune cells had increased fourfold.

One long-term Aids survivor points out that people who die of the disease are known to be severely depleted in nutrients. He takes daily 25,000IUs of beta-carotene, 500IUs of vitamin E, 1g of vitamin C and a multi-mineral tablet that contains useful amounts of selenium and zinc, all of which help to maintain healthy defences despite the onslaught of the immuno-deficiency virus. Indeed, data from the San Francisco Men's Health Study has shown that daily multivitamin use is associated with a reduced risk of Aids.

Dr Raxit Jariwalla of the Linus Pauling Institute of Science and Medicine has demonstrated that megadoses of vitamin C are more effective at suppressing the HIV virus in infected cells than the drug AZT: 10g daily halved virus activity. This was even more efficacious when combined with the amino acid N-acetyl cysteine. Further studies are needed, but early indicators point to a dosage of around 4g daily, with toxicity at 10g. Such treatment needs to be professionally supervised, however.

Some HIV patients suffer neurological dysfunction, often beginning with leg and foot pains, progressing, sadly, to Aids-related dementia. American researchers at the University of Rochester School of Medicine found that one-fifth of such cases had abnormal vitamin B_{12} metabolism. They have proposed that replacement of this vitamin could significantly improve neurological function.

Cancer

Being faced with a life-threatening illness can be terrifying indeed, as I know from my own experience when, in 1986, I discovered a lump in my breast. After plucking up courage to visit my doctor and make a hospital appointment, I spent an agonizing five days waiting for the results of a needle biopsy. At that point, losing my breast seemed more distressing than dying. Luckily, the tumour was small enough to be removed with only minor surgery followed by several weeks of radiotherapy. The daily queues for treatment gave me plenty of time for deep reflection. In my heart of hearts I knew that I had been under severe stress in my work for prolonged periods. I also realized that I had been neglecting my health in the never-ending rush to keep pace with London's hectic life and, much against my own inclinations, had even resorted to convenience foods and a great many cheese sandwiches – high in fat, of course. If I wanted to stay alive I knew instinctively that it was vital to make some fundamental changes.

The decision then followed to visit the Cancer Help Centre in Bristol, where there was promise of new insights and sound guidance. I was not disappointed. Indeed, the love and care and sensible recommendations prompted me to cut down dramatically on stress and adopt a low-fat, low-sugar, mainly vegan wholefood diet, abundant in raw or just lightly steamed vegetables. Despite scares of possible secondary tumours and pressure from the hospital to have my ovaries irradiated, I decided against further intervention and concentrated on natural therapies. Since then I have never felt better!

A great deal of scientific evidence has now accumulated showing the link between cancers and inadequate nutrition. Indeed, Dr Sandra Goodman, PhD, has identified 5,000 such references published during the last 15 years or so (see Bibliography). These come to the following conclusions:

- An American study of 11,000 men (Enstrom et al., 1992) showed that high vitamin C intake is strongly correlated with low cancer deaths;
- A 19-year study (Shekelle et al., 1981) of 3,000 men showed that people with low levels of beta-carotene (pro-vitamin A) have a seven- to eight-fold greater risk of lung cancer than those with high levels;
- The National Cancer Institute of Canada (Howe et al., 1990) predicted that dietary modification (more fruit, vegetables, vitamin C and less saturated fat) could reduce breast cancer incidence by 24 per cent in post-menopausal women and 14 per cent in pre-menopausal women;

and so on. Particularly heartening are the results of a large-scale collaborative study between the United States National Cancer Institute and the Chinese Cancer Institute involving 30,000 Chinese people in Linxian, an area of that country where cancer mortality is high. In the group given supplements of vitamin E, beta-carotene and selenium in doses roughly double the US RDA (see chapter 3), deaths from stomach cancer were cut by 21 per cent and from all cancers by 13 per cent over a five-year period – a striking result.

So convincing is the evidence that in November 1993 Dr Hendrik Bueno de Mesquita, head of cancer epidemiology at the Dutch National Institute of Public Health, stated that a quarter of cancers affecting Europeans could be prevented simply by switching from a diet high in meat and animal fats to one with more vegetables and fruit. He told a conference in Brussels that the protective effects of fruit and vegetables were most marked against cancers of the digestive system and throat and lungs, and probably also of the breast. He estimated that as many as 50 to 60 per cent of all cancers of the stomach could be prevented by more vegetables and fruit and less salt and salted foods. He reckoned that 30 to 40 per cent of cancers of the colon and rectum could be similarly prevented and some 10 to 20 per cent of breast cancers, as long as intake of animal fats and meat was reduced. Such a change in diet would prevent almost 200,000 cancer deaths in the twelve EU countries annually.

A classic symptom of certain cancers, especially of the stomach, lung, pancreas and colon, is sudden weight loss. It seems that some tumours produce a protein called cachetic factor that causes the breakdown of normal body tissue, especially muscle and fat, in order to sustain itself. Scientists working for the Cancer Research Campaign have found that eicosapentaenoic acid (EPA), a substance found in oily fish, not only prevents this from happening, but also causes the tumour to shrink. Professor Gordon McVie, scientific director of the campaign, pointed to the low cancer incidence among Eskimos. This is good evidence that oily fish protects against cancer as well as heart disease.

Of special interest to women is a study completed in 1993 by Dr Aedin Cassidy at the Dunn Clinical Nutrition Centre in Cambridge, which examined the effects on hormone levels of a diet rich in soya protein. Just 60g daily lengthens the menstrual cycle by two to six days, thereby reducing hormonal stimulation to the breast tissue. This could explain why Japanese women are five times less likely to find themselves with breast cancer than those in the West.

Another surprise to the medical profession has been the discovery that Scottish women raised during the Second World War have lower incidence of breast cancer than their younger sisters. During those years they would have been restricted to the 'war diet', low in meat and dairy products

185

and high in fibre from wholemeal bread and home-grown vegetables, with supplements of cod-liver and halibut-liver oils for vitamins A and D and orange concentrate for C. This implies that a diet low in calories is as important as one that is vitamin-rich.

Laboratory researchers at the Bristol Medical School have just concluded that natural by-products of high-fibre diets can cause bowel cancer cells to 'commit suicide' in a process known as programmed cell death. The team found that this is triggered off by short-chain fatty acids that are produced by fibre fermented in the gut by ever-present bacteria. Professor Paraskeva said, 'Our work re-emphasizes that diet is very important.'

An anti-cancer diet Clearly it is wise to take heed of so many research findings which come to similar conclusions. Read the section on immunity-boosting foods above and follow the Health-Giving Diet described toward the end of chapter 2 and at the beginning of chapter 20, with particular emphasis on fresh vegetables and fruit. Carrots and dark-green leafy vegetables containing carotenoids are especially protective. Cut back substantially on saturated fats and avoid salty foods. Eat fish regularly. Adopt the habit of substituting tofu, tempeh and textured soya protein for meat, and don't forget the beans and lentils. Miso and seaweed have protective qualities also, especially against radiation. Do not eat refined carbohydrates such as white flour and sugar, as these will deplete your immunity. Drink herb teas in preference to fruit juices, once again to keep sugar intake low. Stay well clear of food containing carcinogens, such as smoked fish, smoked cheeses and anything burnt.

People living with cancer will benefit from carrot and other raw vegetable juices. Vitamin supplements should emphasize the antioxidants as follows: beta-carotene at up to 37,500IUs (cut back slightly if your palms turn yellow),

186

vitamin C buffered with calcium building from 2g to 6g daily (reducing amounts if there is any sign of diarrhoea), 15mg of zinc orotate, 200mcg of selenium and 400IUs of vitamin E (not for breast cancer patients as it could stimulate oestrogen production); 500mg of vitamin B complex and up to 3g of evening primrose oil with naturally occurring vitamin E are also prescribed by specialists.

Fortified Soya Drink and vegetable soups (see chapter 20) will be useful to those with digestive problems, while a teaspoon of orange- or mint-flavoured fish oil daily should be beneficial to patients suffering weight loss, but be careful not to take in too much oily vitamin A as this can be toxic; follow the directions on the bottle.

Do not drink alcohol. A Norwegian study published in July 1993 (Kjaerheim et al.) demonstrated that abstinence cut cancer risk by 27 per cent.

Candidiasis

Candida albicans, often referred to as thrush, is a fungal disease that can prove troublesome and may take some persistence to eradicate, depending on severity. It has become common in recent years in the West, due in part to antibiotics (including those unseen ones in factory-farmed meat and eggs), the contraceptive pill and anti-inflammatory drugs, also chlorine in drinking water, all of which can disturb the natural flora of the mucous membranes, allowing the candida yeast to take over. It is most likely to appear in the mouth or vagina, under the nails or on the skin. People can become vulnerable to this ailment if immunity is low and it frequently affects Aids patients in its invasive form. In this case the harmless yeast changes into an aggressive fungus with long tendrils that eventually enter the bloodstream, infecting many other parts of the body, such as the lungs and bronchial tubes.

Chronic candidiasis can produce a very wide variety of symptoms and for this reason can be difficult to identify.

They may range from lethargy, migraines, joint or muscle pains, recurrent cystitis or irritable bowel syndrome, to hypersensitivity to certain foods and chemicals.

Milder versions respond very well to an immunity-enhancing programme, so follow the recommendations at the beginning of this chapter. It is important not to eat any refined carbohydrates because these are just what the candida most likes to feed on! Also eliminate all yeasty foods including bread, yeast extract, cheese, grapes, raisins and sultanas, orange juice and all alcoholic drinks, which may worsen symptoms. If you are taking B vitamins, choose only those that are yeast-free.

Emphasize foods that have natural anti-fungal properties, that is garlic and raw green leafy vegetables. Marigold tea is often suggested by herbalists for similar reasons. Well-cooked free-range eggs will provide biotin, which is known to discourage candida growth. Oleic acid from cold-pressed olive oil is equally effective. The nutritional supplements Capricin, made from coconuts, and sorbic acid from mountain ash berries are both proven treatments. Your doctor will probably prescribe Nystatin, which is itself made from a fungus and is well tolerated.

To reinstate the natural balance of good bacteria in the intestine, include in your diet plenty of live natural yoghurt made from the *Lactobacillus acidophilus* culture.

Herpes

The herpes virus frequently lies dormant in the body cells, but as soon as the immune system is depressed, perhaps due to stress, lack of sleep, drugs, polluted environment or unsatisfactory diet, then it will have the opportunity to reproduce itself and symptoms will appear, often as the familiar cold sore on the lip. This is a sign of Type I, *Herpes simplex*, which affects mainly the mouth and face. Type II, *Herpes genitalis*, is sexually transmitted. It is prudent not to touch the sores, nor to share towels, as the infection can be easily spread.

Boosting the immune system nutritionally, as described above, and by taking plenty of rest, is the surest way of overcoming the infection. Supplements will also help. Take at least 1g of vitamin C with bioflavonoids daily in divided doses with meals and 15mg of zinc. This has been shown to halve the duration of the illness. The amino acid L-lysine is markedly antagonistic to the herpes virus, so take around 1g daily during the outbreak and increase consumption of fish and chicken. At the same time decrease intake of arginine, which seems to support its growth, in the form of nuts and seeds, wheat and oats, and peas.

Prick vitamin E capsules and apply directly to the lesions. Ointments that include either iodine or lithium will also speed healing.

Glandular fever

Along with chicken pox and shingles, this is yet another form of the herpes virus, and the suggestions earlier in the chapter regarding the need to boost immunity apply equally well here. Young people are particularly vulnerable to this infection, also called mononucleosis, the main symptoms being swollen lymph glands, sore throat, feverishness and fatigue. These can be very persistent.

Take a vitamin B complex tablet daily that includes biotin, and 10,000IU of beta-carotene to help repair the mucous membranes of the throat. Extra vitamin C at around 1g daily together with about 15mg of zinc are excellent for fighting infections. Make sure that protein intake is generous for the building of antibodies. Evening primrose oil can also be an effective treatment at up to 3g daily.

Post-viral syndrome (ME)

Having been a sickly child, Frances became a fitness fanatic and trained as a PE teacher. Despite the rigorous exercise, she was still prone to respiratory infections, especially during the winter, and was frequently put on courses of antibiotics. One winter she was feeling very depressed after her boyfriend had left her and she came down with a vicious attack of 'flu. After about ten days, conscience-stricken, she staggered back into work, but had to return home again before the day was out and collapse into bed. When she woke up the next morning she was aching all over and felt utterly dreadful. The doctor prescribed yet more antibiotics, but the condition became even worse. Feeling a total failure, she was forced to take the remainder of the term off and cope as best she could with blinding migraines that kept recurring, increased joint pain and above all a debilitating exhaustion. There were many days when it was impossible to stand upright because she felt so weak.

Eventually the doctor diagnosed ME (myalgic encephalomyelitis) and advised Frances to rest as much as possible and to take multivitamin tablets. There was nothing more he could do. Plunged into complete despair, Frances realized that she would have to seek help elsewhere and consulted a nutritionist. In addition to the ME, he diagnosed a yeast infection and put her on to a raw vegetable diet similar to the one described under Candidiasis above, avoiding yeast-containing foods. He said it would be advisable to come off the contraceptive pill. An exclusion programme (see under 'Allergies' later in the chapter) proved that she was allergic to wheat and dairy products. He explained that her immune system had become weakened from too much fast food and prolonged use of antibiotics, combined with emotional stress.

Sweat analysis showed very low zinc levels and Frances was put on 30mg daily together with yeast-free B-complex tablets with extra vitamin B_6. She also took 1g daily of buffered vitamin C with bioflavonoids in divided amounts and 2g of evening primrose oil. After several weeks of a healthy wholefood diet combined with the supplements, Frances began to notice improvement and she was able to halve the zinc intake.

The following term she was well enough to return to work, but she now realized that she would have to maintain a healthy diet indefinitely and that multi-vitamin tablets plus extra zinc and vitamin C would help her safely through the winter months.

Auto-immune diseases

One of the main problems with transplant surgery is rejection of the new organ, despite the sophisticated methods recently developed. The body's immune system recognizes this as 'foreign' and immediately goes on the offensive. In order to prevent this from happening, potent immuno-suppressive drugs have to be administered to the patient.

Somehow the elements of the immune system know the difference between self and non-self, but the precise process remains a mystery although various theories have been put forward. Bearing in mind the vast numbers of foreign organisms, the accuracy of the immune response is truly astonishing. Occasionally, however, the lymphocytes make a mistake and produce antibodies against the body's own cells. Serious damage can result.

Women are more prone than men to auto-immune diseases, but it is not known why. There are two main types: in the first the cells of just one organ are damaged, for example the pancreas as in diabetes (see chapter 10); in the second, parts of tissues of more than one organ are affected, as in multiple sclerosis.

Multiple sclerosis

If you turn to chapter 16 you will read about the nervous system. Just like electrical wiring, our nerves are sheathed in an insulation material and the name of this substance is myelin. During the course of the disease the body's own white scavenger cells attack the myelin so that the electrical impulses can no longer travel normally. Scarring results, giving the illness its name, which means 'many scars'. Loss of coordination or poor balance may therefore occur, together with tingling or numbness in the extremities, while blurring of vision, poor bladder control, and especially fatigue and depression are other likely symptoms. There is no medical cure, but nutritional therapy can make a significant difference to the course of the disease, especially if instigated at an early stage.

Since there may be a number of factors that trigger off MS, nutritional approaches work best if individually designed. Often a food intolerance can aggravate symptoms and this should always be checked out. (See under 'Allergies' below.)

Most MS patients, however, do seem to have difficulty in metabolizing fats, so a wholefood diet that is low in saturated fats, as described in chapters 2 and 20, is an essential starting-point. At the same time evening primrose oil at around 3g daily, or two tablespoons of linseed oil, will assist many patients; others may improve with the help of fish oil.

The symptoms of MS are similar to mercury poisoning and for this reason it is sometimes suggested that amalgam fillings be replaced. The process must be very carefully carried out, however, if further toxicity is not to occur. Mercury also depresses the immune system. Remember that vitamin E together with selenium protect against mercury poisoning, so take wheatgerm daily plus cold-pressed plant oils (for example in salad dressings) and consider supplements. (In this respect vitamin C is not recommended as animal studies indicate that it may actually assist in mercury absorption.)

In a double-blind trial in America, 49 out of 50 MS patients improved substantially after treatment with the amino acid D-phenylalanine, so it is worth trying this for

192

a few weeks (but not if you have high blood pressure). Non-meat food sources include peanuts, sesame seeds and almonds, low-fat yoghurt, oats and wheat, soya beans, peas and fish.

Low intakes of magnesium can produce symptoms similar to MS, such as twitching and muscle fatigue, so plenty of dark-green vegetables and whole cereals are a must. This mineral is also involved in the synthesis of fats and other food constituents – another good reason to increase consumption. Furthermore it is needed for the manufacture of lecithin, along with B vitamins (especially B_6, choline and inositol) and essential fatty acids, found to be seriously deficient in the brains and myelin sheaths of MS sufferers; as a natural emulsifier of fats, lecithin obviously has special significance in the treatment of this disease. Derived from soya beans, it can be bought in granules and sprinkled on foods; take three tablespoons daily. At the same time replace meat portions with soya protein (see chapter 20 for recipe ideas).

Another nutrient vital to the nervous system is vitamin D. In a few cases there may be an inherited tendency towards poor absorption or increased need. Young patients may therefore benefit from supplementation at around 10mcg (400IU) along with calcium, together with dietary emphasis on fish and free-range eggs: small amounts of fish-liver oil, especially in winter, are likely to be beneficial. Fresh air and sunshine will be good for all patients.

In some cases symptoms involving coordination have been lessened on the administration of vitamin B_{12}, prudent in any event for those on vegan diets.

Since alcohol worsens symptoms it is best to refrain from drinking. There is good reason for this because it destroys those B vitamins that MS patients need so desperately and it interferes with the metabolism of unsaturated fats, already a serious problem for people with multiple sclerosis.

Lupus

Lupus erythematosus means 'red wolf' in Latin, descriptive of the rash across the nose and cheeks, typical of this disease. For some unknown reason, nearly all patients are female and many tend to be high achievers. In the systemic variety, the patient's own immune system forms antibodies against DNA, the genetic blueprint inside every cell. Thus, the disease can penetrate to all parts of the body, harming many organs.

A nutrient-dense diet that accentuates pantothenic acid (vitamin B_5) from wheatgerm, free-range eggs and lentils, fortified with brewer's yeast and desiccated liver (for non-vegetarians) and vitamin E from wheatgerm and cold-pressed plant oils, should speed healing. PABA (para-aminobenzoic acid), a constituent of folic acid, helps in the assimilation of pantothenic acid and has been used successfully to clear symptoms. Brewer's yeast is rich in this, but if you decide to take a B-complex formula check the label to ensure that PABA is included. Animal studies have shown that a low-calorie, low-fat diet, that limits dairy and other animal products, is beneficial.

Ulcerative colitis

This disease, in which it is thought that antibodies attack the colon, can be horribly tenacious, as Michael discovered, having suffered from it for three years. He linked the onset with the stress stemming from his work as an insurance salesman. He was unhappy with his high-pressure job, wishing he had gone into some sort of social work. The symptoms of pains in the abdomen, with frequent diarrhoea sometimes accompanied by bleeding, were exceedingly uncomfortable, and he felt constantly drained and depressed.

After talking with a nutritionist, he switched to a healthy diet that was high in protein and unsaturated fats, but always eating only small portions at once, especially of fibrous foods such as raw fruit and vegetables. The nutritionist explained that the extra bulk would help to reduce the muscle spasms in the gut, whereas refined carbohydrates would make these worse. He increased his liquid intake to replace lost fluid, learning how to make juices from vegetables that were very rich in nutrients (see chapter 20). Foods containing iron, such as lentils and black molasses, and vitamin C, citrus and berry fruits and salads, were prominent in his diet to offset his anaemic tendencies and he also took a good all-round multi-vitamin and multi-mineral tablet daily.

This approach resulted in noticeable improvement after several weeks, but it was only after finally changing his job and becoming a carer in a nursing home that he had the disease under control.

Occasionally colitis can be caused by a food intolerance, so this should be checked (see under 'Allergies' below). More than half of patients with active disease react to dairy products. Sometimes aspirin or foods containing salicylates can be the culprits – see if the symptoms are worse after taking a dose. If your test is positive, avoid fruits (except bananas, pears and mangoes), spices and herbs (except soya sauce), vegetables (except legumes, Brussels sprouts, cabbage, leeks and lettuce), coffee and tea, nuts (except cashews and sunflower seeds), and all packaged and tinned foods. Seafood, dairy products and whole cereals except sweetcorn are all fine in this respect. Also refrain from eating honey, yeast and peppermint.

Allergies

There is a positive epidemic of allergies at present and women's and health magazines frequently contain articles offering advice to sufferers. As explained at the start of this chapter, our immune defences are generally able to trap unwanted particles such as dust, pollen grains and hairs and then expel them in mucus. Sensitive people may overreact, however, producing excess mucus or histamine along with inflammation, typical of hay fever or asthma, as discussed in chapter 9. Increasing environmental pollutants and additives in foods are putting a heavy burden on our immune defences, constantly presenting them with foreign substances that they are unable to recognize. Many people involved in natural therapies believe that the strain of dealing with this assault increases the likelihood of mistakes in immunological function.

As regards food, a true allergy entails the formation of antibodies against a protein or carbohydrate. Sometimes molecules enter the system imperfectly digested, which trigger off this process. Normally we do not know this is happening because the antigen/antibody complex thus formed is easily metabolized by the liver. In some sensitized individuals, however, histamine is released from the white cells known as mast cells located in the membranes open to the environment, such as in the nose, and in the intestine, causing uncomfortable symptoms.

A food intolerance does not involve the formation of antibodies and is probably due to a lack of appropriate enzymes for proper digestion. The effect can be a general malaise, bloating or intermittent pains and headaches.

To check for a food sensitivity

Surprisingly, the offending food is often one that the person craves and therefore eats regularly, commonly dairy products, wheat, citrus fruits and also artificial additives and colourings. The trouble may have started in early childhood during weaning, showing up as indigestion, runny nose or even earache, symptoms that do not necessarily suggest food sensitivity but rather some sort of infection. The earlier the weaning, the greater the chance of allergic reaction. After a while the immune system adjusts to the culprit and symptoms subside. Later in life the problem recurs, set in motion perhaps by stress, and the food item is not suspected since it has been consumed in the diet all along.

Keep a food diary, noting down what you eat each day and your subsequent reactions. In addition to the above items, other possible allergens may be eggs, seafood, nuts, celery, soya products or even strawberries. Remove suspects one at a time for at least five days each and see what happens. You may experience withdrawal symptoms, so be patient and wait another week at least to see if the problems clear. If they do, then double-check that this is the offender by reintroducing the food on a particular day within the next few weeks in substantial amounts. The test is positive if the symptoms reappear. You must then eliminate the food altogether for many months or even years. It may be possible to eat it again in the future in small amounts.

If you switch to the Health-Giving Diet recommended in this book (see chapters 2 and 20), then you may find that recurring ailments may disappear automatically, since it excludes additives and convenience foods and is low in sugar and fat. If not, then follow the process described above.

The antioxidant vitamins A (as beta-carotene), C and E plus selenium will help protect the body if air pollutants are thought to be causing problems, while bromelaine from pineapples should alleviate digestive troubles. At the same time give your immune system a boost as described in the earlier part of this chapter.

A gluten intolerance

Philippa was at her wit's end. Her baby son, almost one year old, had suffered recurring colic followed by diarrhoea and sickness for nearly three months, was seriously losing weight and failing to grow properly. Despite a stint in hospital for observation and many visits to the doctor, no diagnosis was forthcoming.

In desperation she visited a nutrition consultant who,

after asking detailed questions about diet, suspected an intolerance to gluten, a protein present in wheat, oats, barley and rye, and therefore recommended a diet that excluded these foods. Indeed, simply by cutting out bread, cakes and biscuits, improvement in the child's health was obvious within a week.

The nutritionist suggested that Philippa should ask her doctor to arrange for a proper biopsy to have the diagnosis of coeliac disease officially confirmed, since gluten intolerance can, but does not necessarily, indicate this disorder.

Chapter 12

A Strong Frame

It is easy to imagine that bones are somewhat inert things, since the ones we normally see on our dinner table, at the butcher or scattered in the countryside, have generally been dead for several weeks or even years. The bones of a moving human or animal, however, are very much alive. They are interlaced with narrow canals which carry nerves and fine blood and lymph vessels, which assist in their healthy maintenance and repair.

Our bones have several functions: they provide a framework and support for the soft parts of the body, which would otherwise collapse; their rigidity also gives protection to the vulnerable vital organs, the skull guarding the brain, the ribs shielding the heart and lungs, while the spinal cord is cleverly threaded through the vertebrae. When acted upon by the muscles, our bones operate as levers to create movement, and the way in which they meet at joints provides the body with great flexibility. They also have non-structural jobs to do: in the marrow they manufacture red blood corpuscles and the white blood cells of the immune system that defend the body from disease; additionally they act as a mineral store for calcium and phosphorus which can be used by the soft tissues when the need arises.

A new-born baby's bones are still soft, having been formed from membrane and cartilage, allowing it to emerge through the narrow birth passage. Bones consist of flexible fibrous tissue and hardened crystalline calcium salts, such as calcium phosphate. At first there is twice as much fibrous material as hardened mineral, but in old age the proportions are reversed. This means that an old person's bones are much more rigid and therefore more easily broken, especially if nutrition has been inadequate.

Throughout life two sets of cells are busily at work in our bones: the ones called osteoblasts form the fibrous structure, while those known as osteoclasts break down and absorb the bone. This means that after about 15 years our bones are entirely new! Another risk of ageing is that more bone is broken down than created, with the result that they can become thin and brittle and so lacking in strength that they may collapse or fracture spontaneously. This condition is referred to as osteoporosis.

Osteoporosis

At only 58 years of age, Nancy is 4 inches (10cm) shorter than she used to be. The aching began in her late forties, gradually becoming worse, until the pains in her back were agonizing. Even simple movements such as turning over in bed were excruciating. One morning as she bent down slowly to put on her slippers she felt something go: her spine had fractured. She can scarcely recall the nightmare that ensued, but at least she now had a positive diagnosis – chronic osteoporosis.

One of the problems with this disease is that it cannot be accurately identified until it is already far advanced. X-rays can only detect the damage after at least 33 per cent of the bone has already disappeared and at this stage it is very difficult (although not impossible) to rectify. Bone scans can detect it earlier. Women are particularly prone to bone loss during the years following the menopause, often dropping 8 inches (20 cm) in height due to shrinkage of the skeleton, sometimes accompanied by a humped back in old age. This occurs because bones that carry the weight,

OSTEOPOROSIS

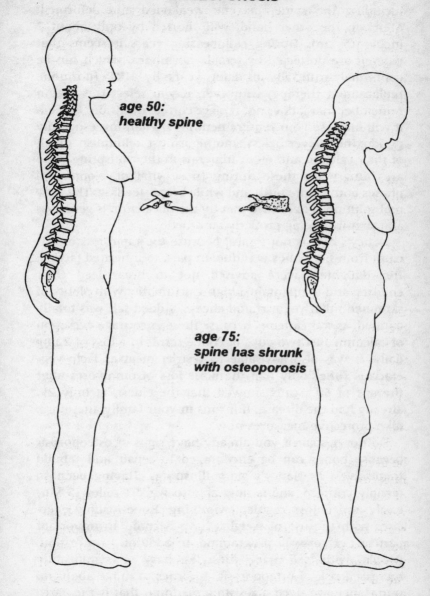

age 50:
healthy spine

age 75:
spine has shrunk
with osteoporosis

Osteoporosis causes shrinkage of the skeleton and deformity in the bones, especially those bearing the weight. Extra calcium, when well absorbed, helps to prevent this disease.

including the spine, become weakened and deformed. Men, on the other hand, will shorten by only about 2 inches (5 cm). During childbearing years it seems that women are protected by female hormones, which can be continued artificially in later years by HRT (hormone replacement therapy). However, if you select this option remember that it does not replace correct nutrition. Indeed, it will increase your requirement for B vitamins, especially pyridoxine. Nevertheless, mothers must relinquish much of their calcium and other minerals to their offspring, who are hungry for these during those vital developmental phases both before birth and while breast-feeding. The only real solution is to ensure that intake of calcium is generous and that it is being properly absorbed.

Nancy's case is not typical because the rapid loss of calcium from her bones was due, in part, to inherited factors. Her daughters were advised not to breast-feed their children and to maintain a high-calcium diet with plenty of skimmed milk, yoghurt and cheese. Added salt was totally banned, as was caffeine, because these encourage excretion of calcium. Just two cups of coffee result in a loss of 22mg daily. It was also advisable to restrict meat as lacto-vegetarians suffer only half the bone loss of omnivores after the age of 60. Scans showed that the eldest, at only 29, already had the disease. If it runs in your family, therefore, take protective measures now.

Do not despair if you already have signs of osteoporosis because bones can be encouraged to repair and rebuild themselves, as Nancy's story illustrates. Having been so terribly crippled, she is now able to walk 3 miles (5 km) easily and enjoys regular swimming. Bone-loading exercises with the use of weights have become an important part of her get-well programme, in addition to nutrition. People with sedentary lifestyles have a significantly increased risk of osteoporosis. In order to move about on our planet, we need a resisting medium, that is the earth when walking or running, or the water when swimming. At the same time, gravity pulls us down into strong contact with this medium. Our skeletons need to be very resilient to defy such pressure, and the more we ask our bodies to do this the more we foster density of bone mass. Indeed, a major hazard of being an astronaut is calcium loss through weightlessness.

After surgery to pin the fracture and natural repair of her bones with nutritional supplements, Nancy's condition gradually improved. Gentle swimming was the easiest form of exercise initially, and with determination she increased the length of her walks until she was able to achieve 3 miles (5 km) three times a week. She is now free of the terrible back pain and the quality of her life has improved beyond all recognition. If only she had known about the importance of calcium in her diet she would never have suffered such appalling agony.

The RDA for calcium of 800mg is now considered by many physicians to be much too low for older women and they would like to see it set at a minimum of 1,200mg daily, preferably 1,500mg. Smoking and alcohol will increase your risk of osteoporosis and hence your nutritional needs. So how can we acquire this amount in our diet? Hard water can give us about 125mg per half-pint (275-ml) glass, while milk contributes a little over twice that. So 1 pint (570ml) of skimmed milk will make up one-third of your daily requirement, as will 3oz (90g) of cheese – but beware the high fat content here. Low-fat yoghurt provides a healthier alternative. This is fine for people who can tolerate dairy products, but those who cannot will have to turn to other foodstuffs such as whitebait, whole sardines and salmon that include the bones, while vegans can select from spinach (one portion will give about 500mg, as will tofu), broccoli or spring onions (about 100mg), or perhaps seaweed, rich in minerals, especially arame, hijiki, kelp or kombu with as much as 1g per 3-oz

(90-g) portion. Even so, it takes some effort to maintain the daily 1,500mg. The obvious answer is a calcium supplement, but many of those purchased in health food shops cannot be digested by the hydrochloric acid in the stomach. Check with manufacturers whether proper tests have been carried out in this respect and how long the tablets will take to dissolve.

The question of absorption is all-important. Magnesium needs to be present at half the level of calcium, and phosphorus in equal amounts (but we already consume more than enough of this in the West), while silicon encourages the formation of collagen and elastin, two proteins present in bones. Boron seems to be involved in maintaining hormonal balance. Supplements are available which combine these essential minerals in the correct proportions. Acid foods will assist assimilation as will vitamin C, also vital for the formation of connective tissue. In the presence of milk sugar, or lactose, calcium absorption is rapid with new bone being laid down within two hours. Other sugars, however, have the reverse effect. Vitamin D is indispensable, so make sure you have sufficient sunshine or take fish-liver oil capsules at the RDA. This vitamin is particularly protective against osteoporosis.

Arthritis

Our joints are ingeniously designed, the ball-and-socket type of the hip and shoulder allowing movement in any plane, while the hinge joint of the knee and elbow gives movement in one plane. Then there are pivotal actions that include sideways motions and also the gliding ability of the ankle and wrist. As a result, our bodies are both useful and expressive, so that we can do heavy manual labour, such as digging the garden, or leap and spin with the beauty and elegance of a gymnast or ballet dancer. Our manual dexterity has been a major factor in enabling us to evolve into the sophisticated humans that we now are.

All our movable joints are held together by ligaments made of strong bands of fibrous tissue that are elastic enough not to impede flexibility. Where bones meet, we have natural shock absorbers in the form of a smooth layer of cartilage, which also protects the ends of the bones from wear. The joint is well lubricated by a slippery liquid called synovial fluid.

Despite this clever engineering, joints can wear out or become painfully inflamed, a condition we refer to generally as arthritis, although there can be a couple of hundred different types and reasons for it. Medical treatment attempts to control pain and inflammation temporarily, but offers no cure, and there may be undesirable side-effects from drugs. On the other hand, healing nutrients can make a pronounced difference without toxicity, often providing long-lasting relief or even cure in some cases. The two most common sorts are osteoarthritis and rheumatoid arthritis.

Osteoarthritis This is usually regarded as a degenerative disease, being associated with old age and roughened and worn-out cartilage, especially in the weight-bearing joints such as the hips. As a result, the ends of the bones tend to thicken and spread out, causing stiffness and pain.

My own mother progressively suffered agonies with this disease. In her youth she had been an outstanding hockey player, captain of London University team, and then centre-forward for the county of Kent. I still have in my possession a diary of the early 1930s which contains a photograph of her energetically striking out at the ball in a county match. Having always been so active, it was a real hardship for her to have to slow down to a stumbling pace, but unfortunately osteoarthritis often affects former sportspeople and dancers due to the extra stress that the joints have endured. It also sometimes develops at the site of an old injury. My mother eventually had the hip joint replaced by an artificial one, but then had to tolerate the development of the disease in the other leg, by which time she was too old to withstand any more major surgery.

Anyone with osteoarthritis in the hips or legs needs to lose weight if they are too heavy, to ease the pressure on the affected joints. The only lasting way to do this is to cut down on saturated fats and refined carbohydrates, and to increase roughage with fresh fruit and vegetables (see chapters 16 and 20).

The other approach is to increase nutrients that have an anti-inflammatory effect and those that assist in cartilage and bone repair. You may have to experiment to discover which ones work best for you, but the following suggestions have been very helpful in many cases. The antioxidant vitamins A, C and E, together with the trace element selenium, will help to reduce inflammation. A combined supplement should prove advantageous. If you are taking aspirin, then extra vitamin C is particularly important as this drug increases requirement. Ascorbic acid is indispensable for all healing and repair work; indeed, connective tissue cannot be formed without it. Be generous with vegetables such as broccoli and Brussels sprouts, but avoid very acid sources such as citrus and berry fruits – more about this under 'Rheumatoid arthritis' below. Instead, take a supplement of vitamin C of at least 1g daily in divided amounts and choose a buffered form such as calcium ascorbate.

Needless to say, calcium is vital for bone repair in correct ratio to magnesium as described under osteoporosis. If you are under any kind of stress, then calcium will be withdrawn from your bones and must be replaced. This mineral is doubly important because it helps to relieve pain. However, try and find sources other than dairy products which are high in lactic acid and no good for your joints. If necessary, take a supplement. Equally, your vitamin E requirements will be increased, so give yourself daily supplies of wheatgerm and vegetable oils. Studies have demonstrated that doses of vitamin E well above the RDA at 400mg are efficacious. Reduce this amount when benefits are noticed. As you raise your intake of poly- and monounsaturated oils, so decrease foods high in saturated fats.

Vitamin A can be obtained as beta-carotene or in the oily form. Many patients have found that fish oil is beneficial, so take cod-liver oil capsules, which are naturally abundant in this vitamin. Do not exceed stated doses, as retinol not immediately required is stored in the liver and can build up to toxic levels. Fish oil is also one of the best sources of vitamin D, which is essential for calcium absorption. Make sure your intake is good. Interestingly, arthritics are often found to be deficient in this vitamin. Include plenty of fish in your diet, such as mackerel, herrings and salmon (not sardines) – at least two generous portions per week. Meanwhile, maintain liberal amounts of those yellow and orange fruit and vegetables and dark-green leafy plants that will provide you with health-giving carotenoids.

The B vitamins are worth exploring therapeutically. Niacin (vitamin B_3) has been given to patients as nicotinamide in doses of up to 4g daily with some success. Pyridoxine (B_6) is a useful adjunct to the antioxidants mentioned above and is necessary for the proper metabolism of magnesium. Some anti-arthritis drugs deplete this vitamin. Pantothenic acid (B_5) has been useful for pain control: try 500 to 1,000mg per day. Remember, however, that members of the B-complex group work in cooperation with each other and too much of one can cause deficiency in another, so do not take unbalanced doses for too long. As soon as you feel relief, reduce the amount and take a complete B-complex supplement alongside or plenty of brewer's yeast. This will help to alleviate the stress that often accompanies arthritis.

Have yourself analysed for trace element and mineral

deficiencies, and make sure you have at least the RDA of zinc, selenium, manganese, iron and copper. Drugs may cause depletion of iron in particular, so have a jar of black molasses in your kitchen cupboard which, if taken daily, at around 3 teaspoons, will fulfil basic needs. Do not drink tea as the tannin forms insoluble salts with dietary iron so it cannot be absorbed. If you are totally unable to give it up, at least buy Luaka tea, which is low in tannin, and drink it weak. Also beware of other items that hinder mineral absorption, including coffee and wholewheat bran. Zinc is very important for healing and manganese is involved in the composition of bone ends.

On the subject of tea, make your own herbal infusion with celery seeds. This old-fashioned remedy has been proved by Dr David Lewis of Aston University to have a 'definite anti-inflammatory action' (see chapter 20 for recipe). At the same time it can help to disperse the uric acid that is often attracted to injured joints. Equally, it encourages the synovial fluid to run smoothly.

Another traditional remedy, that of the copper bracelet, has also been proved to be of value wherever the arthritis occurs. This is because minute traces of the mineral, which have a naturally anti-inflammatory action, are absorbed into the system through the skin. A good food source is lentils, so make yourself nourishing soups (see chapter 20) and cutlets.

For natural pain relief, the amino acid phenylalanine is far safer and usually more effective than drugs. In one study 43 patients, most of whom had osteoarthritis, were given 250mg of D-phenylalanine three or four times daily. After two to three weeks, significant reduction in pain was reported. It is believed that this amino acid is able to encourage our natural built-in pain killers and mood-enhancers, the endorphins and encephalins, to operate more effectively and for longer. It is generally purchased as DLPA; take 750mg half an hour before eating three times daily. If you do not notice obvious relief in three weeks, you can increase the dose up to double, but cease the supplements when the pain goes. No one amino acid should be taken for too long.

Capsules containing a preparation of the New Zealand green-lipped mussel alleviated pain and stiffness in 35 per cent of patients with osteoarthritis in a study which took place at the Glasgow Homoeopathic Hospital in Scotland. They took three every day for six months. Clearly this is well worth a try.

Food intolerances seem to have an adverse effect even on osteoarthritics, so it is important to check for these. Try excluding plants of the nightshade family for a few weeks and see if you notice any improvement. These are tomatoes, aubergines, peppers and potatoes. See also chapter 11 under 'Allergies'.

Rheumatoid arthritis What you eat can have a most significant effect on the course of this disease. At the least symptoms can be reduced and at best the condition can be completely cured. Unlike osteoarthritis, rheumatoid arthritis often afflicts comparatively young people and is more likely to affect the hands and feet rather than the hips. It is auto-immune in nature. In other words elements of the immune system make the mistake of treating the body's own cells as foreign material and attack them. The result is inflammation and damage to the joints, with accompanying pain and stiffness. No one knows what prompts the immune system to behave in this way, but one theory is that a bacterium triggers the process. Certainly the ailment is associated with stress. Women are twice as likely to be sufferers of this disease than men.

Barbara first noticed the aching in her wrists and hands some eight years ago. At first this was slight and occasional, but after her son was involved in a serious motor accident there was a real flare-up of the symptoms. These prompted her to visit her doctor who eventually diagnosed rheumatoid arthritis. Since she was a professional seamstress this was a considerable blow, because on bad days it was impossible to grip a needle or pin, or even guide the material accurately under the foot of her sewing machine. The doctor warned that her fingers could become permanently swollen and bent and suggested that she think about an alternative source of income, especially as the medication he prescribed was causing the side effects of nausea and headaches. There was no cure, although she may have periods of remission. This was devastating news to Barbara.

Not to be defeated, she made an appointment with a naturopath recommended by a friend. He explained that the acid/alkaline balance in her body had been upset due to long-term poor nutrition, subsequently exacerbated by the worry over her son's injuries. If she kept strictly to a diet low in acid-forming foods, then the balance could be restored. After about six weeks she should notice a lessening of the pain and inflammation as the build-up of uric acid in the joints was dissolved away. Iron-rich meat may in any case be causing problems, as rheumatoid arthritis patients have difficulty in metabolizing this mineral.

Hope renewed, Barbara gave up all refined flour and sugar, red meat, dairy products, citrus fruits, salt, chocolate, coffee and tea. Instead she ate fish (not the roes), whole grains (except wheat) including brown rice, buckwheat, millet and quinoa, soya products, nuts and seeds and some poultry, also vegetables and gentle fruits such as bananas. Instead of bread she ate rice cakes and pumpernickel. Additionally she took 3g of evening primrose oil daily, a 500mg tablet containing vitamin B complex, 1g of calcium ascorbate in divided amounts and 15mg of zinc.

Within two months Barbara was again holding a needle. While accepting that some of the deformity in the joints could not be reversed, at least the pain and stiffness had gone to such a marked degree that she was once more able to resume her work.

This particular approach may not be right for every rheumatoid arthritis sufferer as different people have individual responses to nutrients. The condition can be triggered by a food intolerance, so if you suspect this follow the exclusion programme described in chapter 11 under 'Allergies'. Culprits can be any of the following: dairy produce, gluten, the nightshade family (aubergines, peppers, potatoes and tomatoes), citrus fruits and rhubarb; sugary and refined foods. Also try any of the recommendations under Osteoarthritis (see previous section), especially those known to have a natural anti-inflammatory effect, including the antioxidants and fish oils. Indeed, studies have demonstrated that oils containing gamma-linolenic acid (GLA) from seeds of the evening primrose and borage plant, or eicosapentaenoic acid (EPA) from fish oils and linseeds, are just as effective as anti-inflammatory drugs without the side-effects. Copper salicylate at 60mg twice daily has also given good results. As for the green-lipped mussel preparation, this showed a 67 per cent success rate among patients with rheumatoid arthritis. Also remember to wear a copper bracelet. For pain relief take the amino acid DLPA, as described in the above section, for about three weeks, then use the herbs feverfew or devil's claw (this last one is not for diabetics) for up to two weeks at a time.

If you suspect that your illness was prompted by stress, then you could well respond to supplementation of pantothenic acid (vitamin B_5) as calcium pantothenate. Take at least 500mg daily in graduated amounts. Its best natural source is Royal Jelly. Researchers found that improvement was significant if combined with the amino acid L-cysteine, for patients with osteo- as well as rheumatoid arthritis (see chapter 3 under 'Amino acids').

Eggs, beans and gelatin contain amino acids high in sulphur which are vital for the formation of connective tissue

211

from which healthy joints are constructed. Emphasize these in your diet, therefore. Also important in this respect are bioflavonoids.

Carpal tunnel syndrome

Rheumatoid arthritis can occasionally trigger the condition known as carpal tunnel syndrome, although there may be other causes. It is characterized by tingling in the index and middle fingers and pain in the wrist and arm, with increasing weakness in the thumb, as the meridian nerve which runs down the forearm becomes compressed. Supplements of vitamin B_6 can be as effective as surgery. Take 100mg daily together with brewer's yeast tablets. You will need to persevere for at least two months.

Gout

This affliction immediately conjures up the image of an overweight Victorian gentleman, leg propped up on a footstool, moaning about the pain in his toe joints. His family and friends are unsympathetic, blaming the patient himself for an over-indulgence in good living – wine in particular. The novels in which this character features generally view him as a figure of fun. This is unfortunate, for the pain of gout can be extreme and disabling. A long-standing friend of my husband, still only in his mid-forties, developed gout last year, and as a result has lost many days from his active job as a fireman.

In this ailment, the excess uric acid forms crystals in the joints, which in turn cause the inflammation and pain. The best way of dissolving these is with cider vinegar which contains malic acid: take one dessertspoonful in a tumbler of hot water sweetened with a little honey three times a day. Malic acid is different from the toxic uric acid and is entirely beneficial. Cucumber is another traditional remedy.

Needless to say, it is essential to follow a healthy wholefood diet (see 'the Health-Giving Diet' in chapter 20) and to cut out all wines, beers and spirits. Foods high in purines, which are various acids excreted as uric acid, must be avoided at all costs. These include offal, sardines, anchovies and fish roes, also yeast and its extract. Spinach, strawberries and rhubarb, which are known to worsen symptoms, are banned, too.

Vitamin C encourages the excretion of uric acid, so take plenty – about 2g daily in divided amounts. Take as calcium ascorbate and include some magnesium and about 15mg of zinc to aid healing.

Chapter 13

Fuel for Muscles

When someone mentions muscles, we immediately bring to mind those that we can see, such as the biceps or the calf muscles. We also associate them with movement and know that the more we exercise them, the stronger and more efficient they become. The rippling muscles of a body-builder may inspire admiration or, at the other extreme, revulsion, depending on our taste, while we may have a keen aesthetic appreciation for the sleek body of a dancer, ice-skater or gymnast. Generally, however, we are not consciously aware of the operation of many muscles vital to our existence, such as the ones in the walls of arteries, or those along the alimentary canal that push food forward in a wave-like motion called peristalsis. Poor muscle tone, therefore, results not only in weakness in the limbs and an increased risk of injury, but also in sluggish blood and lymph circulation, shallow breathing, inadequate digestion, recurring constipation, and sagging internal organs.

Muscles are only able to contract (that is, shorten in length) and relax (return to their original dimensions) and generally work in opposite or 'antagonistic' pairs to move a limb. For example, the biceps at the front of the upper arm contracts and moves the forearm (to which it is attached) upwards. When the triceps at the back of the upper arm contracts, the forearm straightens again. Nerve

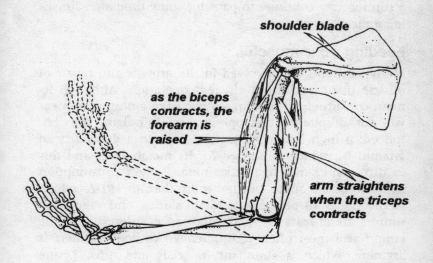

Energy is released for muscle contraction as glucose is broken down to carbon dioxide and water in the cells.

impulses tell them to do this by stimulating the cells and fibres of the muscles.

In order to move at all, however, muscles need energy, and this in turn comes from our food, which arrives in our cells in the form of glucose. There are two stages to the release of energy for muscle contraction: the first is anaerobic in which pyruvic acid is formed from the glucose; and the second is called aerobic because the pyruvic acid is oxidized to produce carbon dioxide and water. If the exertion is considerable, then there may be a build-up of pyruvic acid which cannot be oxidized quickly enough. Instead, it is converted to lactic acid and carried away by the bloodstream to the liver where it is recycled into glycogen, or else oxidized here to carbon dioxide and water. In this case an 'oxygen debt' has been created. This is why a runner may continue to pant for some time after finishing a race.

Feeding your muscles

Many nutrients are involved in the growth and repair of muscle tissue and in its efficient operation. Although its main constituent is protein, eating large amounts of meat will not, despite popular opinion, create bulging muscles. Indeed, a high intake of protein leads to a deficiency in vitamin B_6, which is utilized for its metabolism, and this in turn results in a loss of stamina. Protein consumption needs to be adequate, but not more than the RDA, which in the UK is 10 per cent of total calories, and vegetarian sources are at least of equal importance. Interestingly, the amino acid most often recommended to body-builders is arginine, which is abundant in seeds and nuts. Lysine is suggested for muscle mass, too, and this comes predominantly from meat, poultry and fish. If intake of these amino acids is combined with regular training their effect will soon be noted, and of course they are infinitely preferable to steroids.

The vitamin most needed for durability of muscles is ascorbic acid, mandatory for the synthesis of connective tissue, which holds the fibres together and provides elasticity, especially collagen and to a lesser extent elastin. So it is 'rabbit food' that helps to keep muscles strong: fresh salads and green vegetables as well as fruit.

As far as the sports enthusiast is concerned, the best source of energy comes from complex carbohydrates which require less oxygen for burning than fats or proteins and are therefore less likely to lead to a build-up of lactic acid, which can contribute to painful muscles. Generous helpings of whole grains, peas, beans and lentils, vegetables and fruit, therefore, add up to an effective fuel. Efficient combustion can only occur, though, in the presence of the right nutrients: vitamins from the B complex, especially niacin and thiamine, also biotin and the trace element chromium, are all vital. Strenuous exercise will greatly increase requirements for these, but foods such as whole-meal bread and pasta, brown rice, oats and yeast extract, also free-range eggs, nuts and shellfish, will restore them to the body (see also chapter 3 for food lists). If continued fatigue is experienced, then supplements are indicated.

Fats can be useful for endurance, such as running a marathon, as energy is released more gradually, but carnit-ine from animal protein must be available to shovel the fuel into the cells. Indeed, this amino acid can enhance the ability to tolerate prolonged physical strain and is some-times taken by athletes as a supplement. One of the most important factors for energy release is coenzyme Q10, only recently widely available in capsules. It is naturally present in the membranes of the mitochondria, the minute gener-ators inside cells. Without it the body cannot extract energy from food. Although it is produced in the body by the liver, this is frequently in insufficient quantities, especially as we grow older, and we have to acquire extra from food such as nuts, spinach, broccoli, soya products, fish, chicken and beef. After taking this coenzyme as a supplement for a month, the triathlon veteran, 72-year-old Holger Riise from Denmark, improved his time by 50 minutes, breaking the world record. Vitamin E is a beneficial adjunct, since it prevents the destruction of Q10. Fresh wheatgerm is always a reliable source. Another vitamin important for the burn-ing of fats is ascorbic acid, which augments aerobic capacity as well as muscular endurance. So keep eating that rabbit food and don't forget the oranges!

Vitamin E, along with selenium, delays the disintegration of red blood cells, the body's transport system for the oxygen. The constant oxidation of the red cells in an ath-lete's bloodstream shortens their lives, especially if these two nutrients are lacking. Many more vitamins and minerals are needed to create new red cells, iron in particular, which must be available in a good supply, otherwise anaemia and muscular weakness will be the outcome. Besides lean meat, black molasses, parsley and lentils are all excellent sources.

In order to receive signals from the nerves so that they can contract and relax, the muscles are dependent upon the correct balance of electrolytes (minerals held in a solution of water), including potassium, sodium, chloride, magnesium and calcium. If any of these are in short supply, then several complaints can arise, including muscular cramps, exhaustion and heat stroke, and in severe cases even death.

Muscular cramps

Greg was a karate enthusiast, training three times a week for an hour and a half. After two years of this he felt extremely fit, but sometimes the sessions were harsh and the more he progressed, the harder the exercises became, demanding fast reactions, looseness of the joints and strength for the punches, blocks and high kicks. Sometimes exercises were repeated to the point of exhaustion and the kata (or long series of combined movements) performed at the end of the evening demanded considerable stamina. Although intensive training was always preceded by thorough warming up, Greg would sometimes wake in the night with agonizing cramps in his calf muscles.

After a chat with his instructor, who had studied sports nutrition, Greg decided to make his own special drink which would replace the essential electrolytes which he sweated out during training. This contained twice as much potassium as sodium, together with some carbohydrate for instant energy in the form of honey (see recipe for Sports Drink in chapter 20). He drank this before and immediately after the workout, with a quick sip at halftime. Additionally, he increased his potassium and magnesium intake in his food by eating plenty of dark-green vegetables, nuts and dried fruits, soya products, bananas and jacket potatoes. He also took brewer's yeast tablets and switched from white to wholemeal bread and pasta, and was liberal with skimmed milk. His cramps quickly disappeared and he was not troubled with them again. He also noticed that his muscles were less sore.

Cramps can occur spontaneously, regardless of exercise, if the muscles are not receiving all their sustaining nutrients. In addition to the electrolytes described above, ensure that vitamin E is adequate by eating wheatgerm daily. Extra vitamin B_6 may also be helpful. If recovery is slow, it may be worth checking for food intolerances (see chapter 11 under 'Allergies').

Fibrositis

Since muscle fibres are held together by connective tissue, any strain can cause damage to this, bringing about swelling and inflammation. The muscle tissue itself can similarly become inflamed (myositis). The problem often occurs among menopausal women when the need for calcium and vitamin E is increased. Changing to a health-giving, nutritious diet (see chapter 20), with supplements of vitamin C to mend the damaged tissue, plus extra E and calcium can quickly bring relief. If the patient has been under any stress, then brewer's yeast tablets are an excellent antidote.

Chapter 14

Looking Your Best

Millions of pounds are spent every year by the cosmetics industry on research into some wonder cream that will banish frown lines, crow's feet and wrinkles and guarantee lifelong youth and beauty, while yet more millions are earned through the sale of make-up that will hide the blotches, blemishes and other imperfections. The fact remains, however, that beauty begins within. Or to put this the other way, many nutritional deficiencies will quickly show up on the body's exterior in the form of, for example, dry and flaking skin, cracks at the corners of the mouth, dull, splitting hair or spots on the nails. Indeed, nutritional therapists are trained to notice such signs as indicators of internal disharmony or ill health. Equally, correcting nutritional imbalances will soon be evident on the surface with clear skin, strong nails and lustrous locks.

The skin

Surprisingly, the outermost layer of the skin consists of flattened dead cells, which wear away and fall off only to be replaced by more as the cells beneath move towards the surface. You may notice them as a powdery grey dust on your dressing table! Yet this cornified layer of the epidermis is very useful to us because it reduces evaporation of moisture and deters bacteria from invading the body. Immediately below, in the dermis, is a fine mesh of capillaries that supply the skin, including the hair follicles and sweat glands, with oxygen and nutrients and take away the wastes. Opening into the hair follicles are the sebaceous glands that keep the skin well oiled. There are many nerve endings in the skin which constantly give us information about our surroundings, such as changes in temperature, sources of danger or comfort, objects that can be manipulated and so on.

Like other parts of the body containing a high proportion of connective tissue or muscle, the skin consists largely of protein, so must receive the correct amino acids for the creation of those rapidly dividing cells. Also mandatory are essential fatty acids, many vitamins and minerals and plenty of fluid. Despite a wholesome diet, there are environmental factors that can damage the skin, especially sun, wind and pollutants, so it needs a certain amount of protection to avoid early ageing and more serious health problems such as skin cancer.

Acne

At 15 years of age Tom was basically a good-looking fellow. He was already quite tall and muscular, having a liking for sports, but recently he had suffered an eruption of blackheads and pimples on his face that became red and angry, eventually producing yellow pustules. Worse, some of them were leaving scars, and creams that his mother bought at the chemist seemed ineffective. Poor Tom felt like a leper. Whenever he looked in the mirror all he could see was the spots. He had begun to take an interest in girls but feared that his ruined complexion would simply be an object of ridicule or revulsion if he tried to form any friendships. He began to lose confidence in himself and became withdrawn and depressed.

Sadly, this story is all too common among adolescents, with as many as 80 per cent showing some signs of acne, one-quarter of these with a severe form of the condition.

Occasionally it lingers on into adulthood, although usually it clears up spontaneously at the end of the teens.

The increase in the levels of sex hormones from age 13 stimulates the sebaceous glands to produce more oil, or sebum, than usual, which has a tendency to be too acidic. This irritates the skin, causing small swellings that block pores, trapping the sebum which may then dry out and produce a blackhead. Bacterial infection generally ensues and a pustule will develop. Since the face, neck and shoulders have the greatest density of sebaceous glands, these are the areas most prone to acne.

The only effective cure is to prevent the pimples from forming in the first place. Many teenagers notice that their complexion is worse after eating sweets. There is good reason for this. Researchers at Alabama University discovered that the ability of white cells to destroy invading bacteria declined significantly only one hour after volunteers had consumed a sweet soft drink. Difficult though it may be, it is essential to give up all confectionery, sweet cakes, soft drinks high in sucrose and sugar in tea and coffee. This will give your immune system a better chance to fight the infection. Sugar-free goodies made from whole ingredients are fine (see chapter 20) and fructose from dried fruits such as dates will provide instant energy.

It is also necessary to replace all refined, processed and junk food with whole grains and fresh fruit and vegetables. Cut down on all animal fats, especially red meat (which can be replaced with fish or poultry), butter, cheese and creamy milk (skimmed is best), but increase the intake of polyunsaturated and monounsaturated plant oils, by eating more nuts and using olive oil for cooking and safflower or sunflower oils to make salad dressings. Avoid any hydrogenated fats found in chocolate and most margarines as these will cause a depletion in essential fatty acids; seek out the non-hydrogenated type from health food shops. Bad cases of acne will respond well to 500mg of evening

222

primrose oil three times daily, which will provide the much-needed linoleic acid, frequently in short supply in people with erupting skin.

Doctors often prescribe antibiotics to help clear skin infections, but these are not a good idea as there may be unpleasant side-effects and resistance can develop over time. Researchers have found that supplements of zinc are just as effective as these drugs, without their dangers. Indeed, the skin of healthy individuals supports some 20 per cent of this mineral. Rapid growth during adolescence combined with early sexual activity can leave young people, especially males (because semen is zinc-rich), much too low in this essential trace element. It is also lost in perspiration and needs to be constantly replaced in the diet: shellfish, wheatgerm, pulses and soya products are all efficient sources (see also chapter 3), but beware of too much bran which can prevent the absorption of zinc. Take 15–30 mg of zinc sulphate daily, depending on the severity of the infection, reducing this amount when improvement in the skin is noticed.

Also important for fighting infections are vitamins A and C. Patients with acne have been found to have low levels of vitamin A in the blood, so this should be increased with generous portions of orange and dark-green vegetables and yellow and orange fruits, together with cod-liver oil (follow the directions on the bottle) and a supplement of beta-carotene, adding up to around 12,500IU of vitamin A. (Do not exceed recommended doses of the oily retinol as toxicity can result if intake is prolonged.) This vitamin is required for the building of the epithelial layers of the skin and will help to prevent the pores from becoming clogged up. The fresh fruit and vegetables will contribute vitamin C, but a further 500mg daily will assist in healing and will keep the connective tissue immediately under the surface in good condition.

Sometimes acne can be an indication of stress, in which

case the B vitamins will help to alleviate this. Yeast extract in the form of Marmite or similar, is rich in these. Especially beneficial is brewer's yeast, which also contains chromium known to be effective against acne.

To prevent scarring, use vitamin E. This can be applied directly to the skin by pricking a capsule. Check the evening primrose oil as this will probably also include vitamin E to offset any possible rancidity. If not, take a supplement of about 50IU. Selenium will increase its effectiveness, so include 25mcg.

Keep the area very clean with unperfumed soap and pat over with an infusion of lavender flowers. Exercise will increase the circulation to the skin, maintaining a fresh supply of nutrients and helping to keep the pores clear. Remember to take in copious amounts of fluid in the form of filtered water, herb teas and fruit and vegetable juices.

Dry, cracked or oily skin

Dryness of the skin invariably results from a lack of the essential fatty acids which keep it naturally moist. Make sure, therefore, that your intake of plant oils is adequate: safflower- and sunflower-seed and linseed oils are particularly rich in EFAs. Check also that your consumption of vitamins A, C and B are above RDA levels (see chapter 3), especially if you are under any stress. Liberal amounts of water are needed by the skin so drink lots of fluid.

Oily skin and hair are sometimes symptoms of B_2 deficiency, especially if whiteheads are evident: 5mg twice daily of riboflavin should correct this. A lack of B_2 can also show up as cracks at the corner of the mouth, dry patches in front of the ears, or even swollen lips or tongue. If you are taking B_6 as a supplement, this can create a B_2 deficiency since they work together, so take B_2 also. B vitamins are best derived from natural sources such as brewer's yeast or yeast extract, where they occur in balanced proportions (see also chapter 3).

224

Eczema and dermatitis

The National Eczema Society of the UK blames stress, pollution and the effects of modern lifestyles on the continuing increase in cases of this skin problem, currently affecting 1 in 8 children and 1 in 12 adults. Although there are 14 different types, atopic eczema is the one most commonly associated with infants. Generally there are other allergic conditions troubling the child or close family members, such as hay fever or asthma, and this is an indication that something in the environment has been the trigger. Very often it is a food intolerance.

Six-year-old Ben had suffered from eczema on and off for much of his young life, horribly blighted by the nasty rashes, blistering and weeping skin and intense itching, often leaving him crying in the night and very short of sleep. Creams recommended by the family doctor relieved the symptoms temporarily, which then recurred. Ben's mother was in despair until she contacted the National Eczema Society which suggested that a food allergy could be the cause and advised taking him off dairy products. The effect was remarkable. After switching from cow's to soya milk, cutting out cheese and using unhydrogenated margarine, while replacing the calcium with a chewable supplement, there was a noticeable improvement in Ben's skin after only ten days. Eventually it cleared up altogether, but his mother was careful to keep him on a healthy diet. Other common allergens are eggs, wheat, sugar or any food additives.

As we have seen, essential fatty acids are an integral part of the structure of skin, and there is considerable evidence to suggest that eczema sufferers may have difficulty in metabolizing these. When tested, patients are frequently found to be short of GLA (gamma-linoleic acid). Since evening primrose oil is a rich source of this substance, 1g three times daily generally clears the dry patches and

225

rashes. It can also be rubbed directly into the skin. Healing will be assisted if animal and hydrogenated fats are excluded from the diet, while increasing the intake of safflower, sunflower and olive oils.

Sometimes a multifaceted approach is needed to clear obstinate cases. In addition to testing for food intolerances, following the Health-Giving Diet outlined in chapter 20 and balancing the EFAs, take a supplement of zinc sulphate (30mg reducing to 15mg daily as required) together with brewer's yeast tablets (at least three with every meal), and, as long as you are wheat tolerant, have a serving of fresh wheatgerm daily. The nutrients supplied will assist in EFA metabolism as well as healing. Premenstrual women will also benefit from extra magnesium and vitamin B_6. Multivitamin and -mineral tablets, with plenty of A from food (see chapter 3), will give the skin an extra boost. Meanwhile keep steroid creams for emergencies only as they can be damaging if used to excess, and apply aloe vera gel to alleviate itching and soreness.

The symptoms of dermatitis can be similar to eczema, but the cause is nearly always external and can usually be tracked down to detergents, perfumes, certain fabrics and so on. In addition to avoiding the offending substance, you can improve your resistance by following the Health-Giving Diet in chapter 20, and taking a multivitamin and -mineral tablet daily together with two teaspoons of cold-pressed linseed oil.

Psoriasis

Emily was planning a holiday on a Greek island with her boyfriend, but the excitement was clouded by her embarrassment over the scaly patches which had appeared on her elbows, knees and scalp. How could she possibly wear a swimsuit looking like this? Her worst fear was that her boyfriend would be so disgusted by her psoriasis that he would not wish to be near her.

She was surprised when her doctor assured her that a holiday in the sun was just what she needed, as the ultra-violet light would assist healing and, since the condition is worsened by stress, a long rest should help to clear it. Emily realized that stress must be a factor, as the disease had first appeared when she was 16 at the time when her parents were going through a divorce. Since then it recurred if she was working too hard or was unduly anxious about something.

The coal-tar preparations that her doctor prescribed were horribly messy and smelt awful, so Emily went to see a naturopath for advice. She had little interest in cooking and generally bought ready-made frozen meals, tending to rely on chocolate bars for instant energy. As there was a free supply of coffee and tea at the office, she was rarely without a mug of one or the other steaming away on her desk. During the hour-long consultation, the naturopath persuaded her to take her diet in hand, which meant cutting out all white flour and sugar, animal fats and fried food, anything containing additives, all confectionery especially chocolate, also alcohol and vinegar. Instead she must place the emphasis on fresh fruit and vegetables, salads, soya products, nuts and pulses, whole grains, fish and a little poultry, with fluids from herb teas and spring water. Sulphur, present in eggs, onions and garlic, was also important as a cleanser and detoxifying agent, while yogurt would contribute healthy bacteria. In addition 30mg of zinc sulphate daily, reducing to 15mg after four weeks, was prescribed, plus brewer's yeast tablets for the B vitamins and an extra 50mg of B_6, also 200IU of natural vitamin E. To help regulate the blood fats, 3 tablespoons of granular lecithin had to be sprinkled into her food each day, while 500mg of evening primrose oil was to be taken orally with each meal, with the same amount rubbed directly into the scaly patches. A herbal ointment, Phytolacca cream, was recommended to ease the itching.

227

The naturopath warned that this was a difficult condition to cure but, since she wanted to look good for her holiday, Emily reckoned it was all worth a try. She also joined a yoga class for relaxation. By setting time aside specially to take care of herself she managed to stick to her new programme and, after summoning up courage to tell her boyfriend, she was overjoyed to gain his support. By the time she returned from her holiday her skin was clear.

Sunburn sensitivity

Fair-skinned people are better able to tolerate sun without burning if their diet is well supplied with the more recently recognized B vitamin PABA (para-aminobenzoic acid). Eat plenty of whole grains, take brewer's yeast and include molasses with meals: recipes in chapter 20 will give you some ideas. An ointment containing this vitamin can also be applied to the skin. At the same time check that your levels of the antioxidant nutrients A, C and E are adequate to give extra protection against the damaging effects of ultraviolet rays.

Warts

These can be a real nuisance, but fortunately they can disappear just as suddenly as they arrive, indicating that the body's own immune system is fighting the infection. The Health-Giving Diet outlined in chapter 20 will help boost your natural immunity and you will find more detailed information concerning the immune system in chapter 11.

Dandelion sap helps to get rid of them. Squeeze a little from the stem and rub into each wart, taking care to avoid the surrounding skin.

Nails

Since nails are formed largely from protein, of which the chief one is keratin, it is important that your daily food

228

includes all the essential amino acids (see chapter 3). Those containing sulphur, found in eggs, onions, garlic and mustard, encourage healthy growth.

Thin or brittle nails

Problems with the nails can indicate early anaemia, especially if they become thin or flattened. If you can eat liver, this will fulfil your iron needs, but make sure it is organic otherwise it may be full of toxins. Have jumbo oats in your muesli and eat lentils and beans frequently. Also make good use of black molassses in cooking (for example 'Pumpernickel' described in chapter 20), or spread on wholemeal toast. Additionally, consider taking a multi-mineral supplement. Avoid tea and coffee and pitta bread, all of which diminish iron absorption significantly.

Evening primrose oil is also excellent for the nails: take 2g daily in divided doses.

White spots

These can indicate a dearth of zinc, so eat a wholefood diet rather than refined or processed foods, which are lacking in this mineral. If you have access to unpolluted shellfish, eat these regularly, and have a serving of wheatgerm each day. You may be losing zinc through perspiration, in which case take a supplement of around 15mg of zinc sulphate daily until you notice improvement.

Athlete's foot

This is notoriously difficult to cure, especially if the fungal infection is under the nails. Plenty of live yoghurt will keep it at bay together with B vitamins from brewer's yeast (at least three tablets three times daily) and wheatgerm. Some people have sprinkled vitamin C powder directly on to the affected area with some success. Tea tree oil is usually recommended by herbalists.

Growth of the fungus will be discouraged if the nails are washed frequently, kept very dry and exposed to the air.

Hair

Although the cosmetic industry makes a fortune selling shampoos, conditioners and artificial colourings, thick, glossy hair that retains its hue is based on sound nutrition. At the bottom of each follicle, cells keep dividing to add new ones to the base of the hair, making it grow. A whole-food diet that incorporates sufficient protein is indispensable for healthy hair, providing the nutrients needed by the newly forming cells. Around 12 per cent of the hair consists of the amino acid cystine, available, besides animal sources, in seeds, nuts and whole grains, so eat plenty of these with added wheatgerm.

Hair loss

Female clients of mine who have experienced sudden hair loss in isolated patches have all connected the onset with stress. This may have been family troubles, such as worry over teenage children, or career concerns. Whatever the emotional problem, it makes sense to return to the body those nutrients that the stress has been soaking up, in particular B complex and C. Wheatgerm and yeast extract need to be in generous supply, and organic liver if you eat meat; alternatively take brewer's yeast tablets or a B complex that includes inositol, folic acid and biotin. PABA, which occurs naturally in these foods as well as in whole grains and black molasses, can prevent balding. If you are able to buy it, take a supplement of around 300mg daily; you may need to ask for a prescription. Eat good portions of fresh fruit, salad and vegetables for the ascorbic acid and add a supplement of at least 500mg daily. Zinc has significantly helped alopecia patients: take 30mg every day for four weeks, then reduce the amount by half. Hair loss may also indicate a lack of iron, so increase your consumption of pulses and have black molasses regularly. Make sure, too, that your diet is adequate in vegetable oils.

Certain drugs including the contraceptive pill can affect the growth and thickness of hair; vitamin B_6 with magnesium will assist in counteracting the negative effects of the Pill. Do, however, check with your doctor if you suddenly lose hair, as an underactive thyroid could be the cause.

Greying

Here again, vitamin B deficiencies, particularly of B_5, B_{12} and biotin, may bring about early greying of hair, although predisposing factors may simply be hereditary. Brewer's yeast tablets will restore the balance and supply PABA, which is excellent for the hair. Check also that your consumption of copper is at RDA levels, because this mineral is involved in hair pigmentation. A wholefood diet that includes lentils, nuts and fish should meet your requirements, but remember that zinc supplements will reduce your uptake of copper.

If you have to resort to dyes, choose henna or those extracted from vegetables. Chemical dyes have been linked to cancer and could do you serious harm.

Dandruff

The latest research implies that a fungus may be at the root of this common problem. Selenium, when included in shampoo, has anti-fungal properties, so seek this out from your health-food store. Also take low-fat live yoghurt daily and follow the suggestions made above under 'Dry skin', putting emphasis on cold-pressed sunflower and linseed oils.

If you can cope with the mess, rub linseed oil into the scalp and leave on as long as possible before washing out.

Chapter 15

The Five Senses

While thinking about this chapter I wandered into the garden in the late afternoon, gasping as the cold air hit my nostrils. The autumn light was beginning to fade with the sun low over the adjacent fields, just turning from gold to red and catching the coppery hues of the beech tree. Here and there berries glowed deep crimson among the shrubs and in between stretched the damp green grass. The fresh sweet smell that still lingered reminded me that my husband had just mown it. Everything was very still and quite breathtakingly beautiful. Suddenly, a large bird flew overhead, flapping its wings energetically, accompanied by a raucous quacking. I deduced that it was a village duck aiming for our pond. Shortly afterwards I was aware of the low drone of an engine and the crunch of wheels on gravel indicating that my neighbour was home early from work. Turning back towards the house, I inhaled the perfume of one of our late roses, catching myself on a thorn as I did so. As I lingered under the porch, our cat rubbed herself against my boot and I bent down to stroke her soft, warm fur. Just then an acrid smell warned me that I had left some scones in the oven and I rushed inside to rescue them. Only a few minutes had passed, but my senses had been bombarded with hundreds of stimuli, providing me with interesting and useful information together with a prick of pain and a variety of pleasures.

Without sight, smell, touch, taste and hearing it would be impossible for us to orientate ourselves in the world. Loss of even one of these faculties leaves us either badly disabled or with a reduced quality of life. How important it is, therefore, to safeguard our senses! We can do this with sound nutrition and with regular exercise that will encourage the circulation to carry the nutrients and the oxygen to the receptor organs. By following such a pro- gramme, there is every chance that we can retain them in good working order into our ninth or even tenth decade.

Eyes

Because our two eyes are positioned either side of the nose, they each receive a somewhat different image on the back of the retina. By merging the two pictures into one, the brain forms a fully three-dimensional image, giving us a sense of size, shape and distance. The retina contains liter- ally millions of specialized light-sensitive cells of two types, rods and cones. The cones enable us to distinguish colour while the rods allow us to see shapes in dim light.

The retina depends on both vitamin A and zinc for accu- rate functioning and, if healthy, will contain a considerable amount of these nutrients. The retinol combines with pro- tein to form visual purple, a pigment in the retina, which allows us to see when light levels are low.

Vitamin A deficiency has very serious consequences for the eyes, causing drying up of the tear ducts (xerophthalmia) and ulceration of the cornea at the front of the eye (keratomalacia), leading to blindness. Up to a quarter of a million people in south-east Asia alone go blind as a result of inadequate intake of vitamin A and, sadly, most are growing children who have higher retinol requirements than adults. Because vitamin A in its oily form is stored in the liver for future use, a programme of injections is now beginning to save the sight of many of these children.

SECTION THROUGH THE EYE

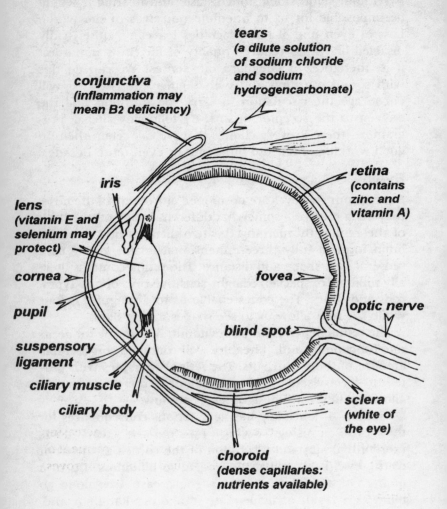

tears
(a dilute solution of sodium chloride and sodium hydrogencarbonate)

conjunctiva
(inflammation may mean B2 deficiency)

iris

retina
(contains zinc and vitamin A)

lens
(vitamin E and selenium may protect)

cornea

fovea

pupil

optic nerve

blind spot

suspensory ligament

ciliary muscle

ciliary body

sclera
(white of the eye)

choroid
(dense capillaries: nutrients available)

The eyes are a mirror of the health: cracking at the corners may indicate a deficiency of vitamins B6 or B2; an inflamed conjunctiva signals a possible lack of B2, while dry eyes can denote a food intolerance or a dearth of vitamin A. Night blindness is a symptom of low zinc and vitamin A levels. Cataracts suggest poor sugar or calcium metabolism, or UV radiation damage.

Night blindness

If you eat raw carrot each day you will not suffer from this condition, as the beta-carotene contained in the vegetable will convert into vitamin A in the body and form the visual purple in the retina that allows you to see in a poorly lit environment. Night blindness can be a hazard, especially to drivers. It is also a warning sign that vitamin A levels are too low in the body and need to be quickly replenished before more serious eye problems occur. Make sure therefore that you obtain at least the RDA (800mcg or 2,650IU). Organic lamb's liver is exceedingly high in vitamin A, while the same weight of carrots has one-tenth this amount, still more than twice the RDA. Fish oil is another food rich in retinol. If you are a vegetarian aim to eat at least two sources of beta-carotene daily, especially in winter when dark-green vegetables are less readily available: for example a good portion of broccoli and of goat's milk cheese plus 1oz (30g) of butter should add up to the RDA. Parsley grown on your windowsill offers an instant supply. And don't forget the leaves of that despised weed, the dandelion. To begin with you will probably need to take a supplement of about 10,000IU of beta-carotene daily, or a couple of teaspoons of cod-liver oil.

It is thought that zinc in some way assists in the metabolism of vitamin A. Certainly it is necessary for the health of the retina. If the condition persists despite increasing levels of beta-carotene or retinol, then take a supplement of zinc at 15mg daily until your vision in dim light improves.

Cataracts

A colour photograph of mountain sheep completely blinded by cataracts caused by over-exposure to UV radiation, a direct effect of ozone depletion, remains implanted in my memory. How can we be so stupid and uncaring as to go on destroying our fragile ozone layer with chemical pollutants to the point at which our own eyes and those of innocent creatures can become permanently damaged?

Humans can protect their eyes with polaroid sunglasses, those who are able to buy them, that is. Otherwise, unprotected exposure to the sun's rays causes gradual clouding of the lens until the person can no longer see, a situation that is becoming increasingly common. The lens can be removed by surgery and the vision restored with glasses, but prevention is obviously a better course of action.

It is not clear to what extent excellent nutrition can influence the degeneration of the lens as a person ages, but there is some evidence that the antioxidant nutrients vitamin E and selenium, if maintained at more than adequate levels, especially through middle age, may help to keep cataracts at bay. So keep a constant supply of wheatgerm in your fridge for daily helpings, as well as cold-pressed plant oils for salad dressings. Also make sure that you have plenty of riboflavin from foods such as free-range eggs, yoghurt, broccoli, yeast and soya products.

Diabetics need to be particularly careful and additionally increase vitamins A and C together with bioflavonoids. Any upset in the metabolism of sugar or of calcium can lead to eye damage and must be balanced out with a special dietary approach (see chapter 10). Strangely, there appears to be a link between high milk intake and cataract formation, especially among elderly diabetics, while yoghurt has a protective effect – but it is not known why. Expert nutritional advice needs to be sought to suit individual cases.

Conjunctivitis

If a foreign body accidentally finds its way into your eye, there is no danger that it will disappear round the back of the eyeball because the conjunctiva will prevent that from happening. It is the thin epithelium that lines the inside of the eyelids curving round to attach itself to the cornea in a continuous piece. Sometimes this becomes inflamed or irritated, perhaps due to an infection, or an allergy or maybe even a food intolerance. Any infection can be better fought with good doses of vitamin C, which will also help combat hayfever symptoms. Take 2g daily in divided doses. This can also be put directly on to the conjunctiva in the form of potassium ascorbate eye drops.

If the conjunctivitis is a recurring problem, especially if accompanied by puffiness, then a food intolerance is suspect. Try to discover the offending items by excluding likely foods and then reintroducing them one by one. See chapter 11 under 'Allergies' for a suggested programme.

Over-sensitive, sore or tired eyes

If you find yourself screwing up your eyes whenever they are exposed to bright light, then you could be short of riboflavin (vitamin B_2). Although this is available in many foods, the amount is frequently small. For example a 100-g (3.5-oz) serving of broccoli provides just one-eighth the RDA, while a similar amount of free-range eggs or cheese gives a little under one-quarter. Liver and kidney supply more than you need, but vegans must seek it from a number of sources. Brewer's yeast tablets combined with a B_2 supplement of about 30mg daily are advisable for sensitive or sore eyes, particularly if any redness appears as a ring, or for eyes that are quickly fatigued.

Another symptom of riboflavin deficiency is cracking at the corners of the eyes, which also indicates a lack of vitamin B_6. In addition to yeast, therefore, have a liberal serving of wheatgerm daily which should supply you with the RDA of pyridoxine. You will almost certainly require a B_6 supplement of about 50mg as well until the disorder clears. Keep in mind the need to keep riboflavin and pyridoxine in balance with each other; too much of one leads to a deficiency in the other.

Any of these eye problems are always assisted with a

generous and regular supply of vitamin A. A glass of carrot juice before your dinner will work wonders!

Ears

Have you noticed how your ears 'pop' whenever you go up in a lift or aeroplane or climb a mountain? As the air pressure falls on the outside of the ear drum, so the pressure inside the middle ear adjusts itself via a narrow tube connected to the nasal cavity which can open or close to admit or release air as required. The middle ear contains three tiny bones that receive vibrations from the ear drum, a thin membrane rather like a drum skin that covers the end of the tube-like outer ear. Nerve endings in the inner ear transmit impulses to the brain, which interprets these as different sounds.

Yet the ears are not just for hearing. They also regulate our balance by detecting tilting and twisting movements which disturb fluid in the semicircular canals of the inner ear. Nerve fibres from their bases send appropriate messages to the brain. This in turn informs the muscles what to do to keep the body upright. At the same time gravity acts on grains of calcium carbonate (chalk), pressing them against sensory cells connected to these nerve fibres. So the brain can enable the body to become aware of its position.

Ear infections

Because of the connection with the nose, germs can easily move into the middle ear and cause trouble. A build-up of fluid in this area can lead to the condition known as glue ear, common in small children. Any ear infections should be immediately reported to a doctor as they can seriously impair hearing, but supplements of vitamins C and A will certainly help and can be safely taken in conjunction with prescribed medication. A multivitamin and -mineral supplement is recommended for children prone to recurring

238

infections. Always check for food intolerances, following the guidelines under 'Allergies' in chapter 11, and possible allergens such as house dust mites or grass pollen, all of which can cause ear irritation.

If there is a build-up of mucus, cut out dairy products and reduce all starchy and sugary foods. Gargling with beetroot juice or salty water will help to clear it.

Make sure that nutrition is especially sound during cold winter months, with plenty of fresh fruit, dark-green vegetables and salad for vitamin C, regular wheatgerm for zinc, iron and B vitamins, and the inclusion of yeast extract and black molasses in cooking or as a spread. Nutrients thus provided will help to keep infections away.

Tinnitus

A persistent ringing in the ears bothers many people, but causes can be hard to determine. A recent Israeli study links it with low levels of vitamin B_{12}, so eat Marmite regularly or take brewer's yeast as a supplement. Fish oils may also be helpful.

Check for any food intolerances as described in chapter 11 under 'Allergies'.

Travel sickness

Holidays, excursions and business travel can be made miserable through sickness caused by motion. Yet there is a simple remedy. In a properly controlled trial in America, ginger root was found to be more effective than a commonly prescribed drug. This is available in tablet form from herbal suppliers (see Addresses), or else you can make your own Ginger Brew and take it with you to sip as necessary (see recipe in chapter 20).

Nose

Can you describe how you recognize different smells? We know that the top of the nasal cavity is lined with groups of sensory cells referred to as chemo-receptors. These are stimulated by airborne chemicals and accordingly send messages via nerve fibres to the brain, which can somehow distinguish one from another, but we are not yet certain precisely how it does this.

Human sense of smell is nothing like as acute as that of many other creatures: bloodhounds can follow a trail for many miles over rough mountain terrain, while an insignificant creature like a frog is able to smell its natural habitat, a pond, well over a mile away. Nevertheless, restricted as this sense is, we find it both useful and evocative. The perfume of a flower can be a real delight and the scent of a lover's skin highly erotic. We also use our noses to detect mouldy, bad or burnt food and to warn us away from fire or toxic fumes. The ability to remember smells can be a matter of survival.

Recently I met up with my classmates at our former boarding school, having not visited the place for some decades. Adjacent to the building there is still a bank of wild garlic. We all exclaimed as we walked past it, saying that we think of the school every time we smell the plant.

Loss of smell

This can occur when the nose is stuffed up or runny. If it happens repeatedly then test for food intolerances, starting with milk (see chapter 11 under 'Allergies'). Also check out wheat, eggs, chocolate and sugar and avoid additives and preservatives. Boost your immune system if you are prone to colds. You will find details about how to do this in chapter 11. Infections can be more quickly banished with the assistance of 2g of vitamin C daily and regular doses of garlic.

Sometimes the smell receptors can be permanently damaged from a severe attack of influenza. This happened to my mother when in her seventies. I recall the many occasions when she bent down to smell something with keen anticipation and the subsequent disappointment at being reminded that she had lost this faculty. All the more reason to keep your immune system well fed so that you are less likely to succumb to passing viruses.

Tongue

Our taste-buds, which are mainly arranged in groups in the grooves of our tongues, are the receptors that can sense different chemicals when they are dissolved in saliva. We classify these as sweet, sour, bitter or salty. The sensation we call 'flavour' is more subtle and also involves smell, as vapours rise and reach the chemo-receptors in the nose.

Loss of taste

Because of the close connection with the sense of smell, a stuffed-up nose can reduce the ability to taste. In this case follow the recommendations described in the above section.

However, impaired taste is a classic symptom of zinc deficiency, so foods rich in this mineral should be supplied. Shellfish, wheatgerm, lean lamb, soya products, lentils and other foods listed in chapter 3 will help to fulfil needs. Keep miso in your fridge and use this regularly in soup. To achieve the RDA of 15mg you will need to eat several zinc-rich foods each day, although a liberal serving of wheat-germ on muesli with a base of jumbo oats should give you this. To make sure, take 15mg of zinc orotate daily until your sense of taste returns.

Chapter 16

The Body's Computer

Have you looked up into the night sky recently and marvelled at the splendour of the Milky Way with its 100 billion stars? No less miraculous is the human brain, which, although weighing only 3 to 4lb (1.4 to 1.8kg), contains this same vast number of nerve cells, or neurons, so that information can be stored, retrieved and used, and so that emotions can be experienced and movement controlled.

If the two corrugated cerebral hemispheres of the brain were laid out flat, the surface area would be in excess of one square metre. The left and right hemispheres are roughly symmetrical and straddle a central core that extends down to the spinal cord. The brain and spinal cord together are known as the central nervous system and nerves carry electrical impulses from here to all other parts of the body, giving signals to muscles and glands, and carrying other messages back from the sense organs.

Neurons receive signals via branching fibres called dendrites and send information to others along an axon or nerve fibre. A single nerve cell could have a fibre attached to it that extends for a whole metre to carry instructions, for example, to the little toe. Hundreds of these microscopic axons accumulate to form complete nerves, rather like highly complex telephone cables, which can carry many

HOW NEURONS SEND MESSAGES TO EACH OTHER

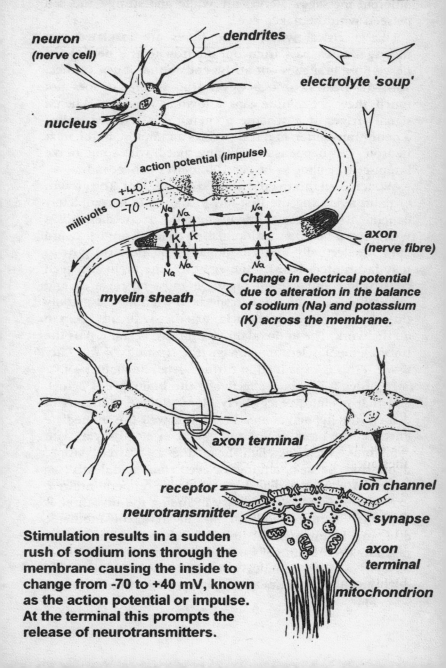

neuron
(nerve cell)

dendrites

electrolyte 'soup'

nucleus

action potential (impulse)

+40
millivolts 0
-70

Na Na   Na
K   K   K
    K
Na Na   Na

axon
(nerve fibre)

*Change in electrical potential
due to alteration in the balance
of sodium (Na) and potassium
(K) across the membrane.*

myelin sheath

axon terminal

receptor

ion channel

neurotransmitter

synapse

**Stimulation results in a sudden
rush of sodium ions through the
membrane causing the inside to
change from -70 to +40 mV, known
as the action potential or impulse.
At the terminal this prompts the
release of neurotransmitters.**

**axon
terminal**

mitochondrion

different messages. Nerves are white and stringy and can be seen with the naked eye.

Like electrical wires, nerve fibres are insulated, yet messages must pass from one neuron to the next. Each nerve fibre branches out at the end so that it can connect with the next neuron at several places. Yet it does not touch: there are minute gaps, known as synapses. When a signal arrives at a synapse a chemical is released, called a neurotransmitter, and this triggers an impulse in the next neuron. This happens at lightning speed, with some nerve impulses travelling as fast as 100 metres per second.

What has all this to do with food? Quite a lot. The growth of neurons during the first few years of life is completely dependent upon the nutrients supplied in the diet. It is a well-known fact that malnourished children are backward both intellectually and emotionally and physical growth may be stunted, too. By the age of 7, the brain has been constructed, but like all organs it must be repaired and maintained and in these respects B vitamins, especially thiamin (B_1), B_{12} and folic acid, together with zinc, help to do the work. The antioxidant vitamins A, C and E plus the trace element selenium prevent the 'rusting' of the fatty tissue. (This is explained in further detail in chapter 19.)

In order to operate effectively, the brain needs a fuel, and that is almost exclusively blood glucose. Sufferers of diabetes or hypoglycaemia know full well the immediate effect on the brain of ups and downs in blood sugar, with symptoms such as light-headedness, blurred vision, depression, nausea, fainting, or even coma and death (see chapter 10). Yet, so that this fuel can be properly utilized, various nutrients are necessary including the first three B vitamins, thiamin, riboflavin and niacin, also pantothenic acid and biotin and the minerals chromium and magnesium. Then brain cells must have a constant supply of oxygen, or they will quickly die. This arrives via red blood cells which in turn are reliant on protein, iron, zinc and copper plus vitamins B_6, B_{12} and folic acid for their creation. A generous supply of vitamin C will assist in the absorption of iron.

So that the electrical impulses can be conducted and signals thereby passed on, the brain and other body cells are immersed in an 'electrolyte soup' consisting of dissolved sodium, potassium, chloride, calcium and magnesium. These minerals also come from the diet and, as far as the brain is concerned, it is vital that the ingredients are correctly balanced. This is often not the case because we in the West eat far, far too much salt which seriously depletes the potassium.

The chemicals called neurotransmitters that allow communication between one neuron and the next are all constructed from food items. For example, acetylcholine is derived from the nutrient choline, while serotonin is derived from the amino acid tryptophan. Another amino acid, pyroglutamate, which is found in fruit and vegetables, is the main ingredient for the production of 'nootropics', prescribed by doctors to patients with memory problems.

It is obvious that the brain cannot perform at its best without a reliable supply of all these essential nutrients. At the same time the delicate and complex mechanism of this organ can be easily obstructed by alcohol, drugs, environmental toxins and food intolerances, all of which are best shunned.

Anaemia

In chapter 8, a description was given of the way in which oxygen combines with haemoglobin in the red blood cells for transportation to the body's tissues. Haemoglobin is a protein that contains iron and it is synthesized for new red blood cells from ferritin stored in the bone marrow. Each red cell lives for about 120 days. After destruction the iron is recycled and stored before being used again. Despite this, a plentiful amount of this mineral must be supplied in the diet, otherwise anaemia can be the result, especially among growing children and menstruating or pregnant women. Even before anaemia has been identified, a lack of iron can bring about electrical irregularities in the brain, often showing up as listlessness, dizziness and even difficulties with learning. Pallor, little appetite, irritability and muscle fatigue are other signs of iron deficiency. This is surprisingly common in the West, with 30 per cent of children and menstruating women absorbing less than the RDA, and of these 2 per cent are anaemic.

Supplements of iron gluconate can be taken at up to 30mg daily, but above this amount upset in the bowels can occur. An equal quantity of zinc should be consumed otherwise absorption will be impaired (particularly important for pregnant women). Desiccated liver is a natural alternative, but vegetarians will acquire the RDA of 12mg of iron from a serving of lentils or haricot beans, one free-range egg and two slices of wholemeal bread, especially if spread with black molasses. Children should only take iron supplements under medical supervision as poisoning can ensue. Tea and coffee need to be avoided by iron-deficient people as these beverages hinder its absorption.

Yet iron supplements alone may not dispel anaemia. The red blood cells themselves must be both healthy and numerous, reliant on protein, zinc and copper plus various B vitamins, as explained in the introduction to this chapter. Although vegetarians do not eat meat, the main source of iron for most people, they do at least include plenty of fruit and vegetables which in turn are high in vitamin C and this aids absorption and retention of any available iron.

This mineral has to be dissolved by hydrochloric acid in the stomach, which requires the following nutrients for its secretion: vitamins B_1, B_2 and B_3 plus pantothenic acid and choline. A lack of any of these can lead to anaemia. (See chapter 3 for food sources.)

Vegans and old people are at risk of pernicious anaemia

arising from a vitamin B_{12} deficiency. This can be fatal as the number of red blood cells decreases and there can be severe damage to the nervous system. Treatment will involve injection of this vitamin. Desiccated liver along with brewer's yeast are recommended to aid recovery together with a diet rich in nutrients and protein. Vitamin E from wheatgerm and plant oils will help protect the membranes of the red blood cells from damage and thereby increase their longevity.

Migraine and other headaches

Years ago while living in London, I shared a flat with a migraine sufferer. A natural redhead, her complexion was normally pale, but when an attack came on she turned deathly white and broke out in a sweat. She complained of flashing lights and severe pain which nothing could alleviate except prolonged rest. Sometimes the migraine lasted for several days and was extremely debilitating. The only way I could help was to be very quiet, as any noise made her feel worse.

Even in those days her doctor knew of the connection with foods containing tyramine, a toxin derived from the amino acid tyrosine. This occurs naturally in chocolate, yeast extract, cheese, liver and sausages, also broad beans and pickled herrings, all of which should be avoided by the migraine sufferer as they can trigger an attack. The pain is caused by the blood vessels in the brain alternately constricting and dilating. Normal dilation is dependent on the availability of B vitamins, so make sure you have sufficient, especially niacin (see chapter 3 for sources). Yeast-free B-complex tablets are available from health food stores.

Other food intolerances can also provoke migraine headaches and the patient needs to go on an exclusion diet to discover what these are (see 'Allergies' in chapter 11). Apart from the above foods, tea, coffee, cola and alcohol (in particular red wine) must be cut out, also sugar and any food additives. Coffee actually prevents the brain's own natural pain-relieving hormones from working effectively. Other suspects can be wheat or milk, or even citrus fruits or bananas. It makes sense not to risk smoking.

More recent research has indicated that the blood platelets of migraine patients are unusually sticky. Eat plenty of fish therefore and take at least 500mg of vitamin C daily, also evening primrose oil (about 2g) or linseed oil plus a little vitamin E, all of which will help to thin the blood, as will ginger.

Some migraines may be initiated by low magnesium, so supplements of this mineral will alleviate this type.

Cluster headaches, in which the pain is often experienced on one side behind the eye, can also be induced by the food intolerances described above.

Premenstrual women sometimes suffer headaches due to water retention in the brain tissues. Supplements of vitamin B_6 can relieve this. Equally, women on the contraceptive pill need more pyridoxine.

A headache can often be a symptom of stress, so it is always important to practise deep relaxation and meditation which can provide relief. Acupressure on points at the nape of the neck below the skull either side of the spine, and beneath the eyebrows towards the inner corners of the eyes, can also be successful.

A natural way to control pain is through the amino acid phenylalanine, which enhances the effect of the body's own morphine-like substances called endorphins. It is best taken as DLPA complex with vitamins B_1, B_2 and B_6 and C, all of which help the body to use it efficiently. It is also well worth trying the herb feverfew, *Tanacetum parthenium*, which helps to maintain a correct balance of the hormone-like substances known as prostaglandins. These control many body functions, including blood flow. Patients have reported a reduction in nausea and vomiting on 50mg daily (or $2^1/_2$ fresh leaves), also fewer, less severe attacks. Take

248

with food for up to 14 days only. Neither of these remedies is recommended for pregnant women, however. Supplements of bioflavonoids have been found to reduce the pain of some sufferers.

For headaches brought on by colds or other infections, see chapter 11.

Anxiety and panic attacks

Enid had always been highly strung, but after her husband left her, her anxiety became all-consuming. Her waking life became full of dread. Each time she got into the car she was convinced she would have an accident, and whenever she left the house she imagined it being invaded by burglars. Shopping became a real nightmare. One day, as she was wheeling a trolley around the supermarket, she was overwhelmed with a terrible sense of impending doom. The packets on the shelves blurred into a crazy jumble of colours and her chest felt constricted so that she could scarcely catch her breath. She felt dizzy and clung on to the trolley for support, convinced that she would collapse on to the floor and die of heart failure. A kind shop assistant noticed that she looked ill and found her a chair, but it was a good quarter of an hour before she recovered sufficiently to stand up again. After that she became terrified of going out on her own, fearful that another panic attack would overtake her and that she would be unable to reach home.

Such attacks are the result of an over-stressed system and it is exceedingly important to identify and reduce sources of strain, at the same time practising deep physical relaxation and meditation to lower overall stress levels. A counsellor can help with difficult problems. It is also important to understand that a panic attack will not of itself cause death and that any chest pain is generally the result of tension. Knowing this will at least lessen the fear of an attack. Nevertheless it is sensible to see a doctor for a check-up.

When the body goes into a state of alarm from some sort

249

of stress signal such as fear, adrenaline and other hormones are released into the bloodstream which increase the heart rate and make extra energy available for instant action. Modern life offers little in the way of physical outlet for stress, however, since you can rarely run away from your problems, nor can you attack people who cause you the anxiety. So the stress becomes directed inwards and physical ailments can result from the damage, some very serious. Because the metabolic rate increases, the demand for nutrients goes up, especially for ascorbic acid, also potassium, phosphorus and calcium. Vitamin C can be protective against stress and a supplement of at least 500mg daily is recommended. It is prudent to eat a very healthy diet (see chapter 20) when under any strain.

Certain nutrients have a calming effect, especially vitamin B_1 (thiamin) and pantothenic acid: wheatgerm and brewer's yeast are therefore good anti-anxiety foods. Magnesium and calcium in a one-to-two ratio will help you feel more relaxed and a combined supplement should be of assistance. Soya products, nuts, dark-green vegetables, whitebait and whole sardines, cottage cheese and figs are all good foods for anyone suffering from anxiety or stress.

It is inadvisable to take caffeine-containing beverages, as these will increase anxiety. Drink camomile tea instead which has a mildly tranquillizing effect. Although alcohol is often taken to mitigate stress, it merely depletes the system even further and adds to the overall burden.

Insomnia

If you were brought up on the stories about Peter Rabbit by Beatrix Potter, as I was, then you will remember those famous lines: 'It is said that the effect of eating too much lettuce is "soporific" . . . They certainly had a very soporific effect upon the Flopsy Bunnies!' There they are on the opposite page depicted fast asleep under a huge lettuce plant. Even Hippocrates, the father of medicine, prescribed

250

this plant for its sedative qualities. Wild lettuce (*Lactuca virosa*) is a mild narcotic and is often used in herbal preparations. You can make your own Lettuce Tea to help you to go to sleep (see recipe in chapter 20).

Since sleeplessness is often caused by worry and anxiety, the recommendations in the previous section apply equally well here. Other herbal preparations that offer more refreshing sleep include ingredients such as valerian root, hops and pulsatilla (see Addresses for mail order).

Between 1971 and 1978 Dr Ernest Hartman of Boston State Hospital carried out a series of experiments on the amino acid tryptophan under double-blind conditions. These showed that it enabled the subjects to go to sleep more quickly and that the sleep was deeper. This amino acid is converted into the neurotransmitter serotonin which is concerned with sleep. Most protein foods contain tryptophan, including milk, cottage cheese, almonds, peanuts, sesame, sunflower and pumpkin seeds, poultry, pheasant, tuna and beef. However, it needs the presence of vitamin B_6 and a small amount of carbohydrate to work. Therefore the ideal bedtime snack consists of, say, a slice of wholemeal sunflower-seed bread with peanut butter and a cup of warm skimmed milk with a little honey; buy your peanut butter without salt as the sodium acts as a stimulant on the adrenal glands. Otherwise a handful of pumpkin seeds mixed with sultanas and almonds, together with lettuce or camomile tea, is suitable for vegans. Do not drink ordinary tea or coffee after 5pm, if at all.

Depression

Very often depression is the reaction to a stressful situation, such as loss of a job, a divorce or death of someone close. In such cases it is very important to eat nutrient-dense foods and take extra care of the immune system as described in chapter 11, otherwise resistance to disease may be lowered. Equally the advice about counteracting the effects of stress in the earlier section about anxiety and panic attacks should be helpful. If depression is deep, then assistance must be sought quickly from your doctor or a qualified counsellor.

Sometimes there seems to be no particular reason for feelings of lethargy and gloom, in which case a nutritional deficiency could be the cause. Shortage of B-complex vitamins, especially thiamin, pyridoxine and folic acid, or of magnesium, can produce such feelings. If you are on the contraceptive pill and feeling generally low, then this is an indication that you are in need of vitamins B_2 and B_6. Supplements of pyridoxine will also alleviate premenstrual depression.

It is well worth having blood-sugar levels checked, as hypoglycaemia is a surprisingly common cause of depression and frequently undiagnosed. See chapter 10 for further information on this disorder.

Check also for possible food intolerances, which can often make you feel grim. See under 'Allergies' in chapter 11 for foods to exclude. Wheat is a particular suspect.

If certain neurotransmitters in the brain are at a low ebb, then depression can follow. To boost their levels the amino acids that act as their precursors can be taken, namely tyrosine or L-phenylalanine. Try around 500mg daily for a fortnight and maintain a good protein intake, especially fish. You will need extra vitamins B_6 and C to aid in the conversion process, so take wheatgerm and eat plenty of citrus and berry fruits, also fresh salads.

Remember that exercise can shift moods because endorphins, our happiness hormones, are released into the bloodstream.

Hyperactivity

The prevalence of sweets and soft drinks in vending machines and at check-out points is a real menace to parents who are trying to encourage their youngsters to eat healthily. Sugar and artificial colourings and other additives affect certain mechanisms in the central nervous system, resulting in behavioural problems in children, especially hyperactivity. The child is unlikely to be able to concentrate or sit still, is always restless and maybe aggressive and easily frustrated. It is very important to resist refined and junk foods and drinks totally and switch to a wholefood diet, but even so it may be some months before real improvement is noticed.

If the child drinks a lot of milk, a magnesium deficiency is suspect since this mineral must be in balance with calcium intake. Junk-food diets can also lead to shortages of B vitamins, especially B_1, B_3 and B_6 and of the minerals zinc and iron. A daily multivitamin and -mineral tablet will therefore boost the effectiveness of the wholefood programme.

Supplements of evening primrose oil at between 1.5 and 3g daily have led to improvements in many cases.

Epilepsy

Epileptic fits are caused by an electrical disturbance in certain neurons. They can be very dramatic and frightening to witness as the sufferer collapses unconscious on to the floor and then goes into convulsions. In such cases obstacles should be moved out of the way to avoid injury and the patient laid on his or her side so that the tongue is not swallowed.

The nutritional status of the patient needs to be checked, as deficiencies may make seizures more likely. There is a particular connection between low manganese and convulsions, so the diet needs to be rich in green leafy vegetables, legumes and whole cereals. Shortages of vitamin B_6 and magnesium are also suspect, which can be corrected by the inclusion of brewer's yeast, yeast extract, wheatgerm, oily fish, nuts and soya products. If pyridoxine is taken in supplementary form, then it must be balanced with the other B vitamins, especially B_2, and pantothenic acid.

Since hypoglycaemics are more susceptible to epilepsy, they should follow the diet recommended in chapter 10. Note that evening primrose oil should not be taken by epileptics as it may very occasionally trigger fits.

Psychotic disorders

Each thought and feeling that we have generates chemical and electrical changes in the brain. It stands to reason, therefore, that if the chemistry of the brain is upset, or if it is not given the nutrients it needs, then distortions in the workings of the mind may occur. Cases have been reported in which vitamin therapy has helped to lessen the symptoms of psychoses, but it is vital that any such treatment is carried out with a doctor's support. Drugs should never be stopped suddenly as psychotic episodes could recur with renewed ferocity. They should only be gradually withdrawn as real improvement is noted in the patient.

Schizophrenia

Someone wryly said, 'If you pray to God, they call you a Christian, but if you hear God speak to you, they call you a schizophrenic.' Definitions of madness vary from culture to culture, but the auditory and visual distortions that occur with true schizophrenia can be utterly nightmarish.

Charles was a gifted young violinist studying music at a college in London. Friends and teachers had noticed that he was becoming increasingly withdrawn, but only realized there was something wrong when he failed to turn up for his first-year examinations. He was discovered cowering in his room, convinced that someone was plotting to torture him. At first these episodes were sporadic and, surprisingly, his playing was unaffected, so he was able to stay on at college, although it took him considerably longer than three years to complete the course.

It was in his late twenties that he began to hear voices telling him to do crazy things. Once he was discovered at the zoo climbing over the high fence of the lion's enclosure. Only quick action on the part of the warden prevented mauling. Hospitalization followed and treatment with a dopamine-blocker, since schizophrenics have been found to generate too much of this neurotransmitter. It suppressed the delusions and hallucinations and enabled him to return home, but at the end of each episode he was left feeling chronically depressed and often contemplated suicide.

It was Charles's sister, Helen, who had an interest in nutritional medicine and she read about the work of Dr Michael Lesser. While in New Guinea he happened to meet a paranoid schizophrenic woman in a small village. Since antipsychotic drugs were unavailable, he left her with niacin supplements together with B-complex tablets and vitamin C and told her family to keep her on a high-protein diet. After several months the paranoia disappeared. Helen encouraged Charles to try this approach and, although he wasn't cured completely, the psychotic episodes were less frequent and usually brought on by some sort of identifiable stress. His mood generally was more buoyant and he became better able to live with the disease.

Various studies have shown that probably one-quarter of schizophrenic patients are low in folic acid and 2mg daily may be helpful. However, this must be professionally monitored, as too much can exacerbate psychotic symptoms.

Since individuals respond differently to particular nutrients, it is essential that the nutritional status of any patient is properly assessed. In addition to B and C vitamins, schizophrenics are often low in zinc, magnesium, manganese and chromium, while being too high in copper, and any such imbalances need to be corrected. Fish oils (2g daily) to provide essential fatty acids can also help to alleviate symptoms, as can evening primrose oil (3g daily), but this should be used with caution because of its association in rare instances with fits. It is best to follow the hypoglycaemic diet described in chapter 10 and eat niacin-rich foods, for example yeast extract, wheatgerm, avocados and fish, together with live yoghurt which helps the body to make its own B vitamins. It is also prudent to test for any food allergies which may aggravate the condition, as will caffeine which affects certain neurotransmitters in the brain, including serotonin and dopamine.

Manic depression

Phases of mania, in which the person apparently has no need to eat or sleep, but may pursue a task obsessively, or talk or move unceasingly, have sometimes produced outstanding works of art or literature, or genius in military or political leadership. Many famous people are thought to have had some form of the illness, including William Blake, Robert Schumann, Virginia Woolf and Winston Churchill. Like other psychotic conditions, it can be inherited.

Hair samples from manic-depressive patients were analysed at the University of Dundee and these showed a high level of the trace element vanadium, which later dropped with recovery. Foods that contain this mineral include vegetable oils and the seeds from which they are made, seafood, eggs, soya products, oats and certain vegetables such as carrots, tomatoes, garlic, cabbage and green beans. Intake of these should therefore be restricted. Evening primrose oil must not be taken as certain essential fatty acids can worsen the symptoms. Eat plenty of fruit: improvement has been hastened with vitamin C supplements of at least 1g daily in divided doses. Also test for any food intolerances (see chapter 11, under 'Allergies').

Eating disorders

These are very common, especially among women, and present major risks to health, so they must always be taken very seriously. In addition to nutritional approaches, support from a good counsellor must be found as soon as possible since these disorders are often symptomatic of underlying psychological problems.

Anorexia nervosa

Approximately 1 per cent of adolescent girls become anorexic. TV adverts and women's magazines are filled with images of super-slim models, most of whom weigh no more than $7\frac{1}{2}$ stone (47.6kg) despite their above-average height, encouraging young women to go on to unhealthy crash diets in the hope of attaining this sought-after shape. Of 494 American schoolgirls aged 9–18 years who were tested in 1992, 58 per cent perceived themselves to be overweight, whereas only 15 per cent actually were by objective standards.

Marilyn was training to be a classical ballerina. Each day she was surrounded by mirrors, which were a constant reminder that she must be as light and ethereal as a fairy. If there was even a hint of a tummy she believed herself to be disgustingly fat and immediately stopped eating. She dreaded the weighing session each week at the school. One of the teachers had told her that she would never find work if she put on any extra pounds. After a while the pressure became so great that she was barely eating at all. Her periods stopped and her weight ultimately dropped to a pathetic $5\frac{1}{2}$ stone (35kg). The only way to save her was to put her in hospital and force-feed her.

Anorexia is notoriously difficult to treat and death from starvation is not unusual. Needless to say, strong support from a psychotherapist is crucial. There is one nutrient that can be of considerable benefit and that is zinc, which is often too low in growing adolescents. Supplements can improve the appetite and help to reestablish normal eating patterns; try 30mg daily of zinc orotate, reducing this to half with recovery.

Fortified Soya Drink, vegetable juices and nourishing soups (see chapter 20) can all provide much-needed vitamins and minerals as the stomach readjusts to solid food.

Bulimia nervosa

Cosmopolitan magazine asked 7,000 women about their eating habits and a staggering 14 per cent admitted that they kept their weight down by vomiting. Some revealed that they could then binge on favourite, fattening foods such as cream cakes without having to worry about the extra pounds. The condition is often accompanied by extreme swings in mood, making the bulimic difficult to live with.

Since bulimics generally have low levels of endorphins, the brain's own 'happiness hormones', and these can be raised by improving copper intake, such an approach is worth a try. Seafood, legumes, nuts, raisins, black molasses, and desiccated liver as a supplementary food, need to be plentiful therefore to ensure recommended daily allowance. A daily multivitamin and -mineral tablet that includes copper is a valuable addition. Taking this mineral on its own is not advisable, but a copper bracelet could be worn.

Obesity

Being overweight constitutes a considerable risk to the health as it is associated with many serious illnesses ranging from coronary heart disease to breast cancer. Millions are spent each year on books and tapes that advocate this or that slimming programme, but most are a complete con.

The principles of losing weight are straightforward: cut down on calories by eating less overall and by selecting nutritious foods that are not fattening. This means avoiding saturated fats from meat and dairy products (including cheese), which are very high in calories, as well as giving up sugar and all refined carbohydrates, especially sweets, cakes, biscuits, puddings and jams. Replace salt with a seaweed seasoning, or use cider vinegar in cooking. Protein intake needs to be mainly from plant sources plus fish. In addition eat plenty of vegetables, fruits and salads, preferably raw. Whole grains are also fine unless you are intolerant of them. Indeed, if you follow the Health-Giving Diet recommended in this book and outlined in chapter 20, which is low in fat and sugar and high in fibre, you will certainly lose some pounds initially and then settle to a weight that is natural for your frame. Using smaller plates and dishes will prompt you to serve yourself slender portions.

Some seriously overweight people have been helped by supplements of evening primrose oil at between 2–4g daily, while around half have been found to be deficient in co-enzyme Q. This quasi-vitamin is involved in the release of energy from food.

Sometimes food allergies stimulate weight gain, especially wheat and possibly other grains or dairy products, and it may be beneficial to exclude these if the above approach is not as successful as it should be. (See 'Allergies' in chapter 11 for further information.)

Often people eat too much for psychological reasons, to comfort or calm themselves, or as a replacement for lack of love. In such cases support from a group or a counsellor will be necessary.

Exercise will boost the metabolic rate and burn up food faster, as well as providing a feeling of well-being. Choose something that you really enjoy, then you are more likely to stick at it.

Food for a healthy brain

The brain is highly sensitive to environmental poisoning, especially from heavy metals, so stay well clear of lead, aluminium and mercury. If pollutants are unavoidable, then take the nutrients recommended in chapter 4. Follow the Health-Giving Diet outlined in chapter 20, taking

259

especial care to avoid all food additives such as colourings and to resist soft drinks, alcohol, caffeine and all refined sugary junk foods.

You may like to consider a combined antioxidant supplement to prevent 'rusting' up of the fatty tissues in the brain. At any rate, make sure that vitamins A, C and E plus selenium are well supplied in the diet by eating plenty of yellow/orange fruit and vegetables, dark-green vegetables, fresh citrus and berry fruits, wheatgerm and cold-pressed plant oils and whole grains.

Keep the 'electrolyte soup' of the brain in top condition by cutting back salt and increasing potassium intake from plenty of dark-green vegetables, mushrooms, dates and bananas. Juices made from fresh vegetables are mineral-rich, and remember that fruit and vegetables are the source of that 'smart' nutrient pyroglutamate. Also drink plenty of water.

Make sure protein is adequate, especially from seafood, free-range eggs and lentils, which incidentally are also rich in the mineral zinc – all good brain foods. Eat soya products and take extra lecithin in the form of granules for making that vital neurotransmitter acetylcholine.

Brewer's yeast will provide all those essential B vitamins as well as pantothenic acid and chromium; wheatgerm is equally beneficial. Live yoghurt will help the body to produce its own B vitamins. And don't forget black molasses for the iron content.

Pregnant women and mothers with children below seven years should read chapter 18 to ensure that their offsprings' brains develop properly during those vital formative years.

Remember that problems relating to the nervous system may be due to food sensitivities.

Chapter 17

Food For Loving

Love Bomb, a herbal preparation for enhancing sexual desire, was recently put on display in the window of a health food shop. When the manageress arrived the next morning to open up she discovered that the window had been broken and dozens of bottles had been stolen! The story leaves you wondering whether the thief intended them for personal use only or whether some kind of orgiastic party was being planned.

Aphrodisiacs have been popular since time immemorial: they were even found buried in King Tutankhamen's tomb, presumably to ensure his virility in the afterlife. The most impressive one I have ever seen was a *coco de mer*, a huge double coconut with the shape of a female pelvis. These can weigh as much as 50lb (23kg), although the one my friend staggered home with from his holiday in the Seychelles was considerably smaller. Washed up on distant shores, they were highly prized by Indian moguls.

But do they really work? Some so-called remedies such as bananas, cucumbers and asparagus clearly have no particular lust-enhancing properties apart from their phallic shape. Of the 120 South and Central American herbs recommended to boost flagging desire, just three have been approved by the World Health Organization: catuaba, muirapuama (both ingredients of Love Bomb) and damiana. Catuaba is a stimulant which acts on the central nervous system, while damiana increases blood flow to the capillaries and is mildly euphoric. Since sexual energy droops in line with the amount of stress and fatigue experienced, so certain herbs that have a general revitalizing effect are likely to heighten interest in love-making.

Ginseng is a root that is not only phallic in shape, it actually contains substances similar to male and female sex hormones. Research in Hong Kong has shown that vitality, mood and concentration are all augmented by this herb and that it is an excellent antidote to stress. Its reputation as an aphrodisiac therefore has real substance. As for garlic, this has an organic chemical among its constituents that resembles one released by females when sexually aroused. As long as your passion isn't deflated by the fumes, it could be worth a try! In any case it has numerous health-giving properties and can only do you good.

Most people know that alcohol increases desire but reduces performance so, while a glass or two of best plonk may well help to relax partners and diminish inhibitions, too much is likely to dampen activity altogether. It is obvious that poorly or marginally nourished people will have reduced libido. On the other hand an over-stuffed stomach will snatch the blood supply for digestion, so a heavy dinner is never conducive to love-making. Eat light food, with the emphasis on vegetables and fruit. Sharing a globe artichoke can be an intimate way to start the evening as you both pull off the leaves and chew the succulent heart. Raspberries are recommended for afters. Include carbohydrate from pasta or potatoes for the main course to boost energy for instant action.

Oysters have traditionally been regarded as an aphrodisiac. Since loss of libido is associated with low levels of zinc and these shellfish are its richest source, there is real wisdom in this belief. If you are not keen on seafood, then wheatgerm is almost as good, although rather bitter in flavour. Refer to chapter 3 for other foods high in zinc to

262

give your libido a boost. You may choose to take a supplement to ensure that your intake is adequate. On the subject of nutrients, a comprehensive multivitamin and -mineral tablet each day can do wonders to heighten feelings of well-being.

While certain foods really can enhance one's sex life, so carefully planned nutrition can significantly assist with sexual and reproductive problems.

Infertility

Human fertility in the West has declined significantly over the last half century, with the average sperm count dropping by 50 per cent. In 1940 the average man produced about 113 million sperm per millilitre, but by 1990 this figure was down to just 66 million. In the UK one in six couples have difficulty in conceiving. Is something in the environment or in our food damaging our reproductive capabilities? Some people point their finger at pesticides. As soon as you start to plan conception, therefore, give your body a thorough clean-out with the detox programme in chapter 4, and switch to organically grown produce.

Many nutrients are required for the production of healthy sperm. Up to 400 million may be contained in a single ejaculation and these need to be energetic enough to find their way through the cervix, wriggle into the uterus and then the oviduct, where, with a bit of luck, some of them may manage to meet an egg, or ovum, and stick to its surface. One then has to be sufficiently persistent to enter the cytoplasm of the ovum so that its nucleus fuses with that of the female egg – the moment of fertilization. Since very few sperm manage this arduous journey, manufacture has to be excessive. Their ability to move is also crucial to fertility.

Of the amino acids, arginine is especially important as it is involved in the production of sperm and is found in the head of the sperm in large supply. Several experimental studies have shown that supplements of L-arginine substantially increase numbers of sperm as well as their motility. In one study, 63 per cent of infertile men showed marked improvement after taking 4g daily of this amino acid for 3 to 6 months. Just 1.5 to 2g should be sufficient for most cases. Nuts and seeds are rich in arginine, as are poultry and fish (see also chapter 3). Carnitine, a derivative of lysine, is also contained in the testes and in sperm and supplements may prove helpful: try 500mg of L-lysine daily. Vegetarians in particular will benefit from supplements as this amino acid is obtained mainly from meat, poultry and fish.

Of the trace elements, zinc is essential for reproductive health. Zinc deficiency is linked with low sperm count as well as low levels of the male sex hormone, testosterone. In the male, its main storage place is the prostate gland, part of the urogenital system, which adds fluid to sperm. Fertility will increase in zinc-deficient males if the mineral is taken as a supplement for at least three months; you will have to be patient as new sperm needs this amount of time for its creation. Try 50mg of elemental zinc, cutting back to 25mg daily after 12 weeks. Also eat plenty of zinc-rich foods, especially shellfish, wheatgerm (which should be on the daily menu), soya products, lentils and brown rice. Avoid processed and refined foods altogether.

Sperm-clumping can be a cause of infertility. Vitamin C prevents this from happening in a large percentage of cases at just 1g daily taken in divided doses. This approach will be enhanced by eating citrus and berry fruits and fresh green vegetables and salads.

Semen is abundant in prostaglandins, potent, short-lived substances involved in many body systems including reproduction. They are derived from polyunsaturated fatty acids, so an increase of these in the diet could theoretically help some cases of infertility. Include plant oils, therefore, which also happen to be replete with vitamin E, another nutrient

264

that affects fertility. Additionally, you may consider taking evening primrose oil, three 500mg capsules daily, but these are expensive.

Other nutrients helpful in boosting fertility are vitamin A and the trace elements chromium and selenium. Keep up your intake of carrots, therefore, and any other orange-yellow vegetables and fruit. If you have included the shellfish and wheatgerm as suggested, then these will also contribute the other two trace elements. Consider taking brewer's yeast for extra chromium and to improve all-round health with the B vitamins.

Western women can frequently suffer from malnutrition as a result of faddy diets or, in more extreme cases, anorexia (see previous chapter). Inadequate food can seriously affect fertility. Sometimes ovulation and menstruation may cease altogether. So if you wish to conceive, a healthy wholefood diet, as described in chapter 20, is a basic essential. It is also important to give up alcohol and tobacco both for your own sake and that of the baby.

As with males, zinc needs to be in plentiful supply, and in addition to foods rich in this mineral you may like to take a supplement of zinc orotate at 15mg daily.

Of the vitamins, B_6 is of special significance to women as it affects the balance of the hormones progesterone and oestrogen. It is widely available in yeast extract, oily fish, many vegetables and dried fruits. If you decide to take a supplement, remember that it needs to be in the correct ratio to other B vitamins, especially riboflavin, so also take a B complex or brewer's yeast.

Other helpful vitamins in preparing the body for conception are C and E: bountiful fruit, vegetables, salads, plant oils and wheatgerm should supply your needs and, to be extra sure, you may like to take supplements at 500mg and 200IU respectively.

Sometimes the cervical mucus is hostile to sperm due to excess acidity. Emphasizing alkaline-forming foods may be helpful in such cases, especially vegetables and grains, while avoiding meat, dairy products, citrus fruits and tea and coffee, all of which are acid-forming.

Always seek expert guidance in cases of infertility, as the cause may not be nutritional. Since accumulated toxins may harm sperm, women should have a good detox and switch to organically produced food at least three months, preferably six, before conception. Also read the important advice in the next chapter concerning the health of your baby.

Impotence

Probably as many as 10 per cent of men suffer from this unfortunate condition. The cause is frequently psychological and can be successfully treated by looking at the underlying problem with a sympathetic sex therapist. Occasionally, however, it can be physically based.

Rex was one such case. He had always had a somewhat macho image of himself, being proud of his manhood, and at 42 finding himself suddenly unable to function was a terrible blow. Admittedly he had been under too much stress recently. He was the sort of businessman who had survived successfully on his wits, wheeling and dealing in property. Over the last few years, however, the recession had caught up with him and he was now seriously in debt with a double mortgage on his house. To ease the worry he had taken to drinking rather too much. Ruth, his wife, had always been very caring and supportive, but now she wept quietly into her pillow, believing that Rex didn't love her any more. Additionally there had been other symptoms: Rex had been suffering badly from hay fever that summer and the doctor had put him on antihistamines.

Rex had always been somewhat cynical about any complementary therapies, but Ruth managed to persuade him to let her see someone on his behalf. As it happened, a consultant nutritionist held a surgery in collaboration with their local health food shop every so often and Ruth made an appointment. He pointed out that it was vital to see her husband personally in case of any heart disease, a frequent cause of impotence in middle-aged males. He explained that the same fatty deposits that cause heart attacks can also block the blood vessels that lead to the erectile tissue of the penis. Meanwhile, he made the following suggestions: Rex must come off alcohol and refined carbohydrates, especially sugar, completely, also all animal fats, and replace the antihistamines with vitamin C and magnesium, since certain drugs can result in impotence in some individuals. At the same time Rex should increase his zinc intake, which would boost the level of testosterone in his bloodstream; he prescribed 30mg of zinc gluconate, to be reduced by half as soon as there was any improvement. He cautioned that doses in excess of that amount should not be taken without personal examination in case of any arterial disease. He also gave Ruth a list of zinc-rich foods, especially emphasizing wheatgerm. Brewer's yeast tablets would assist with the stress.

Rex was astonished to find his libido returning after eight weeks of this treatment and thereafter became a convert to sound nutrition. At the same time he had the good sense to have his blood pressure checked, which turned out to be fine. (Anyone who has cardiovascular problems should read chapter 8.)

In addition to certain antihistamines, some hypertensive drugs can also have the side-effect of impotence. You will see from chapter 8 that many patients are able to keep their blood pressure normal through correct nutrition alone, but of course it is essential to consult your practitioner before coming off any prescribed medicines.

Oral contraceptives

During the years when I was on the contraceptive pill, I remember how low my prevailing mood was. It always seemed amazingly hard to generate any enthusiasm, even for things that had previously excited me. It never occurred to me that the Pill could be the reason. Indeed, it was then not recognized how much oral contraceptives altered the body's need for particular nutrients, nor had the link been made between low vitamin B_6 levels and depression. If only I had known that a mere 50mg daily of pyridoxine could have made me feel happier!

As with all drugs, the benefits have to be carefully weighed against unpleasant side-effects and more serious risks. While the hazards of being pregnant could be considerable, the extra hormones ingested from the contraceptive pill may threaten the health of the cardiovascular system, in particular by increasing the likelihood of blood clots, as well as raising the chances of developing breast, liver and other cancers. It may also upset glucose metabolism resulting in diabetes, and then there is a probability of lesser problems including migraine, a gain in weight and thrush. Fortunately, carefully planned nutrition can minimize these risks.

Apart from a deficiency in vitamin B_6, most probably you will also suffer from low levels of B_1, B_2, B_{12} and folic acid. Yeast, wheatgerm and organically produced liver are undoubtedly the richest food sources of the B complex vitamins, but not everyone can stomach liver – myself included. Remember that these nutrients cannot be stored in the body and need replacing daily, so also maintain your consumption of nuts and seeds, green vegetables, soya products and fish. If you feel debilitated by symptoms such as depression, stress or anxiety, tingling or numbness in the limbs, water retention, poor concentration, migraine or raised blood pressure, these are all warning signs that levels of B vitamins are too low and you must take brewer's yeast tablets or a good B complex supplement. Aim for at least 10mg of B_1, B_2 and B_3, 50mg of B_5 and B_6, 150mcg of B_{12} and 400mcg of folic acid.

A warning: depletion of folic acid can result in inefficient formation of blood cells, which in turn can damage an unborn child. When planning pregnancy, therefore, allow at least three, preferably six, months after coming off the Pill before conception and eat lots of green vegetables. A supplement of 500mcg of folic acid will also help your body to return to normal.

Another vitamin you will need more of is ascorbic acid, so also eat lots of fresh citrus and berry fruits and regular salads. It is not advisable to take more than 1g as a supplement, however, as it could boost your oestrogen level and therefore actually increase related health risks. Women who take oral contraceptives are often found to be low in vitamin E also, so here again select foods such as plant oils and wheatgerm to ensure a good intake.

By contrast, vitamins A and K are both found to be raised in the blood of those on the Pill. As far as K is concerned, this means that the blood is more likely to form clots, while too much A could harm an unborn child – another definite reason to come off the Pill several months ahead of any pregnancy.

Minerals to watch are zinc and magnesium. Check that your intake of these is better than usual (see chapter 3 for food sources), otherwise you may be short. Zinc in particular is an important safeguard against disease, helping to ensure that the immune system is operating effectively.

Scanty or heavy periods

Women who are persistently going on to slimming diets are often short of both calories and nutrients and menstruation may become irregular or scanty as a result. It is quite possible to eat healthily and not put on weight simply by cutting down on all saturated fats, giving up salt and sugar, and switching from refined to wholefoods which add fibre. You will find further details in the previous and last chapters. Once healthy eating patterns are established, periods should return to normal.

Heavy periods sometimes indicate that your body is in need of more vitamin A and supplements can therefore reduce bleeding. Aim for around 10,000IU (3mg) of beta-carotene to begin with, adjusting this amount up or down as necessary, meanwhile including oily fish, carrots and apricots in your diet. You may be losing iron, so step up lentils, beans and oats; also take black molasses, and replace Indian tea with herbal varieties. Additional supplements of zinc and vitamin B_6 can also be helpful.

Even food intolerances can affect menstruation, so test yourself for these by following the guidelines in chapter 11 under 'Allergies'.

PMT and dysmenorrhoea

The old-fashioned term 'the curse' always seemed to me to be an apt description of a monthly event that for some women is only to be dreaded. A full fortnight ahead of the due date the first symptoms would hit me: breast tenderness and swelling, generally followed by a downward swing in mood into depression and an anxious, jumpy, often snappy state. During the last week, my usually excellent coordination turned into uncontrollable clumsiness, sometimes stumbling or tripping over, with things dropped and spilt, all of which only added to the irritability. Worst of all was the build-up in tension, until it felt as if all my cells were standing on edge and screaming – for what? I never knew, but it was accompanied by extreme restlessness and food cravings, in the vain hope that something would alleviate it. On some days it became so bad I thought I was going crazy. It was all made far worse by the terrible fear of what might be to come – pain so appalling that I sometimes found myself on the floor writhing in agony and shivering violently with cold, but with sweat pouring off me. With a bit of luck I might pass out altogether – which occasionally happened – but generally the diarrhoea and vomiting took over and I spent hours alternately trying to get the right end over the loo. These experiences were very distressing, but the vomiting did have one salutary result: the heaving sometimes eased the pain for about ten minutes – until it started all over again.

I still feel hugely angry at the reactions of doctors: 'Go for a walk', 'Have a hot bath', 'Drink some warm cocoa', 'Take an aspirin', 'It's a natural event, you'll just have to put up with it', and so on. How is it possible to follow such advice when you can't even stand upright because of the pain and when anything taken by mouth comes straight back up again? None of those doctors took the syndrome seriously. Perhaps they thought I was exaggerating. No tests were ever suggested nor was I ever asked about my eating habits or my lifestyle. In the end I gave up going.

As usual, my own research and experimenting eventually paid off. One magic ingredient was evening primrose oil: the recommended dose of 1,500mg daily had no effect and I nearly abandoned this approach, until I read somewhere that a study in Newcastle had used double this amount with success. Indeed 3g did the trick and immediately eased breast swelling and tenderness and much of the tension. Vitamin B_6 and zinc proved to be two other important nutrients, at 50mg and 15mg daily respectively. While the first helped to ease the symptoms of the premenstrual tension, the second definitely reduced pain. Not only is zinc important for reproductive functions, it is involved in the metabolism of essential fatty acids, and it seems that PMT sufferers have difficulty with this.

The other vital nutrient is magnesium. Like zinc, it takes part in the conversion of linoleic to linolenic acid, which in turn soothes the symptoms of PMT. In the past calcium has sometimes been recommended, but too much is bad practice as it unbalances the absorption of magnesium. The warm drink of milk is therefore not helpful as it contains very little magnesium and, unless skimmed, is high in fat.

This brings me to another subject: animal fats. It was only after cutting these out of my diet for other purposes that I noticed the easing of PMT symptoms – and for good reason. Saturated fats enhance the production of a substance called arachidonic acid, which then causes excess levels of the prostaglandin PGF. This suppresses the release of the much-needed female hormone progesterone. In addition to PMT and dysmenorrhoea, it is now known that women with inadequate progesterone levels are almost $5\frac{1}{2}$ times more likely to develop breast cancer – what better justification to give up animal fats? Remember that chunks of cheese and hydrogenated margarine are just as damaging from this point of view as red meat.

Diet, indeed, plays a crucial part in this syndrome. If the sugar cravings are satisfied, blood-sugar levels are immediately affected, as is mood. At the same time, the sucrose will cause loss of magnesium, which you actually need more of. Instead, eat nourishing snacks of raisins, nuts and seeds. Also resist caffeine cravings as too much coffee worsens breast tenderness and anxiety and indeed is linked with benign breast disease. Tea reduces iron absorption. Keep to herb teas, such as camomile, which is soothing. Salt cravings are also a hazard since the sodium will contribute to fluid retention. Try to find other harmless flavourings. If you give up salt, diuretics should be unnecessary. Women who live in countries where vegetable consumption predominates are less likely to have to face the misery of PMT, so eat lots of these every day. Also include complex carbohydrates, with the emphasis on peas, beans and lentils and whole grains. Fish and poultry, which are low in saturated fat, are fine. Wheatgerm and yeast extract will provide extra B vitamins, important if you are on a supplement of B_6 as nutrients from this complex need to be in balance. They also help to mitigate the effects of

272

stress. The vitamin E available in the wheatgerm and also in cold-pressed plant oils helps some women with breast tenderness. Have small meals regularly to keep blood sugar stable.

As always, regular exercise and stress reduction are of benefit. I found that leg swings from the hip helped to relieve the pain of uterine contractions.

Menopausal symptoms

If you have been unlucky enough to endure the wretchedness of PMT and dysmenorrhoea, then you will welcome the menopause with extreme relief! It is sad that this period of a woman's life is so often viewed in a negative light, frequently equated with loss of youth, beauty, vitality and sexuality. On the contrary, it can prove to be a most rewarding and creative time, released at last from the burden of childcare. Moreover, sound nutrition will ensure lasting good looks as well as lustiness. Nor need you put up with any of those awkward symptoms such as hot flushes as hormone levels diminish.

Adhering to the Health-Giving Diet as outlined in chapter 20 is a basic necessity. Please also refer to chapter 12 for advice concerning the health of your bones. If amounts of essential fatty acids absorbed from plant oils and evening primrose oil together with the mineral zinc are more than adequate, then menopausal symptoms should not occur. I still take at least 2g of evening primrose oil per day and 15mg of zinc orotate, together with an all-round multivitamin and -mineral tablet, plus at least 500mg of buffered ascorbic acid with bioflavonoids. Hot flushes and night sweats have never bothered me. Nor have I noticed any decline in sexual interest – on the contrary, no longer having to worry about contraception allows far greater spontaneity!

Of the bioflavonoids, hesperidin has been shown to be the most effective in relieving hot flushes and other menopausal symptoms – even more so than oestrogen replacement. Take 500mg of hesperidin together with 1g of buffered vitamin C daily. Vitamin E is especially useful for assuaging night sweats and alleviating aches and pains: 200IU should do the trick. Siberian ginseng is also excellent for counteracting all symptoms, at about 500mg.

The best herb tea is purple sage, which has oestrogenic properties. Make your own infusion from fresh or dried leaves (see chapter 20 under 'Infusions').

Women who continue with an active sex life are unlikely to have problems with vaginal dryness and thinning and shrinking of the walls, which can occur as oestrogen ebbs. However, if you do experience this, a simple answer is to use Replens gel, a non-hormonal way to restore moisture. Vitamin E oil is also beneficial.

If you look after yourself in this way and adopt a positive attitude, you will have an easy transition through the years of 'the change' to the next epoch, now referred to by some American women as 'post-menopausal zest'!

Chapter 18

The Next Generation

After the moment of fertilization, the ovum divides and subdivides repeatedly to form a tiny embryo. Within a week to ten days this passes down the oviduct and implants itself into the lining of the womb. Here the production of cells continues, some forming the placenta and others the tissues and organs of the new human, the head region first becoming identifiable along with the spinal cord and heart, which is soon pumping its own blood supply. At six weeks the brain is growing quickly, eyes and ears and limb buds are all forming. After only another six weeks it looks just like a miniature baby and is now referred to as a foetus.

This amazing process depends on a liberal supply of the correct raw ingredients taken in by the mother in the form of air, food and drink and passed on to the embryo via her bloodstream. These substances include oxygen, glucose, amino acids, vitamins and mineral salts. At the same time her bloodstream carries away the waste products from the embryo, such as urea and carbon dioxide. The blood vessels of the developing foetus are so fragile, they remain separate from the mother's circulation, but nutrients and wastes can pass from one to the other through the fine capillary walls and very thin membranes in the placenta, which is attached to the embryo by the umbilical cord.

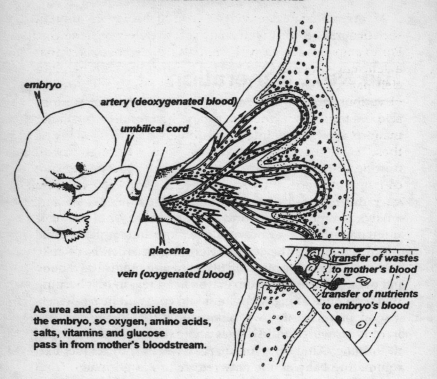

embryo

artery (deoxygenated blood)

umbilical cord

placenta

vein (oxygenated blood)

transfer of wastes to mother's blood

transfer of nutrients to embryo's blood

As urea and carbon dioxide leave
the embryo, so oxygen, amino acids,
salts, vitamins and glucose
pass in from mother's bloodstream.

Before conception

The importance of preparing for conception has already
been outlined in the previous chapter. Indeed, many professional nutritionists now believe that what you eat in the
months prior to pregnancy is just as important as your
intake of nutrients while the foetus is forming, both for the
sake of the mother's continued good health as well as
the baby's. It is well proven that optimum nutrition helps
to prevent birth defects, lessens the chance of spontaneous
abortion, greatly reduces risks to the mother in terms of
hypertension, toxaemia and other serious problems, as well
as offering the newborn well-developed organs that can be
better than merely 'normal'.

276

At present approximately 1 in 100 babies in affluent societies will be born with some sort of defect or handicap. For example, research with animals has demonstrated that a deficiency in vitamin A has led to offspring with harelips, cleft palates, blindness and deafness as well as deformities of various vital organs. A poor supply of vitamin B_2, folic acid, vitamin E, zinc or manganese has resulted in similar malformations including fused fingers and toes. Many of these could be entirely avoided simply through sound nutrition. Refined sugary diets and junk food just do not contain sufficient nutrients to give a new baby the best start in life.

Yet it is astonishing how nature can find ways of compensating even when diet is inadequate, and a healthy child will appear nevertheless, but caring parents will not take any such risks. So a wise mother will already have done her best to clear her body of toxins, will have given up smoking and alcohol and any drugs (unless absolutely essential), all of which can damage the embryo, and will have switched to a fresh, balanced wholefood diet, preferably organic and without additives, that does not contain refined carbohydrates (especially anything made from white flour and sugar). It needs to be plentiful in protein, essential fatty acids (from plant and fish oils), carbohydrates (fruit, whole grains, potatoes and legumes), and all known vitamins and minerals, in particular the following: vitamins A, B (including folic acid), C, D, E, K and the minerals zinc, calcium and magnesium, iron, iodine and selenium. To make sure she is well supplied with all essential nutrients a good multivitamin and -mineral tablet each day that includes iron, zinc and folic acid is recommended. Additionally, her body weight needs to be healthily in line with her height.

While it is important to have generous supplies of nutrients, it is equally essential not to consume any one to excess. Vitamin A in particular should not be taken in supplement form at more than 10,000IU daily as this can be toxic and actually cause congenital abnormalities.

Parents living in polluted environments, especially in cities, are advised to have hair samples analysed for heavy metals, as lead, cadmium and mercury are all associated with birth defects and poor mental development as well as miscarriages. Other pollutants including pesticides can also be extremely hazardous to the unborn, as we have already seen. Chapter 4 explains the nutritional means of reducing their impact and ways of clearing them from the body.

Miscarriages

Valerie desperately wanted to have a family of her own. Sadly, her mother had suffered recurring psychiatric problems, necessitating extended hospitalization, so that Valerie's childhood had been spent largely with her grandmother. A secure family unit was what she most longed for, especially now that she was married. Her unsettled upbringing had left its mark in the form of a nervous disposition and she had suffered bouts of anorexia in her late teens and early twenties. At only $7\frac{1}{2}$ stone (47.6kg), she remained underweight for her height.

When she eventually became pregnant, therefore, she was very excited. However, she suffered dire bouts of early morning sickness, and eating became increasingly problematic. During her fourth month she began to experience periodic pains in her lower abdomen, followed by bleeding. Although the doctor came as soon as he was called and treated her with hormones, he was unable to save the baby.

Valerie was devastated by this experience and it was a full year before she felt able to try again. This time she decided to consult a nutritionist first to see if she could improve her weight and general state of health. Hair analysis showed that she was extremely zinc-deficient, which partly accounted for her loss of appetite. She also learnt that shortage of this mineral and of other nutrients such as manganese, essential fatty acids, folic acid and vitamin E can equally cause miscarriages. She was therefore prescribed 30mg of zinc orotate daily, which was to be gradually reduced to half that amount as her appetite improved. At the same time a nutritional programme was worked out for her that was very rich in protein and essential nutrients. The nutritionist explained that protein and calories were the most crucial factors affecting the health of both mother and baby and, like any woman planning a child, she must aim to eat 50g of good-quality protein each day before conception, increasing to 75g during pregnancy, equal to three or four generous servings of cheese, free-range eggs, soya beans, fish, skimmed milk, poultry or lean meat; nuts, grains and legumes could also be combined as alternative or additional sources of all the essential amino acids, the basis of the new baby's body structures.

Plenty of wheatgerm and cold-pressed plant oils featured in Valerie's diet. These are abundant in vitamin E, which is involved in the successful division of cells. A lack of this appears to be a common cause of miscarriage, so Valerie was also prescribed 200IU as a supplement.

The nutritionist explained that daily fresh vegetables eaten raw or just very lightly cooked must form part of Valerie's new eating programme, as these contain that vital B vitamin folic acid, all too easily lost through overheating or thrown out with the cooking water. She also recommended brewer's yeast, which along with the wheatgerm is a prime source of all B vitamins. To make sure that Valerie would not lose her next baby through lack of folic acid, she also prescribed a 500mcg daily supplement. This nutrient is needed for the formation of the nucleic acids DNA and RNA which bear the hereditary material for the next generation.

Essential fatty acids were already plentiful in the diet from plant and fish oils and manganese available from the whole cereals and vegetables. Additionally Valerie was to give up tea to ensure that iron from the diet was being absorbed. Gentle herb teas and fruit juices were far better options.

After six months of this programme, Valerie's appetite had improved noticeably and she had been able to gain weight and looked much healthier. She felt confident enough to try for another baby and this time she carried it full term and at the end of nine months was the happy mother of a beautiful baby girl.

Cleft palate

This all-too-common defect can almost certainly be avoided by eating nourishing food at least three months ahead of conception as well as during pregnancy, together with a daily multivitamin and -mineral tablet. It is essential not to smoke, as the combined effect of toxins in the tobacco plus the nutrients destroyed by it contribute to this kind of abnormality.

Animal research has shown that diets deficient in vitamins A and B_2 and folic acid have resulted in abnormalities including harelip, clubfoot and cleft palate.

Spina bifida

A study of Welsh women completed in 1982 found that those who ate a diet of convenience and fried foods, white bread and sugar, with virtually no fresh vegetables or fruit, were most likely to bear a child with neural tube defects including spina bifida.

Supplementation with 500mcg daily of folic acid before and at the time of conception and through pregnancy greatly reduces the risk of having an infant with this distressing condition, even if the mother has previously produced a baby with neural tube defects. Because the spinal cord begins to form at only three weeks after fertilization, it is obvious that supplementation must start ahead of conception. A multivitamin and -mineral tablet daily that includes B_{12} and zinc, together with excellent diet as outlined in chapter 20, with an emphasis on dark-green leafy vegetables, will enhance the effectiveness of this treatment.

Pregnancy

It is natural to gain weight during pregnancy as the expectant mother will be taking in at least an extra 15 per cent of food to satisfy her baby's requirements; another $15\frac{1}{2}$lb (7kg) is regarded as the very minimum amount, even for heavy women, and up to 30lb for those of average weight (depending on height and build). The mother can safely lose the excess after the baby is weaned, when it no longer has to rely on her for its food supply. Demands for the main nutrients will soar once conception has taken place, by as much as 100 per cent for some, so diet must be very good indeed; your doctor will in any case prescribe supplements, especially of iron and folic acid. Unfortunately it is not generally recognized that if zinc is not included the mother will become deficient in this mineral, because both iron and folic acid will take up the available absorption sites in the intestine. A supplement of zinc at 10mg is quite safe and indeed advisable.

Many familiar problems of pregnancy can be averted or treated with the right nutrients, as described in the following pages. Common complaints such as constipation, varicose veins and haemorrhoids are discussed elsewhere in the book (see Index).

Early morning sickness

The medical profession tends to regard this as one of the inevitable hazards of being pregnant, but nutritional therapists see it as a symptom of nutritional or hormonal imbalance, sometimes accompanied by swings in blood sugar. Happily, vitamin B_6 and magnesium can often rectify the problem. Requirements vary, so you will need to experiment with doses. Try 25mg of pyridoxine with each meal

281

to prevent nausea, along with 50mg of magnesium. Have a protein snack before going to bed, for example a peanut-butter or chicken sandwich made with wholemeal bread, plus a glass of skimmed milk, as this will help to keep the blood sugar even next morning. See also the recommendations regarding hypoglycaemia in chapter 10. It is very important to avoid sweet things and all refined food as these cause chaos with blood sugar, which itself contributes to the nausea. Camomile tea is very soothing.

Dyspepsia

As the baby gets bigger it can sometimes press against the abdomen, causing dyspepsia. Avoid antacids as these prevent absorption of phosphorus and generally contain aluminium. A natural remedy is dill tea (see 'Infusions', chapter 20). One teaspoon of crushed seeds to 1 pint (570ml) of boiling water should provide the right strength.

Anaemia

If you are taking iron supplements prescribed by your doctor (generally 30–60mg daily), then you are unlikely to suffer from this type of deficiency anaemia. Make sure that they are from an organic source, as inorganic iron destroys vitamin E. Remember not to drink tea as the tannin binds with iron and prevents its uptake; on the other hand orange juice will aid its absorption. Never take more than the recommended amount as too much iron can be harmful.

Your daily requirement for iron will at the least double as you make new blood for the baby and the placenta. It is of crucial importance not just for the health of red blood cells, but also for the developing brain. It is just as well, therefore, to seek out food containing iron. Be careful of eating too much liver, the richest source, because this is also full of oily vitamin A which can be toxic in large amounts. Black molasses used in cooking or spread on wholemeal bread or Ryvita for a snack is quite safe. Also make a point of having oats and lentils regularly.

Vegetarians and vegans need to be extra careful. In addition to sufficient iron they must ensure a good intake of vitamin B_{12}, generally lacking in their diet. Brewer's yeast taken daily will guarantee an adequate supply and yeast extract, tempeh and miso are other natural sources. Yeast-free B complex supplements that include vitamin B_{12} are also available. This vitamin is crucial for the growing infant as any deficiency could result in brain damage or other defects.

A different type of anaemia results from too little folic acid and an early symptom of this is a grey-brown pigmentation that appears on the upper part of the face and neck. It is sometimes referred to as 'pregnancy cap'. Here again a diet high in fresh dark-green vegetables, wheatgerm and soya products plus an extra 500mcg of supplemental folic acid with each meal will ensure that the skin returns to normal in three weeks or so.

Stretch marks

These are far more likely to occur if the diet is at all lacking in necessary nutrients, or if the tissues become swollen due to fluid retention (see Oedema below). A well-nourished woman will have elastic tissues which will stretch easily and return to normal without leaving scars. Plenty of protein and vitamins C and E are particularly important in this respect. Eat regular amounts of fresh citrus and berry fruits and daily helpings of wheatgerm and cold-pressed plant oils in salad dressings, together with supplements of 250mg of vitamin C with each main meal and 200IU of vitamin E daily.

Oedema

Swellings, especially around the ankles, often occur in pregnancy, due to retention of fluid in the tissue spaces.

Do not be persuaded to take diuretics as these can be harmful, causing loss of vital nutrients along with the water. When you understand the cause of this condition you will realize how easily it can be corrected nutritionally.

A protein in the blood called albumin draws the fluid from the tissues back into the circulation, after which its waste products are extracted by the kidneys. Thus oedema is often a sign of protein deficiency. As soon as the intake becomes adequate, any swelling is likely to go down.

Because vitamin B_6 helps with the synthesis of albumin, a lack of this vitamin can also result in oedema. Eat plenty of oily fish and fresh vegetables and take a supplement of 20mg of pyridoxine daily. If necessary increase this amount, but do not exceed 100mg.

Also check that your consumption of vitamin E and choline (another of the B vitamins) is up to scratch. Free-range eggs, daily servings of wheatgerm, fresh vegetables and plant oils should fulfil requirements.

If the oedema is due to raised blood pressure, which can sometimes occur, then you may like to read about 'Hypertension' in chapter 8.

Toxaemia

This term means that toxins have entered the blood which can lead to the dangerous illness of eclampsia, a state of convulsions and coma, possibly even death. The earlier symptoms of pre-eclampsia usually begin after the twenty-eighth week of pregnancy, with a rise in blood pressure, an increase in weight, puffiness of the face or hands, and protein in the urine. Early detection is essential, so always attend those antenatal check-ups regularly. If the illness progresses, then the birth will probably have to be induced.

Toxaemia appears to be linked with a deficiency of vitamin B_6. Indeed, just 10mg daily of pyridoxine will protect most women throughout their pregnancy. Eat plenty of oily fish and fresh vegetables too.

As was explained in chapter 8, high blood pressure can be associated with poor intake of the minerals calcium and magnesium. During pregnancy the need for calcium rises by 50 per cent and magnesium must increase accordingly to maximize absorption, remaining in a 2 to 1 ratio. Total intake must therefore be 1,200mg of calcium and 600mg of magnesium. Rich sources of calcium, such as milk, are sometimes low in magnesium and must be balanced by soya beans, whole cereals and dark-green vegetables. It is unlikely that you will be absorbing sufficient of these two minerals from your diet, so take an extra 600mg of calcium and 300mg of magnesium in the form of supplements.

Additionally, in order to avoid hypertension and the serious problems associated with it, essential fatty acids must be liberally supplied from fish and plant oils. Evening primrose oil at 3g daily has successfully treated pre-eclampsia.

Premature labour

The minerals calcium and magnesium are thought to help prevent and treat this unhappy situation. Indeed, a lack of magnesium can cause spasms in the womb. At least 1g of calcium daily and half this amount of magnesium should prove of value. Essential fatty acids must also be abundant and 3g each day of evening primrose oil should be taken.

An easier delivery

The two minerals calcium and magnesium can be of assistance here also as they both ease pain and help to relax the muscles. Taking 2g of calcium and 1g of magnesium after the onset of labour has given many women easier deliveries. Choose a combined mineral supplement that also includes vitamin D to aid absorption.

If your nutrition has been excellent all along, especially with regard to vitamin E (which increases elasticity), zinc, protein, potassium and essential fatty acids, then your delivery should be quicker as well as less painful.

Postnatal depression

This is often due to a depleted body after giving birth, particularly to low supplies of B-complex vitamins and calcium. Increasing your consumption of these (see chapter 3 for foods), along with emotional support from family, friends or a counsellor, will aid quick recovery.

Protecting the infant

Most mothers are quite naturally anxious in case their child may in some way be imperfect. The question 'Is the baby all right?' is usually their first after giving birth, and the reassurance that it is totally normal provides huge relief. By feeding herself really well, the mother is doing her utmost to prepare the new infant for life on earth, both mentally and physically, with the best chance of optimizing its potential. As we have already seen, certain deficiencies can result in a retarded or abnormal child.

Cretinism

Towards the end of pregnancy, the woman's basal metabolism goes up by about 25 per cent, under the control of the thyroid. Healthy function of this gland is dependent upon the trace element iodine and the mother needs an extra supply to meet rising demands. Any deficiency can result in a child with poor coordination or low intelligence.

Include seaweed and seafood in your diet (see recipes in chapter 20), also yoghurt, free-range eggs and cheese. If you are taking a multivitamin and -mineral tablet, check that iodine is included.

Foetal alcohol syndrome

Because drinking continues to be a socially acceptable pastime, few people realize how poisonous alcohol is.

Although the placenta can protect the foetus from a number of toxins, alcohol is not one of them and the effects on an unborn child can be disastrous: up to 70 per cent of babies born to mothers who have consumed around five drinks a day will have severe abnormalities, including an imperfectly formed skull, along with limited mental development, a hairy body, compromised immunity, possibly even deformed limbs.

Do not drink at all if you plan to become pregnant or if there is any chance that you might have conceived. Alcohol is especially harmful in the very early stages while the cells of the fertilized egg are dividing and becoming differentiated. If you are unable to give up drinking then do not have children. The legacy for the next generation can be terrible indeed.

Stillbirth

Some stillbirths have been associated with heavy-metal poisoning, especially from cadmium and lead. If you live in a contaminated environment, then it is doubly important to increase your intake of zinc, which helps to get rid of toxic metals from the body. Take 10mg of zinc daily in addition to eating seafood, wheatgerm and soya products regularly. See also chapter 4.

Breast-feeding

There is no question about it: breast is best. Human milk fulfils the new baby's needs far better than any manufactured formula. Not only does it come at the correct temperature and consistency, it is packed with nutrients – more than 200 all told – many not available in cow's milk. For optimal brain growth there must be an abundance of polyunsaturated fatty acids, yet infant feeds do not contain arachidonic and docosahexaenoic acids. Also important is the thin colostrum produced during the ten days following the birth which contains special immune bodies that help the baby defend itself against the multitude of pathogenic organisms in its surroundings.

It is scandalous that infant formulae contain sucrose! Some soya preparations are also aluminium contaminated which interferes with the absorption of calcium, magnesium and iron. This can lead to osteomalacia.

A breast-fed baby is less likely to suffer from colic and allergic reactions, although some infants can be intolerant of substances the mother is eating which are absorbed into her milk. So if the baby is wheezing or has eczema or problems with digestion or sleeping, then keep a food diary to identify the culprits. These are most likely to be cow's milk, wheat or possibly citrus fruits. If you then have to cut any of these items out of your diet, make sure that you are obtaining the equivalent nutrients elsewhere. Indeed, it is very important to maintain your healthy eating programme during nursing to manufacture high-quality milk. Only consider slimming after the baby is weaned, ideally not before six months.

Weaning

At six months, in addition to breast-milk, give one feed a day of freshly puréed fruit, such as bananas, or green or orange vegetables. Gradually introduce rice or millet flakes made into a thin porridge and scrambled free-range eggs, also live yoghurt. Be sure to seek out iron-rich foods such as puréed lentils or lean minced meat (if you eat it), which can be added at eight to nine months; tofu is also a suitable protein-rich option that is easily digested. Be careful about offering dairy products or wheat, first checking for allergic reactions.

By 12 months the baby will probably be weaned to a cup and happily eating mashed foods from the family's table, no doubt making a wonderful mess in the process! Avoid very salty or fibrous foods. The selection will surely be nourishing. It can now include beans and peas, and such items as raw fruit and vegetable sticks, avocado, or rice cakes spread with nut butters.

Eating for two
Nutritional guidelines before and after conception

Follow the Health-Giving Diet outlined in chapter 20, but note that the RDA for the following nutrients increases with pregnancy and lactation: vitamins A, B_1, B_2, B_3, B_6, B_{12}, folic acid, C, D, E, K and minerals calcium, iodine, iron, magnesium, phosphorus, selenium and zinc. The following foods are particularly rich in these essential nutrients and need to be emphasized both before and after conception:

Dark-green vegetables (A, B_6, folic acid, K, calcium, iron, magnesium, phosphorus); use the cooking water for soups and sauces

Yellow-orange fruit and vegetables (A)

Citrus and berry fruits; alfalfa sprouts, tomatoes and peppers in salads (C)

Dried fruits and cherry juice (iron)

Pumpkin and sunflower seeds (phosphorus, zinc) and sesame seeds/dark tahini (phosphorus, selenium)

Peas, beans and lentils (B_1, B_2, B_6, iron, phosphorus, zinc)

Nuts (B_1, B_2, magnesium, phosphorus)

Sea vegetables: spirulina and kelp (B_{12}, iodine)

Soya products: tempeh, tofu and miso (B_{12}, K, zinc)

Whole grains, including brown rice (B_1, B_2, B_6, folic acid, magnesium, phosphorus, selenium)

Wheatgerm (B_6, E, selenium, zinc)

Cold-pressed oils (E) including safflower (K)

Molasses (B_1, B_2, B_6, K, calcium, magnesium, iron)

Brewer's yeast (B_1, B_2, B_6, B_{12}, folic acid, selenium, zinc)

Milk, cheese and live yoghurt (A, B_{12}, folic acid, calcium, phosphorus)

Free-range eggs (A, B_1, B_2, B_{12}, D, K, iron, phosphorus, zinc)

Fish (B_1, B_{12}, folic acid, D, iron, phosphorus, selenium)

Seafood and shellfish (calcium, iodine, magnesium, phosphorus, zinc)

Poultry (B_1, iron, phosphorus)

Lean meat (B_1, B_6, iron, phosphorus)

NB Avoid liver and liver pâtés during pregnancy as the amount of oily vitamin A is too high for the foetus and could cause malformations: just 3½oz (108g) of lamb's liver gives a massive 74,000IU. It is safer to take this vitamin in the form of beta-carotene from vegetables.

Also avoid the following: tea and coffee, unleavened bread, alcohol, tobacco, any drugs (come off the contraceptive pill at least three months ahead of conception), refined and junk foods, artificial sweeteners and additives.

Be extra careful about food hygiene, and avoid cook-chill foods, coleslaw and soft cheeses, as listeria can be fatal to the foetus (see chapter 5).

Seasonings: use Biosalt or Losalt for correct potassium/sodium ratio, plus sea vegetable seasonings for the iodine.

Supplements: always check with your doctor first to ensure correct ratios. Take extra zinc to balance iron and folic acid. You will need twice as much calcium as magnesium.

Protein: increase intake by 10g daily above the normal amount during the first three months of pregnancy, then add a further 20g. Keep this up during lactation. (See table opposite to work this out in terms of food.)

Calories: up to a maximum of an extra 300 per day (equivalent to a jacket potato with beans, or two thick slices of wholemeal bread and margarine).

Calculating protein intake

Food source	Serving	Amount of usable protein
Complete proteins		
Skimmed milk	8 fl oz/225ml	7g
Powdered skimmed milk	1oz/30g	8g
Yoghurt	8 fl oz/225ml	7g
Cottage cheese	4oz/125g	13g
Cheese (Cheddar)	1oz/30g	5g
Egg	1 medium, 2oz/ 60g	6g
Wheatgerm	2 tablespoons	2g
Soya flour	3oz/90g	16g
Soya beans (dry)	2oz/60g	10g
Tofu	4oz/125g	5g
Fish	4oz/125g	14g–19g
Poultry	4oz/125g	15g–22g
Meat	4oz/125g	13g–19g
Incomplete proteins		
Wholemeal bread	2 slices	3g
Peanut butter	2 tablespoons	9g
Nuts	1oz/30g	2g–3g
Oatmeal	1½oz/45g	4g
Brown rice	3oz/90g	4g
Lentils	2oz/60g	4g
Beans (mung, kidney etc)	2oz/60g	4g–7g

Chapter 19

The Golden Years

During the 1980s, a team of archaeologists worked in absolute secrecy in the vaults of a church in Spitalfields, East London. The task was gruesome. They had to excavate the decaying remains of 1,000 parishioners, buried between the years 1729 and 1852 in lead coffins, sealed to keep the bodies intact in anticipation of the day of resurrection. They had paid handsomely for their final resting places, yet what they had not reckoned with was the power of bacteria and fungi to destroy their bodies, causing the flesh to putrefy. The stench from the rotting corpses was sickening and the risk to the health of the archaeologists considerable, but the significance of their finds made this ghoulish assignment worthwhile. Because the burials were comparatively recent, the records of the occupants were all intact and the exact age and cause of death known.

Of great interest to those of us involved in natural health care was the discovery that the skeletons of octogenarians were in surprisingly good shape, with fewer marks of ageing than on those of today. The team anthropologist, Theya Molleson, commented: 'They aged later and they aged more slowly, so that they got to old age in better condition than us. Their bones didn't start thinning until their fifties, whereas now the process starts when women reach their thirties.' It became clear that those who survived the hazards of childhood maladies generally lived into a vigorous old age. Here we have real proof that, although our modern way of life is more comfortable and convenient, it also encourages the early onset of degeneration, so that old people today are frequently crippled with arthritis, suffer from hypertension or heart disease or diabetes, or the unpleasantness of diverticulosis or indeed innumerable other afflictions of civilization.

In this respect, cars are one of our worst evils. Our bodies evolved to be used, not to be carried everywhere on wheels. Before the motor vehicle people either rode on horseback, if they could afford to own one, or else they walked – invariably many miles each day. An elderly neighbour in our village once described the life he remembers from his childhood. Farmworkers were up at six, some having to walk four miles before beginning their labours in the fields. At the end of a long day there was another four miles home. Regular vigorous walking keeps the bones strong and the heart pumping efficiently.

Then the food was local, fresh and unpolluted. Nearly everyone in this neighbourhood grew their own vegetables, the cabbages and leeks mingling with the flowers in the cottage gardens, while healthy chickens pecked about in the yard. Wild food such as cob nuts, blackberries and crab apples was a regular part of their diet, as was wild game, since few people could afford to buy much meat. You had to go out and shoot or trap it yourself.

Because old people today have such low energy levels from years of sedentary living, they can hardly be bothered to look after themselves and resort to convenience foods from tins and packages. They may suffer from poor digestion so imagine, mistakenly, that white bread will be better for them. The resulting lack of nutrients contributes, alas, to their overall deterioration, and so their condition becomes worse. Because they are then prescribed various medications these deplete the body of nutrients even further.

Today, ageing sets in early, from 30 years or even sooner,

and the long list of its physical effects makes dispiriting reading. The heart loses up to 30 per cent of its efficiency and the lungs more than 50 per cent. The resting metabolic rates falls by about 20 per cent and fewer calories are needed, so unless the diet is adjusted the person will put on weight. Cells can generally only divide up to about 55 times and after that they are lost and not replaced. The kidneys are particularly vulnerable, losing about half their nephrons, with a resulting decline in filtering ability. As many as 30 brain cells per minute may die and short-term memory often fails. Cell replacement in the skin and blood gradually slows down, with the epidermis becoming thinner and the hair wispy. As the tissues lose their elasticity and the muscles waste away, the skin becomes wrinkled and the body weaker, with diminished bladder capacity. Bones lose minerals, resulting in brittleness and deformity of the skeleton together with reduction in height which can be as much as 8 inches (20cm) in women. Changes occur to the eye lens, causing long-sightedness. Furring up of the arteries has long since set in, with imminent risk of heart attacks or strokes. Nerve transmission slows down by around 15 per cent, so that reflexes become sluggish. Teeth fall out: 80 per cent of today's old people have none of their own. Digestion of food and ability to absorb nutrients is impaired and the number of taste buds declines dramatically.

While a certain amount of ageing is inevitable it is quite possible to delay the ravages of time and anticipate becoming a sprightly nonagenarian with complete retention of one's mental faculties. Vegetarian playwright George Bernard Shaw is just one example. We have to understand that as we grow older, so our nutrient requirements increase, although calorie need diminishes. As long as we meet these requirements, in addition to following the Health-Giving Diet outlined in chapter 20, and of course take regular exercise, keeping stress levels low and not smoking, then the effects of ageing can be postponed. As we have already seen in previous chapters, major degenerative diseases that are currently associated with old age can be avoided altogether by a healthy lifestyle and excellent diet. These include the killer diseases of several cancers, heart disease, hypertension and diabetes, while other disorders such as caries and even dementia are also nutrition-related.

In 1991 researchers examined 88 centenarians from the Okinawa Prefecture in Japan, the world's leading area for longevity. They had all worked into their eighth decade, the main occupation being agriculture. Their diet was well balanced but simple, consisting of rice or potatoes as carbohydrate, with abundant fresh vegetables and protein from either plants or fish.

What actually sets the ageing process in motion? Comparatively little is known about this, but one of the most prominent theories concerns attack from free radicals.

The dangers of free radicals

Although oxygen is vital to life – indeed, we can survive only a very few minutes without it – it is also potentially extremely destructive. A useful analogy can be made with a car. This depends on oxygen from the air mixing with the fuel to make it run, yet at the same time the bodywork must be protected against oxygen attack, which will cause rusting. We are all familiar with the rust spots that appear where stones have chipped the paint. Similarly, it is oxygen that causes essential fatty acids in our bodies to go rancid, that is wherever they are not protected by particular nutrients known as antioxidants. Have you noticed 'liver' or 'age spots' on the skin of older people? These are the marks of this type of rancidity, human rust spots.

You will remember from chapter 3 that essential fatty acids are unsaturated, in other words they are liquid at room temperature. In the same way that essential amino acids join up to make body proteins, so essential fatty acids

295

join up to create flexible structural fats, which are found in cell walls, particularly in the brain and nervous system and in the blood vessels. Chapter 10 explained how important they are for keeping the arteries clear of blockages. It is also obvious that healthy mental functioning and speed of reflexes depend on them to a considerable degree. However, if the EFAs are not protected from oxygen attack by antioxidants, then they will decay. As they do this, they release highly reactive molecules called free radicals which cause even greater destruction by rampaging through the body in an uncontrolled fashion and damaging other cells in the process.

Once the unsaturated fatty acids in the cell membrane have been attacked, a chain reaction is set in motion, spreading from one cell to another. This is known as lipid peroxidation. It is rather like leaving a packet of butter in a warm room and later discovering that it has gone rancid. In the process the cell has lost its self-sufficiency and ability to protect itself.

Free radicals also strike at proteins, including important enzymes. One effect of this is loss of elasticity in the skin, so that wrinkles form. We all know that over-exposure to sunlight causes this to happen, and indeed, like many other substances such as tobacco, alcohol, food additives and drugs, it is a trigger for the release of harmful, ageing free radicals.

If the devastation reaches the centre of a cell, then the DNA with its genetic code will be impaired, so that the cell can no longer behave normally. All of this can happen within a fraction of a second and the result of this can be cancer. Many other diseases are linked with free radicals, including arteriosclerosis, coronary thrombosis, cerebral haemorrhage, arthritis, Parkinson's disease, cataracts and senility.

Free radicals can cause 'cross-linking', in which molecules become welded together, forming hard bonds in the body, making it stiff, another symptom of ageing. Cross-linking is also set in motion by acetaldehyde, a chemical that enters the body from cigarette smoke or that is made in the liver from alcohol. This is yet another way in which smoking and drinking take a toll on your health. On the other hand, enzymes called proteases found, for example, in fresh pineapple may stimulate the body's own enzymes to break down these hard bonds.

So how can we protect ourselves from the mayhem brought about by free radicals? The answer is to increase our intake of antioxidants and the best among the vitamins are beta-carotene from dark-green leafy vegetables and yellow-orange vegetables and fruit, to a lesser extent vitamin A from liver (but take this in moderation only and always organic), oily fish and free-range eggs, vitamin C from citrus and berry fruits, salad and raw green vegetables, and vitamin E from plant oils, wheatgerm and oily fish. Of the minerals, selenium is part of an enzyme belonging to the group known as glutathione peroxidases. These protect the oils in body membranes from damage by free radicals. You can obtain selenium from wheatgerm, oily fish and soya products. There is a synergistic effect between vitamin E and selenium – in other words, by working together, each enhances the effect of the other. Another enzyme from a group called superoxide dismutase (SOD for short) contains zinc (found in oysters and other shellfish); this prevents a chain-reaction of free radicals.

Vitamin B_6 is a useful adjunct to the main antioxidants. Not only does it have slight antioxidant properties itself, but it acts as a catalyst for the others. Unfortunately, many older people have too little of this vitamin in their diets because of their reliance on convenience foods. It is found particularly in whole wheat and oily fish. Also present in whole foods and oily fish as well as soya products, free-range poultry, nuts and green vegetables is the quasi-vitamin coenzyme Q_{10}, another powerful antioxidant.

Forgetfulness

One of the curses of old age is the loss of short-term memory. I can clearly recall my mother writing down every event as it happened, in an attempt to circumvent this loss. But as the deterioration progressed, even this *aide-memoire* became too much to attend to, until she no longer knew where she was or who the people around her were. This was extremely sad to witness, particularly as in her younger days she had been a well-regarded botanist and teacher, with a very able and alert mind.

As described in chapter 16, the chemical messengers called neurotransmitters are indispensable for accurate brain functioning, but with the onset of age fewer are produced. A generous supply of the nutrients from which neurotransmitters are made will, however, enhance their production. One is called acetylcholine which is constructed from choline (found for example in eggs, yeast, wheatgerm and green vegetables) and lecithin (from soya products). This process needs the presence of pantothenic acid (vitamin B_5), brewer's yeast being a prime source for this. If levels of acetylcholine fall too low, poor concentration, sleeplessness and erratic coordination will also be experienced in addition to memory loss. It is often said that fish is good for the brain, and indeed it is, for it contains DMAE (dimethylaminoethanol), which is converted into choline to make acetylcholine.

The amino acids phenylalanine and tyrosine are used by the body to make another neurotransmitter called norepinephrine, which is also involved in learning and memory. Protein foods including cheese, nuts (especially almonds and pistachios), seeds, soya beans, poultry, fish and lean beef are the best sources here. It is very important that the elderly maintain high-quality protein intake to remain mentally and physically alert.

Ageing affects the production of RNA (ribonucleic acid)

which is particularly needed by the brain for memory storage, but its synthesis in the body is encouraged by the presence of vitamin B_{12}. This is found especially in liver, mackerel, yeast extract and free-range eggs (NB battery eggs have barely half the quantity of B_{12} found in free-range ones). Researchers have discovered that vitamin B_{12} deficiency is common among elderly psychiatric patients.

A study carried out in an English hospital in 1982 among elderly patients showed an association between low levels of vitamin B_1 (thiamin) and confused behaviour. Brewer's yeast sprinkled daily on to food should help to rectify any such deficiency.

Alzheimer's disease

When mental deterioration sets in at a relatively young age – that is, before 65 years – Alzheimer's disease is the usual diagnosis. The aluminium theory is still disputed, although this mineral is a known neurotoxin. Research by Professor J. D. Birchall at Keele University has shown that silicon discourages aluminium absorption by the body, so it could be a very valuable protection from early dementia, supposing this theory is correct. At any rate, replacing aluminium pans with stainless-steel ones will lower the risk. Calcium and magnesium supplements (in a 2 to 1 ratio) plus vitamin C will also reduce aluminium uptake in the body.

Since zinc deficiency has been linked with senile dementia, supplements of this mineral are recommended at between 15 and 25mg daily. Good food sources are shellfish, cheese, lentils and beans, wholemeal bread (not white: most of the zinc has been removed), pumpkin and sunflower seeds, tofu, wheatgerm and roast beef; omnivores might consider desiccated liver as an occasional supplement.

The latest studies show that in Alzheimer's patients areas of the brain vital to memory and learning fill up with bundles of protein filaments called neurofibrillary tangles.

Spherically shaped deposits referred to as senile plaques, consisting of beta-amyloid protein, also gradually accumulate in the spaces between cells. This happens when the neurotransmitter acetylcholine is not present. It is crucial, therefore, to maintain generous levels of choline and lecithin in the diet, as described under 'Forgetfulness' above.

In July 1994 a BBC television documentary called 'Poison in the Mouth' made a definite connection between amalgam fillings, which contain mercury, and early dementia. The mercury, a deadly toxin, leaks into the mouth as a vapour. Sweden has now banned amalgam. Look after your teeth and ask your dentist for safer fillings. Also remember that the minerals calcium and magnesium, zinc and selenium, when ingested in food or as supplements, are antagonistic to heavy metals.

There may be other undiscovered causes of Alzheimer's disease, but whatever they are the result is devastating, with gradual deterioration, so that simple forgetfulness becomes chronic loss of memory, leading to confusion and disorientation with a total breakdown of personality. A previously coherent individual may become withdrawn, aggressive or overly cheerful, and talk complete gibberish. Even the simplest task is an impossibility. It is particularly sad for a partner to witness the loss of a loved one in this way.

It is wise to maintain some form of gentle aerobic exercise into old age, especially out of doors, as those who do so score higher on cognitive tests than those who do not. At the least practise deep breathing daily by an open window. Oxygen is of tremendous importance to the health of the brain. Maintaining stimulating mental activity will keep the neurons firing and lessen the chance of early atrophy. Also follow the suggestions under 'Forgetfulness' above.

Poor digestion

Many old folk have problems with eating, either because dentures fit badly or because digestion itself is poor. It is the enzymes in the digestive tract that break food down into molecules small enough to be absorbed into the bloodstream, but the production of these important proteins may decline with age. They can, however, be re-supplied from some foods including pineapple and papaya fruit; alternatively, they can be taken in the form of chewable tablets available from health food suppliers.

The production of hydrochloric acid in the stomach also declines as we age and this, too, is essential for the breakdown of foods. It also activates pepsin, a protein-splitting enzyme. Here again, supplements may be taken in the form of tablets of betaine hydrochloride. Follow the instructions on the bottle.

Foods that are easily assimilated, such as soups made from fresh vegetables and lentils, or juices made from vegetables high in vitamins and minerals, are recommended. Wheatgerm or powdered skimmed milk can be stirred into porridge for extra nourishment. Tofu is a high-protein food that is versatile and easily digested (see chapter 20 for recipes), while alfalfa sprouts are readily chewed and nutrient-rich. Live yoghurt is another food that helps keep the digestive tract healthy. (See also 'Indigestion and dyspepsia' in chapter 6.)

Food for the elderly

Keep to small portions of food that are nutritionally rich but low in calories; never eat until full. Follow the Health-Giving Diet described in chapter 20, particularly avoiding refined, sugary and fatty foods. Do not add salt as the extra sodium will upset the electrolyte soup of the brain. Emphasize foods containing antioxidants, that is yellow-orange vegetables and fruit, citrus and berry fruits and dark-green vegetables, also salads with dressing made from cold-pressed plant oils. Avoid red meat, which contains much iron, an oxidizing metal. Nevertheless, ensure that protein intake from other sources is more than adequate and eat fish at least twice a week, especially the oily sort. Have wheatgerm daily, sprinkled on porridge, muesli or soup. Tofu is easily digested and very versatile for inclusion in either main courses or desserts.

To increase intake of vitamins and minerals naturally, make fresh vegetable juices and have a glass each day. Nourishing home-made soups and vegetable stews are well assimilated.

Fresh pineapple will aid digestion, as will peppermint tea. Instead of jam use yeast extract as a spread and take brewer's yeast for B complex vitamins, while live yoghurt will encourage the body to manufacture its own. Older people often have difficulty in absorbing folic acid and vitamin B_{12}, a deficiency of which can lead to pernicious anaemia (see chapter 16).

Have apricots regularly, as they are rich in antioxidants. This is a staple food of the Hunzas of Pakistan, reputed to live to great ages, even up to 120 years.

Consider taking ginseng to increase vitality – up to 500mg daily is sufficient – and you may like to have a combined antioxidant supplement or multivitamin and -mineral tablet that contains vitamins A, C, E, B_6, selenium and zinc. Also check that it includes vitamin B_{12}, especially if you are a vegan. Evening primrose oil combined with vitamin E at 2g daily will give you the EFAs that your body requires.

Chapter 20

The Health-Giving Diet

The following is a summary of the diet that is basic to good health and long life, described in more detail towards the end of chapter 2 under 'Food for lasting health'.

Emphasize:

- Fresh, organically produced wholefoods that are high in fibre, with as much variety as possible.
- Unrefined cereals, such as brown rice, millet, barley, wholemeal bread and pasta; also uncooked as a muesli base.
- Fresh vegetables in season, raw in salads or just lightly steamed; eat every day. Keep the water for soups and sauces.
- Raw, mixed salads: eat every day.
- Fresh fruit in season, at least two pieces daily, including the skins if suitable. Dried fruits.
- Plant proteins from beans (including tofu and tempeh), peas and lentils, nuts and seeds.
- Fish, especially deep-sea, at least twice a week.
- Free-range eggs and occasional poultry and game; low-fat live natural yoghurt.
- Olive oil for quick stir-frying; cold-pressed plant oils for salad dressings. Margarine with non-hydrogenated oils.
- Herb teas; fresh fruit and vegetable juices; soya milk.

Plenty of filtered or spring water, preferably not with meals.
- Herbs, spices and sea seasonings.
- Yeast extract, tahini, nut butters, black molasses.

Avoid:

- Intensively and chemically farmed foods.
- Refined, processed, packaged, tinned, irradiated and all convenience and junk foods; old, mouldy, reheated or burnt foods.
- Smoked or pickled foods.
- Preservatives, colourings, artificial sweeteners and other additives.
- Saturated fats from red meat and dairy produce (i.e. full-fat milk, butter and cheese); hydrogenated fats.
- Sugar (honey, grain syrups and malt extract are better alternatives), including confectionery, sweet biscuits, cakes, puddings and jams.
- Salt (except substitutes such as Losalt).
- Tea and coffee; all soft drinks and alcohol.

Healthy cooking tips

Soggy, overboiled cabbage not only tastes unpleasant, it has probably lost most of its vitamins during cooking, yet this is the way most vegetables are served, not just in many homes but especially in schools and other institutions including hospitals. Vitamins are best preserved by light steaming only, after which the water should be kept for sauces, soups and gravies. So remember to put that steamer on your shopping list. For maximum benefit from nutrients, eat vegetables newly picked and raw. If you can afford it, invest in a juicer. Recipes below will give you some ideas for serving.

Burnt food does you harm, yet it is surprising how few people realize this. They continue to invite friends to barbecues, offering them blackened sausages and beefburgers, as if they were highly sought-after delicacies. Yet the free radicals that form during the burning process can be extremely injurious, attacking cells and the DNA contained within them, causing faulty functioning, degeneration and even cancer. A fine gift for your friends! Never eat burnt food, including overdone toast and smoked fish. Disregard recipes that tell you to brown onions; simply cook them until they go soft and transparent.

Deep-fat frying is not recommended if you value your heart. Shallow, quick stir-frying is a good way of keeping vitamins, though. Do not use polyunsaturated oils or margarine for this, which again will create free radicals (even if not burnt). Always choose olive oil, which is predominantly monounsaturated, or alternatively a little ghee (clarified butter). You can make this yourself by heating butter until it bubbles and then scooping off the impurities in the form of the foam.

Beans are full of goodness, but they must be properly cooked because certain toxins are naturally present in their raw state which can induce embarrassing flatulence or even, in the case of red kidney beans, diarrhoea and sickness. Raw broad beans may be tempting, especially if tender, but they can be a source of free radical damage if eaten uncooked. On the other hand, freshly picked French and runner beans are quite safe in salads. To guarantee destruction of toxins, after soaking in filtered water boil the beans rapidly for about ten minutes, discard the water and boil again until tender.

Tips on how to store food for maximum retention of nutrients is described in chapter 5.

Eating your nutrients

The value of chewing food well without hurry and in relaxing surroundings cannot be overemphasized. This is considered more fully in chapter 6 for the sake of your digestive system, but thorough mastication also gives your body a better chance of absorbing the nutrients.

It is advisable not to swill your meals down with liquid, because they will rush through you too quickly and once again nutrients will not be so readily assimilated. Just a few sips are sufficient. Have a drink such as a fruit juice half an hour before eating and wait at least another 30 minutes after the meal before making a beverage. This way your food will not be drowned.

Always start your meal with something raw. Many plant juices contain bitter factors and essential oils that enhance the activity of digestive enzymes and encourage more complete absorption of nutrients. Don't worry if you have no time to make a salad. Munching a raw carrot is just as good.

Switching to a wholefood diet may cause flatulence at first, but your system will soon become adjusted to the extra roughage. Chew a few caraway seeds before eating to prevent it.

Health-giving recipes

Included here are suggestions for recipes that may be difficult to find in standard cookery books, simply because they follow the principles outlined at the start of the chapter. You will no doubt enjoy researching your own.

Beverages and herbal remedies

Although many herb teas are now commercially available, quality varies considerably from brand to brand, so it is always worth making your own both for excellence of flavour as well as healing power. A wide variety of herbs can be bought by mail order from the suppliers listed under 'Addresses'.

Pregnant women need to be cautious about drinking too much of any one tea and should especially avoid sage and feverfew. Gentle teas such as camomile, peppermint and lime blossom are quite safe in moderation.

Infusions

To make an infusion, simply pour hot water (just off the boil) on to the leaves or flowers of the herb, cover and leave to stand for at least three minutes. Use approximately 1 teaspoon of herb to ½ pint (275ml) of boiling filtered water.

Teas such as blackberry leaf, sage, peppermint and nettle mentioned in this book can all be made in this way either from the dried or freshly picked leaves. Camomile, lime blossom and marigold are made from an infusion of the flowers. Berries such as blackcurrants and juniper can be similarly infused after first crushing them. A little honey can be added to taste.

To make seed teas, for example celery seed or dill, crush 1 teaspoon of seed and add ½ to 1 pint (275 to 570ml) of boiling filtered water, depending on strength. Allow to stand for five minutes before drinking.

Decoctions

A decoction is made with the roots of the plant, cut or bruised, and then simmered in filtered water for 10 to 15 minutes.

Rosehip Tea Rosehips are very rich in vitamin C. The tea is therefore useful for the alleviation of mild infections.

    2 tbsp freshly gathered rosehips
    1 pint (570ml) filtered water
    1 tsp honey

Chop the hips then place them in the water and bring to the boil. Simmer for 10 minutes. Strain and sweeten with the honey.

Makes 2 to 3 cups

Chicory Tea The chicory plant contains a bitter principle as well as vitamins A and B₃ (niacin) and the minerals potassium, calcium and iron. One cup of the tea daily is traditionally used for the prevention and treatment of gallstones. It is also recommended by herbalists for liver complaints, rheumatism and gout. If desired, sweeten with a little honey.

From the root:

2 tsp shredded chicory root

$^1/_2$ pint (275ml) filtered water

Boil for 3 minutes, cover and allow to stand for at least 5 minutes before drinking.

From the leaf:

1 to 2 tsp dried chicory leaves

$^1/_2$ pint (275ml) filtered water

Bring to the boil and allow to infuse for 10 minutes.

Makes 1 mug

Dandelion Coffee This can be purchased ready prepared, but it is not difficult to make your own and dandelions are a superb source of vitamin A.

Dig up mature roots in the autumn. Wash them and then put in a medium oven for 2 to 3 hours until well roasted. Chop the roots into small pieces or grind them up and make the coffee by decoction (see above).

Chicory coffee can be similarly prepared.

Lettuce Tea Culpeper says of lettuce that it 'procures sleep and easeth the head-ache' and then adds, 'It abateth bodily lust'! It certainly has sedative properties and is recommended for insomnia.

1 large lettuce

1 pint (570ml) boiling filtered water

1 tsp poppy seeds

3 tsp camomile flowers (or 2 camomile tea bags)

Pluck the lettuce leaves into small pieces and put into a

pan with the boiling water and the other ingredients. Simmer for 20 minutes. Cut the stem in several places and put into the pan without losing any milky latex. Simmer for a further 5 minutes. Strain.

Drink while tea is warm, shortly before retiring.

Makes 2 to 3 cups

Ginger Brew Ginger is a natural anticoagulant and therefore excellent for heart-disease patients. Also useful for the prevention of colds, 'flu and cystitis. Instead of the following recipe a simple decoction can be made by simmering 1 inch (2.5cm) of cut ginger root and a pinch of cinnamon in ½ pint (275ml) of filtered water for 10 minutes. Sipping this tea can prevent travel sickness.

    2 tsp grated fresh ginger root
    1 pint (570ml) filtered hot water
    1 tsp honey
    1 tsp vitamin C powder
    slice of lemon

Pour the hot water on to the other ingredients and steep for 3 minutes. Sip while hot.

Makes 2 mugs

Rice Water This is a soothing remedy for digestive troubles or infections of the urinary tract. Small amounts can be safely given to children.

    1 tbsp organic brown rice
    1 pint (570ml) filtered water

Boil up the rice in the water, cover and simmer for about ½ hour. Strain off the water and allow to cool before sipping.

Makes 2 cups

Lemon Barley Water A traditional remedy for catarrh and a calming antidote to fever.

    2 oz (60g) pearl barley

1 pint (570ml) filtered water
juice of ½ lemon
2 tsp honey

Put the barley and water into a pan, bring to the boil, then simmer for ½ hour. Strain and reserve the barley for further use. Stir in the lemon juice and honey and sip while hot.
Makes 2 to 3 cups

Herbal Gargle Very good for sore throats.
1 tbsp honey
1 tbsp sage
1 tbsp cider vinegar
½ pint (275ml) filtered hot water
few drops of clove oil (optional)

Steep the ingredients in the hot water for 5 minutes. Strain before using as a gargle.

Fortified Soya Drink Highly nutritious and easily assimilated when digestion is poor. Extra vitamins and minerals can be added as required.
4 oz (125g) firm tofu
1 pint (570ml) soya milk
1 orange (or 1 banana or 2 slices pineapple, cubed)
2 tbsp wheatgerm
1 dsp cold-pressed safflower or sunflower oil
2 tsp kelp
2 tbsp live low-fat yoghurt
2 crushed Dolomite tablets
15mg zinc tablet, crushed
1 tsp vitamin C powder

Blend all the ingredients together in a liquidizer and consume as required. Can be stored for up to two days in the refrigerator.
Makes 3 or 4 mugs

Sports Drink This drink will help to replace fluid and

minerals sweated out during exercise and will thus prevent dehydration, cramps and sore muscles. It can be sipped during training or taken afterwards. Flavours can be varied.

  2 pints (1 litre) filtered water
  4 peppermint tea bags or equivalent fresh leaves
  1 tsp Biosalt or Ruthmol
  1 tbsp honey
  2 crushed Dolomite tablets
  1 tsp kelp

Bring the water to the boil and pour on to the peppermint leaves or tea bags. Allow to infuse for 3 minutes. Strain and stir in the Biosalt and honey, Dolomite and kelp.

Can be drunk warm or cold and taken to training sessions in a Thermos flask. Shake well.

Makes 4 mugs

Breakfast

This is a most important meal, especially for people with irregular blood sugar, so don't skip it! If you start the day by eating well, you will have lots of energy throughout the morning. Food taken early will be efficiently utilized by the body as fuel for energetic activity and is not likely to be stored as fat.

The classic fried breakfast of bacon, eggs and sausages is, sadly, not at all healthy and is likely to put a strain on the digestive system and damage the arteries in the long term. Included in this section are some healthier low-fat alternatives.

Muesli We make a huge jar of this at home, reinventing the combination of ingredients each time. Here is one variation, but any grain flakes can be incorporated along with different nuts and seeds. It is packed with nutrients, especially B and E vitamins, and is a sound source of dietary fibre, which will keep the bowel in good working order.

  1 lb (500g) oat flakes

3 oz (90g) millet flakes
3 oz (90g) barley flakes
3 oz (90g) rice flakes
2 oz (60g) sultanas
2 oz (60g) raisins
4 oz (125g) dried apricots, chopped
2 oz (60g) dried dates, chopped
2 oz (60g) dried figs, chopped
2 oz (60g) flaked almonds
2 oz (60g) cashew nuts
2 oz (60g) sunflower seeds
1 oz (30g) pumpkin seeds

Mix all the ingredients in a large bowl and store in an airtight jar.

Each serving:
soya milk or nut milk (see 'The complementary dairy', page 326) as required
fresh apple with skin, sliced
banana, sliced
1 dsp wheatgerm
1 tbsp low-fat bio-yoghurt

You may like to soak each serving in the milk overnight, although this is not essential unless jumbo oats are used. Add the fresh fruit, wheatgerm and yoghurt.

Makes about 2³/₄lb (1.38kg)

Millet Porridge This makes a change from oats and has a creamy texture. There is plenty of carbohydrate here for energy, as well as some useful protein, plus vitamin B_3, calcium and potassium.

4 oz (125g) millet flakes
¹/₂ pint (275ml) apple juice
1 pint (570ml) filtered water
2 tbsp sultanas
pinch of cinnamon

Put the millet flakes, apple juice and water into a large pan and cook gently while stirring until the porridge thickens (10 to 15 minutes). Add the sultanas and cinnamon.

Serve hot with Soya Cream (see 'The complementary dairy', page 327).

Serves 4 to 6

Spiced Compôte Really delicious. Hunza apricots are the staple food of the longest-living people on earth. They are a fine source of vitamin A which is protective against cancer.

　　8 oz (250g) mixed dried fruit (e.g. Hunza apricots, prunes, apple rings)
　　1 pint (570ml) filtered water
　　1 tsp mixed spice
　　1 oz (30g) lightly toasted flaked almonds

Soak the fruit overnight in the water. Add the spice and bring to the boil in a medium pan, then simmer gently for 10 minutes or so until soft.

Serve with the almonds and some Soya Cream (see 'The complementary dairy', page 327) for extra protein.

Serves 4

Scrambled Tofu This is a low-fat alternative to scrambled eggs and ideal for anyone concerned about their cholesterol levels. It only takes a few minutes to make.

　　1 tbsp soya milk
　　4 oz (125g) firm tofu, crumbled
　　2 fresh basil leaves, chopped
　　dash of soya sauce
　　1 large slice of wholemeal bread

Warm the soya milk over a gentle heat in a small pan. Add the tofu, basil and soya sauce and stir until well heated. Meanwhile toast the bread lightly. Pile the tofu on the toast.

Serves 1

Tempeh Tomatoes Another low-fat, high-protein food,

313

this is made from cultured soya beans and is bought in a block. Simply cut off the required pieces. Tempeh contains both iron and calcium, especially valuable for vegans, plus several B vitamins.

2 or 3 slices of tempeh
dash of soya sauce
knob of ghee (see 'Healthy cooking tips', page 305)
2 tomatoes, quartered
1 large slice of wholemeal bread

Flavour the tempeh with the soya sauce on both sides. Place the ghee in a medium frying pan and heat gently until melted. Add the tempeh slices and tomatoes and shallow-fry. Turn the tempeh once so that it becomes just golden on both sides.

Toast the bread lightly. Pile the tempeh and tomatoes on.
Serves 1

Nut Sausages These provide good protein, without the hazardous fat and preservatives of meat sausages. Additionally they are rich in nutrients and dietary fibre. Make the mixture in advance to cut down on preparation in the morning.

1 medium onion, finely chopped
1 oz (30g) ghee (see 'Healthy cooking tips', above)
2 tsp mixed herbs
$1/4$ pint (150ml) vegetable stock
1 tsp low-salt yeast extract
5 oz (150g) ground hazelnuts
3 oz (90g) ground almonds
4 oz (125g) wholemeal breadcrumbs
3 oz (90g) oat flakes

Sauté the chopped onion in the ghee until transparent. Add the herbs. Put the stock in a small pan and heat through, dissolving the yeast extract in it. Combine all the ingredients together, apart from the oat flakes, to make a

314

firm mixture. Divide into portions and roll up to form sausage shapes. Roll these in the oats.

In the morning fry the sausages in a little olive oil for a few minutes, turning as necessary, until crisp and golden.
Makes 6 to 8 sausages

Snacks

My favourite way of stopping the hunger pangs is to have a handful of almonds mixed with equal amounts of pumpkin seeds and sultanas. Together these contain folic acid, pantothenic acid and several minerals including potassium, calcium, magnesium and phosphorus – excellent for the bones as well as supplying the basic ingredients for the 'electrolyte soup' of the brain.

Hazelnut Butter Nut butters can be easily made and they will keep in the fridge for up to one week. They are delicious on oatcakes or ricecakes and there is no need to include salt or sugar.

 4 oz (125g) hazelnuts, lightly toasted
 4 oz (125g) sunflower seeds
 $\frac{1}{4}$ pint (150ml) filtered water
 1 clove garlic

Grind the nuts and seeds together, then put them in the blender with the water and garlic. Liquidize to form a paste.

Store in a jar in the fridge.
Makes 1 jar

Tahini Spread Tahini is made from ground sesame seeds and contains many nutrients in addition to protein, including vitamins A and B_3, calcium, potassium, phosphorus and some iron. Traditionally a Japanese spread, miso is a product of fermented soya beans and grains. It is best to buy the 'live' sort which, like yoghurt, has beneficial bacteria. This spread has a slightly cheesy flavour.

 3 tbsp dark tahini

1 tbsp miso
1 tsp lemon juice

Simply mix the ingredients together and spread on bread or oatcakes.

Makes about 8 portions

Seedy Oatcakes These oatcakes-cum-scones with added seeds and fruit provide a sustaining wheat-free, sugar-free snack offering a wide variety of nutrients.

2 oz (60g) oat flakes
4 oz (125g) medium oatmeal
6 oz (180g) brown rice flour
3 oz (90g) currants
2 oz (60g) desiccated coconut
1 oz (30g) sesame seeds
2 oz (60g) sunflower seeds
4 tbsp sunflower oil
$^{1}/_{2}$ pint (275ml) apple juice

Combine the dry ingredients in a large bowl, then stir in the oil gradually. Add the apple juice and mix well to form a firm dough. Sprinkle a little flour on to a flat surface, then roll out the dough until it is about $^{1}/_{2}$ inch (1.25cm) thick. Cut into rounds.

Heat the oven to 350°F/180°C (gas mark 4) and bake the oatcakes on a greased baking sheet for about 20 minutes.

Makes 12 to 14

Soups

Soups that are liquidized in the blender are especially useful if for any reason digestion is impaired, as they can so easily be assimilated. They are also ideal during and after illness, when the patient is unable to take much solid food, or in the recovery from anorexia when the stomach has to adjust once more to regular meals. The variety is endless, according to the mixture of ingredients, and the nutritional content invariably rich. Most are easily prepared, especially those made from vegetables, pulses and cereals. Soups provide a special opportunity to incorporate sea vegetables into the meal, which are extremely healthy for you.

Miso and Onion Soup According to Japanese legend, miso was sent to humanity by the gods to give them good health, happiness and long life. Unfortunately, traditional methods of making it have been largely superseded by commercial production using sugar and preservatives, with a speeded-up ageing process. Do not buy these. Look for the organic sort that has been aged from between one to two years.

Since miso contains a certain amount of sea salt, too much may not be good for people suffering from hypertension. However, the fermentation process enhances the salty flavour, so by using it in cooking instead of salt you will be putting in less sodium overall. In this recipe the sodium is well balanced by the potassium from the onions and seaweed, which also contains calcium, magnesium and iron.

In 1981 the Japanese National Cancer Centre published results of a nationwide survey, which concluded that people who ate miso soup every day had lower rates of cancer and heart disease and other degenerative disorders than those who did not.

> 3-inch (7.5-cm) piece wakame seaweed
> 1 large onion, sliced thinly
> 2 tsp grated root ginger
> 2 pints (1 litre) filtered water
> 1½ tbsp miso
> *To garnish*:
> 3 tbsp chopped spring onions or watercress

Rinse the wakame and slice into six pieces. Put these into a large pan together with the onion and ginger, add the water and bring to the boil. Turn the heat down and simmer for about 15 minutes until tender. Remove from the stove.

Dissolve the miso in a little of the broth, then stir this in

317

to the soup. (Do not boil the miso or the healthy bacteria will be destroyed.)

Serve not too hot, garnished with the spring onions or watercress.

Serves 4 to 6

Lentil Soup Lentils are a wonderful food. Not only are they extremely cheap, they contain good-quality plant protein and many nutrients including iron, while providing dietary fibre. They are low in fat and therefore a useful ingredient for slimmers, as well as being healthy for heart-disease patients. As a complex carbohydrate, lentils will keep blood sugar steady and, according to Dr Mills of Loma Linda University School of Medicine in the US, they are protective against cancer of the pancreas, as are other legumes.

> 1 onion, chopped
> 2 pints (1 litre) vegetable stock
> 8 oz (250g) lentils
> 2 large carrots, scrubbed and chopped
> 1 potato, scrubbed and chopped
> 1 clove garlic
> $\frac{1}{2}$ tsp ground cloves
> 1 tsp thyme
> 1 dsp low-salt yeast extract
> juice of half a lemon
> *To garnish*:
> nori flakes

Put all the ingredients except the lemon in a large pan and bring to the boil. Lower the heat and simmer gently for about 25 minutes until done, stirring occasionally, topping up the water if necessary. Take off the stove and add the lemon juice.

Liquidize in the blender and serve hot, with the nori flakes sprinkled on top.

Serves 4 to 6

Pumpkin Soup Like carrots, pumpkin contains beta-carotene, an important antioxidant, which is protective against cancer and keeps at bay some of the effects of ageing.

    1 small pumpkin
    2 pints (1 litre) filtered water
    1 tsp ginger
    $\frac{1}{4}$ tsp Biosalt (optional)
    1 leek
    To garnish:
    chopped chives

Remove the skin and seeds from the pumpkin, then chop the flesh. Put it into a large pan with the water, ginger and Biosalt and bring to the boil. Simmer for about 25 minutes. Meanwhile, wash and chop the leek, then add this to the pan. Simmer for a further 15 minutes, adjusting the water if necessary, until the vegetables are tender.

Liquidize in the blender and serve hot with the chives sprinkled on top.

Serves 4 to 6

Vegetable and fruit juices

The very best way to take vitamins and minerals is from freshly extracted vegetable and fruit juices. It is well worth investing in a good electric juicer, because the health benefits are considerable. Raw plants contain other vital ingredients such as essential oils and bitters, hormones and enzymes, many of which are destroyed or altered with cooking. It is thought that these factors influence health by, for example, improving digestive function and boosting immunity. Indeed, much has still to be discovered by scientists, but there is no question that they are wonderfully good for you. Since they are highly concentrated, you will need to drink only one small glass at once.

You will have fun inventing different mixtures. Here are some ideas.

Carrot and Spinach Extremely rich in the antioxidant vitamins A (as beta-carotene) and C, therefore offering protection against cancer and ageing. Carotenoids are also important for the health of the eyes: studies at the Human Research Center on Aging at Tufts University in Boston proved that people over 40 years who had high carotenoid levels in their blood were less than one-fifth as likely to develop cataracts as those with low levels. The folic acid present is important for pregnant women.

    2lb (1kg) carrots, scrubbed
    1 dsp lemon juice
    12 oz (375g) spinach, washed
    1 bunch of watercress

Chop the carrots into chunks and feed through the extractor. Add the lemon juice. Then feed in the spinach and watercress along with a little water. Blend together and drink immediately.
Makes about 1 pint (570ml)

Beetroot and Cucumber Beetroot is reputedly good for the blood and is a useful cleanser. The leaves have hormonal properties, in addition to many minerals, that improve fertility and assist women through menstruation and the menopause, so juice these also. The cucumber will help to rid the system of uric acid and is thus of advantage to those with gout or rheumatism. Its high sulphur content promotes hair growth.

    2 lb (1kg) beetroot with tops, scrubbed
    2 medium cucumbers, washed
    4 sprigs of mint

Chop the vegetables into conveniently sized pieces and feed through the extractor. Blend for a few seconds with the mint and drink straight away.
Makes about 1^1/$_2$ pints (845ml)

Cabbage and Grape Cabbage juice is known to be very protective against stomach ulcers.

    1 lb (500g) young cabbage, washed

    1 1/2 lb (750g) grapes

Roughly chop the cabbage leaves and feed through the extractor together with a little filtered water. Juice the grapes and blend together.

Makes about 1 1/4 pints (720ml)

Salads and dressings

A salad a day will surely keep the doctor away. Include raw organic root and leaf vegetables for a wide variety of unadulterated nutrients. Delicious served with one of the pâtés or dips described below.

Vitamin C Salad Marvellous for keeping infections at bay and for its anti-ageing and cancer-fighting properties.

    1 small crisp lettuce

    1/2 bunch of watercress

    2 large oranges

    1/2 green pepper, sliced

    1/2 red pepper, sliced

    2 tomatoes, sliced

    8 oz (250g) broccoli florets

    1 small onion, thinly sliced

Wash the lettuce and watercress, shake dry and arrange the leaves in a bowl. Peel the oranges and place the segments with the other ingredients on the leaves. Add French Dressing to taste (see page 323).

Serves 4

Walnut Coleslaw Walnuts are good for the heart.

    12 oz (375g) red cabbage, shredded

    4 medium carrots, grated

    1 small turnip, grated

    4 oz (125g) walnuts

1 tsp caraway seeds
½ pint (275ml) Tofu Mayonnaise (see page 323)

Toss the vegetables, nuts and seeds in the mayonnaise.
Serves 4

Avocado and Pistachio Avocados, if eaten regularly, reduce blood cholesterol, according to a recent issue of *Doctor* magazine. In a three-week trial involving two groups of women, levels fell by 8.2 per cent in those who were on a high-avocado diet. This salad is a well-balanced meal in itself, containing protein as well as essential fatty acids, vitamins and minerals.

2 heads of chicory
8 young dandelion leaves
2 avocados, peeled and sliced
2 pawpaw, peeled and sliced
4 oz (125g) pistachio nuts
¼ pint (150ml) French Dressing (see page 323)
½ tsp grated root ginger
3 oz (90g) black olives

Wash the chicory and dandelion leaves and arrange in a bowl with the fruit slices. Toss the nuts in the French Dressing along with the ginger. Garnish with the olives.
Serves 4

Sprout Salad It is very easy to sprout beans and seeds in a large glass jar on the windowsill, providing fresh, organically grown, tasty ingredients for salads at a cheap price. They are also packed with nutrients which, due to enzyme activity, increase at an astonishing rate with germination. Just sprinkle some seeds or beans in the bottom of the jar, cover the top with a piece of muslin then secure with a rubber band. Cover with filtered water and leave to soak overnight, drain off, then rinse three times a day. They will soon be ready to eat. Start with alfalfa, which is guaranteed to succeed.

4 oz (125g) alfalfa sprouts

4 oz (125g) fenugreek sprouts
1 box of cress
6 tbsp Yoghurt Dressing (see below)

Mix together the sprouts and cress, then toss them in the dressing.

Serves 3 to 4

Tofu Mayonnaise Increases protein content of salads.

12 oz (375g) silken tofu
2 tbsp cold-pressed sunflower oil
2 tbsp cider vinegar
2 tbsp lemon juice
1 tbsp chopped chives
1 tsp mustard

Put all the ingredients into the liquidizer goblet and blend until smooth.

Makes about $^2/_3$ pint (380ml)

French Dressing Since plant oils are one of the best sources of vitamin E, salad dressings are a useful way to obtain this important antioxidant. In a study of 500 middle-aged men, Dr Riemersma of Edinburgh University found that those with the lowest blood levels of vitamin E were two and a half times more likely to develop angina than the men with the highest levels. As for the cider vinegar, this is a well-tried remedy for gout.

6 tbsp cold-pressed sunflower oil
2 tbsp cider vinegar
1 clove garlic, crushed
1 tsp tarragon

Place the ingredients in a screw-topped jar and shake.

Yoghurt Dressing Gives a tangy flavour.

$^1/_4$ pint (150ml) goat's milk (or soya) yoghurt
grated rind and juice of $^1/_4$ lemon
1 tbsp spring onions, chopped

$^1/_2$ tsp clear honey

Whisk all the ingredients together.

Makes about $^1/_3$ pint (190ml)

Pâtés and dips

These provide protein that is low in saturated fat. See also 'The complementary dairy' for a cheese substitute which is delicious with salads.

Hummus A mineral-rich recipe, valuable for the iron, potassium and calcium.

    8 oz (250g) chickpeas, soaked overnight
    4 tbsp cold-pressed olive oil
    juice of 2 lemons and grated rind of 1
    3 tbsp dark tahini
    5 cloves garlic, crushed
    dash of Tamari

Boil the chickpeas rapidly for 5 minutes in a large pan. Discard the water and boil up again, cover and then simmer until soft (at least 1 hour). Put the other ingredients into a food processor or blender and liquidize, adding the chickpeas gradually and some of the cooking water as necessary to form a smooth paste.

Serves 6

Mushroom Pâté Mushrooms offer worthwhile amounts of niacin (vitamin B_3) – good for the digestion as well as hypertension – folic acid and potassium.

    1 onion, finely chopped
    2 cloves garlic, finely chopped
    2 tbsp olive oil
    1 lb (500g) mushrooms, chopped
    $^1/_2$ tsp nutmeg
    $^1/_2$ tsp ground cloves
    1 tbsp peanut butter
    juice of $^1/_2$ lemon

¹/₄ pint (150ml) soya milk

Fry the onion and garlic in the oil until transparent. Add the mushrooms and spices and continue to cook until done. Put in the blender with the other ingredients and liquidize to a smooth paste, adjusting the soya milk as necessary. Allow to cool.

Serves 4

Lentil Pâté Serve with wholemeal rolls, Ryvita or oatcakes to provide complete usable protein. Lentils are a good source of iron and potassium.

8 oz (250g) brown lentils
1¹/₂ pints (845ml) filtered water
1 onion, chopped
1 tsp sage
8 oz (250g) cooking apples, chopped
1 oz (30g) ghee (see 'Healthy cooking tips', page 305)
1 dsp dark tahini
To garnish:
sprigs of parsley

Check through the lentils for any small pieces of grit. Wash, then put them in a large pan with the water and simmer (partly covered) until soft.

Meanwhile cook the onion and sage in the ghee for about 3 minutes in a large frying pan. Add the apples and continue to cook, stirring, until they fall to a pulp. Combine this with the lentils and stir in the tahini.

Pile into a pâté dish and chill. Decorate with parsley sprigs.

Serves 4 to 6

Fish Terrine Excellent for the blood vessels.

12 oz (350g) kale
1 lb (500g) cooked salmon
grated rind and juice of 1 lemon
8 oz (250g) low-fat cottage cheese

325

Select a few large leaves of the kale and steam briefly. Shred the other leaves.

Oil a 2-lb (1-kg) loaf tin and line it with the steamed kale, leaving some for the top.

Remove the skin and bones from the fish and blend the flesh in the food processor with the lemon and cottage cheese. Add the shredded kale. Spoon the mixture into the lined tin, making a top with the spare leaves. Refrigerate for an hour before turning out.
Serves 6

The complementary dairy

Soya milk is now readily available in many supermarkets as well as health food shops, and it is a useful very low-fat substitute for cow's milk. However, it does contain less calcium, so it is best to purchase the enriched variety.

Soya Yoghurt This can be produced quite easily at home, especially if you have an electric maker that will remain at the correct temperature overnight. Otherwise you can use a large Thermos flask. The most beneficial yoghurt contains the live culture *Lactobacillus acidophilus* or *L. bulgaricus*.

   1 pint (570ml) soya milk
   1½ tbsp starter culture (or 2 tbsp bio-yoghurt)

Boil up the soya milk, stirring, then take off the heat and allow to cool to hand-warm. Add a little of the milk to the culture and dissolve. Stir this back into the pan. Pour into the containers and fit into the yoghurt maker, or fill a Thermos flask. Leave at this same hand-warm temperature overnight.

Nut Milk For anyone allergic to cow's milk, this is a tasty alternative. Nuts, seeds and cereals can be varied: try cashew and sesame.

   3 oz (90g) ground hazelnuts
   3 oz (90g) fine oatmeal

¾ pint (425ml) spring water

Liquidize in a blender and leave for 1 hour. Strain through a sieve and retain the pulp for use in baking.

Makes about 1 pint (570ml)

Soya Cream Really delicious and without cholesterol.

    6 oz (180g) firm tofu
    1 tbsp cold-pressed sunflower oil
    ¼ pint (150ml) soya milk
    2 tbsp apple juice
    1 tbsp vanilla essence

Put the ingredients in the blender and liquidize until smooth. Adjust the consistency as required.

Makes about ⅔ pint (380ml)

Soya Cheese Here is a tasty alternative to normal cheeses without the saturated fat.

    2 oz (60g) soya flour
    2 oz (60g) ground cashew nuts
    4 oz (125g) non-hydrogenated margarine
    1 clove garlic, crushed
    1 tsp low-salt yeast extract
    2 tsp fresh mixed herbs, chopped finely

Mix together the soya flour and ground nuts in a bowl. Gently melt the margarine in a saucepan, then stir in the garlic and yeast extract. Add the flour and nuts and continue to stir until well blended and thickened. Take off the heat and mix the herbs in.

Put into a small greased mould and chill to set. Turn out when required.

Makes ½ lb (250g)

Baking

Allergic individuals will discover that it is very difficult to purchase breads that do not contain any wheat. Rice or millet flours are always nutritious substitutes.

People with a sweet tooth will be surprised how tempting sugar-free goodies can be, as the ideas offered here will prove. Apple juice and dried fruits make excellent sweeteners. Since baking powder destroys B vitamins, these recipes do not contain it.

Corn Bread Pale yellow, with a pleasant taste.

     1 tsp clear honey
     1 oz (30g) fresh yeast
     1 pint (570ml) warm water
     1 lb (500g) rice flour
     8 oz (250g) cornmeal
     2 oz (60g) caraway seeds
     1 tsp Biosalt
     1 tbsp sunflower oil

Dissolve the honey and the yeast in the warm water. Put three-quarters of the rice flour into a mixing bowl, add the yeast liquid and beat to a smooth batter. Cover with a damp cloth and leave to rise in a warm place for 1 hour.

Mix the remainder of the rice flour with the cornmeal, seeds and Biosalt. Stir in to the risen batter with the oil, then knead for several minutes.

Divide the dough into two and place each into an oiled 1-lb (500-g) loaf tin. Cover again and leave in a warm place until doubled in size (another hour).

Bake in a preheated oven at 425°F/220°C (gas mark 7) for 35 minutes then a further 10 minutes out of the tins. Allow to cool on a wire rack.

Makes two 1-lb (500-g) loaves

Pumpernickel This classic German bread is free of both wheat and yeast, and is dense in texture. The molasses provides a substantial amount of iron as well as calcium, of particular benefit to vegetarians.

     1½ lb (750g) rye flour
     8 oz (250g) fine oatmeal

328

1 tsp Biosalt
4 tbsp black molasses
1¼ pints (725ml) hot water

Sift the flours with the salt in a large mixing bowl. Melt the molasses in 1 pint (570ml) of the hot water and stir in to the flours, adding extra water if necessary, to form a soft dough.

Divide the mixture into two and put each half into an oiled 6-inch (15-cm) pudding basin. Tie a round of grease-proof paper over each, putting in a pleat to allow for expansion. Place each basin in a pan of hot water, cover and steam over a low heat for around 4 hours, topping up the water occasionally.

When done, turn out on to a wire rack to cool. Serve thinly sliced.

Makes two 2-lb (1-kg) loaves

Date Squares Surprisingly sweet, but sugar-free.
8 oz (250g) dates, chopped
¼ pint (150ml) apple juice
4 oz (125g) non-hydrogenated margarine
4 oz (125g) ground hazelnuts
2 tbsp clear honey
4 oz (125g) rice flour
6 oz (180g) millet flakes

Put the dates and apple juice in a small pan and gently stir over a low heat until soft.

Melt the margarine and work this into the remaining ingredients to form a crumbly mixture.

Grease a 7-inch (18-cm) square baking tin and press half the crumble into the bottom. Spread the date mixture over this and cover with the remaining crumble. Press down.

Bake for about 35 minutes at 350°F/180°C (gas mark 4). Allow to cool then cut into squares.

Makes about 16

Special Fruit Cake This contains no sugar, eggs or wheat, but is scrumptious nonetheless. Soya flour and arrowroot combined with water have the same binding power as eggs and are equally nutritious.

  4 fl oz (100ml) sunflower oil
  4 fl oz (100ml) clear honey
  2 oz (60g) soya flour
  1 oz (30g) arrowroot
  $\frac{1}{2}$ pint (275ml) water
  1 tbsp sherry
  grated rind and juice of 1 orange
  grated rind and juice of 1 lemon
  2 oz (60g) flaked almonds
  2 oz (60g) apricots, chopped
  2 oz (60g) dried figs, chopped
  4 oz (125g) dates, chopped
  2 tsp mixed spice
  10 oz (310g) brown rice flour
  1$\frac{1}{2}$ lb (750g) mixed sultanas, currants and raisins

Cream together the oil and honey in a large bowl. Mix the soya flour and arrowroot with the water and beat into the oil and honey, adding the sherry and rind and juice of the orange and lemon. Stir in the almonds, apricots, figs and dates.

Sift the spice into the flour and gradually stir into the soya mixture along with the rest of the dried fruits. Spoon into a lined 8-inch (20-cm) cake tin and cover the top with grease-proof paper, making a couple of slits to let out the steam.

Bake at 300°F/150°C (gas mark 2) for 3$\frac{1}{4}$ hours. Cool a while before turning out on to a wire rack.
Makes one 8-inch (20-cm) round cake

Vegetables

Light steaming or quick stir-frying will ensure maximum retention of goodness. Remember that vegetables should form the main part of your dinner and that eating them every day is an important aspect of your healthy food programme. There is no need to add salt as most already contain sodium.

Roast Garlic The flavour softens with the cooking and is wonderful squeezed on to warm wholemeal bread or vegetable sticks. A choice antidote to heart disease.

    2 large whole garlic bulbs
    2 tbsp olive oil

Remove the papery covering at the top of each bulb and place upright on a baking dish. Drip the oil over the bulbs and cook in the oven at 350°F/180°C (gas mark 4) for $\frac{1}{2}$ hour, basting occasionally.

Serves 2

Baked Stuffed Onions When baked in the oven, onions retain all their juicy goodness. Excellent for the cardio-vascular system.

    4 large onions
    3 tbsp olive oil
    4 oz (125g) mushrooms, chopped small
    1 tsp thyme
    1 tsp marjoram
    4 oz (125g) ground hazelnuts
    1 oz (30g) wheatgerm
    dash of Tamari

Without peeling, put the onions in an ovenproof dish, and cover with greaseproof paper and bake at 350°F/180°C (gas mark 4) until soft (about 1 hour 40 minutes).

Meanwhile, pour the oil into a frying pan and sauté the mushrooms with the herbs. Set aside.

Remove the onions from the oven, cut off their tops and take off their skins. Scoop out the centres, chop these and add to the mushrooms along with the other ingredi-

331

ents. Mix well. Stuff the mixture into the onions, replace their tops and return to the oven for 30 minutes.

These are a meal in themselves. Serve with a tomato sauce and crisp salad.
Serves 4

Gingery Greens Dark-green vegetables offer many benefits: they contain folic acid, a must for pregnant women since it guards against abnormalities in the foetus; they are also high in potassium, which protects against hypertension and is important for the nervous system and the muscles; they supply cancer-fighting carotenoids; moreover they contribute fibrous bulk, ideal for slimmers, and very healthy for the colon. Brazil nuts are rich in that cancer-fighting trace element selenium.

8 oz (250g) spring greens
8 oz (250g) purple-sprouting broccoli
8 oz (250g) spinach
filtered water for steaming
1 tbsp dark sesame oil or olive oil
1 tbsp grated fresh root ginger
1 clove garlic, crushed
1 tsp cornflour
1 tbsp Tamari
3 or 4 spring onions, sliced finely
2 oz (60g) brazil nuts, chopped
1 oz (30g) pine nuts

Wash and trim the vegetables, then shred finely. Steam for about 3 minutes and reserve the juice.

Heat the oil in a large pan, add the ginger and garlic and cook for 1 minute. Add the vegetables and stir-fry quickly for a further minute.

Using a small bowl, mix together the cornflour with the Tamari and 4 tbsp of the vegetable water. Pour this into the greens and bring to the boil, stirring all the time. Cover the pan and simmer over a low heat, stirring

332

occasionally, for about 4 minutes until just done. The vegetables should retain their colour and still be a little crisp.

Toss the spring onions and nuts into the vegetables.

Serves 4

Cauliflower Curry Spices contain many minerals, including calcium, iron, magnesium, phosphorus, potassium and sodium, and most offer vitamins A, B$_3$ and a little C. Hot peppers have been a cure for respiratory problems in Chinese traditional medicine for centuries and modern research now bears out their curative powers. Dr Irwin Ziment of the University of California in Los Angeles has noticed that Hispanic populations who eat fiery foods regularly are less likely to develop bronchitis and emphysema. He links this therapeutic effect with the capsaicin contained in the peppers.

> 1 onion, chopped
> 1 clove garlic, crushed
> 2 tbsp olive oil
> 1 tsp ground turmeric
> $^1/_2$ tsp mustard powder
> $^1/_2$ tsp ground ginger
> $^1/_2$ tsp chilli powder
> 3 tbsp vegetable stock
> florets of 1 medium cauliflower
> 1 tsp garam masala

Fry the onion and garlic in the oil, using a large pan, until transparent. Stir in the turmeric, mustard, ginger and chilli powders and cook for 1 minute. Then include the cauliflower and vegetable stock. Cover and simmer gently until nearly done. Sprinkle in the garam masala, stir and continue to simmer for another couple of minutes.

Serve with Dhal (see page 334) and brown rice.

Serves 4

Main courses

These need to provide you with good-quality protein in addition to vitamins and minerals, so refer to the information concerning essential amino acids in chapter 3. Remember that if you are choosing plant proteins, you need to combine at least two types in the same meal, for example beans with rice.

Dhal According to recent research by Dr Ann Kennedy at Harvard University in the USA, legumes contain 'protease inhibitors' that seem to block the activities of certain enzymes that encourage the growth of cancer, especially of the colon, liver and lung. They also consist of complex carbohydrates that help to steady blood sugar.

12 oz (375g) red lentils
1¼ pints (720ml) filtered water
1½ onions, sliced
½ tsp ground turmeric
1 oz (30g) ghee
1 small red chilli, finely chopped
½ tsp cumin seeds
4 cloves garlic, crushed
1 inch (2.5cm) root ginger, grated
2 tomatoes, skinned and chopped
To garnish:
fresh coriander leaves

Remove any grit from the lentils and put them in a large pan with the water, half the onions and the turmeric. Bring to the boil, then simmer until done (about 20 minutes).

Using a small frying pan, sauté the remaining onion in the ghee until transparent. Meanwhile mix the spices to a paste, then add these to the onion and fry for 2 minutes, stirring. Put this mixture into the large pan with the lentils and include the tomatoes. Stir and simmer for a further 5 minutes.

Serve with brown rice. It is excellent with the Cauliflower Curry.

Serves 4

Millet Rissoles with Peanut Sauce Whole grains are extremely versatile and can be eaten at any meal in different forms: in breakfast cereal, baking or as a main course, as here. They are important for their B vitamins as well as dietary fibre. An egg is not necessary to bind the mixture; arrowroot and soya flour mixed to a paste with water are equally efficient.

To ensure protein complementarity, include peas or beans in the meal.

> 8 oz (250g) millet
> 1¼ pints (725ml) filtered water
> ½ tsp each of basil, oregano, sage and ground bay leaf
> 1 small onion, finely chopped
> ½ red pepper, finely chopped
> 2 cloves garlic, crushed
> 2 tbsp olive oil
> 1 dsp arrowroot
> 1 dsp soya flour
> 2 tbsp sugar-free peanut butter
> 1 tbsp chopped fresh parsley
> oatmeal to coat
> *For the sauce*:
> 1 oz (30g) non-hydrogenated margarine
> 1½ tbsp barley flour (or brown rice flour)
> ½ pint (275ml) warmed soya milk
> 1½ tbsp sugar-free peanut butter
> dash of Tabasco sauce

Using a large pan, bring the millet to the boil in the water together with the herbs. Lower the heat and simmer until done, stirring to prevent sticking, and adjusting water if necessary.

Fry the onion, pepper and garlic in 1 tbsp of oil until soft. Mix the arrowroot and soya flour to a paste with a little water, then stir into the millet with all the other ingredients except the oatmeal. Allow to cool.

Form into rissoles and roll in the oatmeal. Fry gently in the remaining oil until golden.

To make the sauce: Melt the margarine in a small pan, sprinkle in the flour and cook for 3 minutes, stirring. Add the soya milk a little at a time, bringing to the boil. Simmer and stir for a further 3 minutes. Mix in the peanut butter and Tabasco.

Pour the sauce over the rissoles and serve hot.

Makes 9

Quorn Stir-fry If you can obtain it, Quorn is a worthwhile protein-rich vegetarian substitute for meat. It is also high in fibre and low in fat. Ask your local supermarket or health food store to stock it. Alternatively the recipe works just as well with a block of tofu cut into chunks.

  8 oz (250g) Quorn chunks
  3 tbsp soya sauce
  2 tbsp olive oil
  1 medium onion, chopped
  2 cloves garlic, crushed
  1 inch (2.5cm) root ginger, grated
  2 courgettes, diced
  1 green pepper, sliced
  1 red pepper, sliced
  4 oz (125g) mushrooms, sliced
  8 oz (250g) beansprouts
  1 tbsp polenta (maize meal)
  5 tbsp filtered water

Marinate the Quorn in the soya sauce for 20 minutes. Meanwhile heat the oil in a large frying pan or wok and fry the onion, garlic and ginger for 3 minutes. Add the Quorn, courgettes and peppers and stir-fry for a further 3 minutes, then include the mushrooms and beansprouts and continue to cook until just done.

Mix the polenta with the water until it forms a smooth paste. Pour into the vegetables and stir until the juices form a thickened sauce.

Serve with a boiled grain, such as couscous or quinoa (but be careful to pick out any small stones first if you use this).

Serves 4

Three Beans Feast Beans are remarkable at regulating blood levels of insulin and blood sugar and are therefore particularly recommended for diabetics. The double boiling should avoid any problems with flatulence. Just to make sure, chew a few caraway seeds before your meal.

  4 oz (125g) haricot beans, soaked overnight
  4 oz (125g) red kidney beans, soaked overnight
  8 oz (250g) French beans
  4 cloves garlic, chopped finely
  1 onion, chopped
  2 tbsp olive oil
  1½ lb (750g) tomatoes, skinned and chopped
  2 tbsp chopped parsley
  2 tsp basil
  1 tsp paprika

Boil up the soaked beans fast for 10 minutes in a large pan, drain off, replace water and bring to the boil again. Simmer until soft (about ¾ hour) and drain when done. Meanwhile cut the French beans into 2-inch (5-cm) sections and steam them for 3 minutes.

In a large pan sauté the garlic and onion until transparent. Stir in the tomatoes, parsley, basil and paprika and cook for 5 minutes. Add all the beans to the pan and cook for a further 5 minutes.

Serve with brown rice, couscous or quinoa.

Serves 4 to 6

Nut Roast Ingredients are the same as for 'Nut Sausages' above.

Mix them together, press into an oiled 1-lb (500-g) loaf tin, cover the top with grease-proof paper, and bake at 350°F/180°C (gas mark 4) for about ¾ hour.

Serve with a Marmite gravy, jacket potato and lightly steamed broccoli.

Serves 3

Tofu Bake A very nourishing high-protein dish that is low in fat.

    1 onion, chopped
    2 cloves garlic, crushed
    2 tbsp olive oil
    3 courgettes, chopped small
    1 lb (500g) firm tofu, crumbled
    4 oz (125g) oatmeal
    3 tomatoes, chopped
    3 tbsp soya sauce
    3 tbsp tomato purée
    ½ tsp cayenne pepper
    1 tsp mustard powder
    1 tbsp chopped fresh basil
    2 tsp rosemary

Sauté the onion and garlic in the oil using a large pan until transparent. Add the courgettes and cook for a further 5 minutes. Stir in the remaining ingredients and mix well. Grease a 2-lb (1-kg) loaf tin and press the mixture into it. Cover with grease-proof paper and bake for 1 hour at 350°F/180°C (gas mark 4).

Goes well with a tomato sauce, jacket potatoes and a lightly steamed green vegetable.

Serves 4 to 6

Oregano Mackerel This is the best fish of all for the heart, containing more of that magic ingredient omega-3 than any other.

> 2 mackerel fillets
> 2 tbsp lemon juice
> 1 tbsp dried oregano

Rub the lemon juice into both sides of the fish and sprinkle the oregano over each fillet. Cook under a medium grill for about 8 minutes.

Excellent with brown rice and a side salad.

Serves 2

Desserts

The simplest and healthiest conclusion to your dinner is a piece of fresh fruit. However, there will be times when you want to present something more interesting, such as the recipes suggested here. Old favourites such as rice pudding can be made more nourishing by using brown rice and sweetening with honey. It is best to avoid sickly concoctions including pastries even though they may look tempting.

Kiwi Delight Kiwi fruits contain more vitamin C than oranges. As for agar flakes, these are derived from seaweed and therefore offer many useful minerals, including iron.

> 3 tbsp agar flakes
> 1 pint (570ml) orange juice
> 2 kiwi fruits, peeled and sliced
> 8 black grapes, halved

In a small pan dissolve the agar flakes in $\frac{1}{4}$ pint (150ml) of the orange juice by bringing it to the boil, while stirring. Reduce heat and simmer for 5 minutes, continuing to stir. Remove from the stove, add the remaining orange juice and mix well.

Place the slices of kiwi fruit into four small glass dishes. Pour the juice over them and allow to set into jellies in the refrigerator. Garnish with the grape halves.

Delectable with Soya Cream (see 'The complementary dairy' page 327).
Serves 4

Peach Crumble Peaches supply a wide range of nutrients including iron, potassium and sulphur (needed for lustrous hair), plus vitamin A and pantothenic acid, both of which are important for immune function. Cinnamon helps to boost the performance of insulin, according to Dr Richard Anderson, biochemist at the US Department of Agriculture's Human Nutrition Research Center in Maryland, so should be of benefit to diabetics.

    6 oz (180g) dried peaches, soaked overnight
    2 pears, sliced
    2 oz (60g) non-hydrogenated margarine
    12 oz (375g) medium oatmeal
    3 tbsp sunflower oil
    1 tbsp clear honey
    3 oz (90g) chopped walnuts
    2 oz (60g) sesame seeds
    1 tsp cinnamon

Simmer the peaches in $^1/_2$ pint (275ml) of the soaking water until soft. Put the pear slices in a greased ovenproof dish and add the peaches, with just enough juice to cover.

Rub the margarine into the oatmeal, then mix in the oil, honey, nuts and seeds. Sprinkle over the fruit. Dust the top with cinnamon.

Bake at 350°F/180°C (gas mark 4) for 25 minutes.

Addresses

Action Against Allergy, 23–24 George Street, Richmond-upon-Thames TW9 1JY

Action on Smoking and Health (ASH), 109 Gloucester Place, London W1H 3PH; tel. 071–935 3519

Action for Research into Multiple Sclerosis (ARMS), 71 Grays Inn Road, London WC1X 8TR; tel. 071–748 8695 (information); 071–568 2255 (counselling)

Alcoholics Anonymous, PO Box 514, 11 Redcliffe Gardens, London SW10 9BQ; tel. 071–352 3001 (or see local phone book)

Alzheimer's Disease Society, Gordon House, 10 Greencoat Place, London SW1P 1PU; tel. 071–306 0606

Arthritic Association, Hill House, Little New Street, London W1X 8HB; tel. 071–491 0233

BACUP (British Association of Cancer United Patients (information and counselling), 3 Bath Place, Rivington Street, London EC2A 3JR; tel 071–613 2121 (information); 071–696 9000 (counselling)

BioMed International (hair analysis), 55 Queen's Road, East Grinstead, Sussex RH19 1BG; tel. 0342 22854

Biolab (nutritional analysis), The Stone House, 9 Weymouth Street, London W1N 6HQ; tel. 071–636 5959

Bristol Cancer Help Centre, Grove House, Cornwallis Grove, Bristol BS8 4PG; tel. 0272 743216

British Association for Counselling (register of practitioners), 1 Regent Place, Rugby, Warwickshire CV21 2JP; tel. 0788 578328

British Diabetic Association, 10 Queen Anne Street, London W1M 9LD; tel. 071–323 1531

British Homoeopathic Association (register of practitioners), 27a Devonshire Street, London W1N 1RJ; tel. 071–935 2163

Complementary Medicine Services (testing for food intolerances), 9 Corporation Street, Taunton, Somerset; tel. 0823 325022

Coronary Prevention Group, Plantation House, Fenchurch Street, London EC3M 3DX; tel. 071–626 4844

Eating Disorders Association, Sackville Place, 44 Magdalen Street, Norwich NR3 1JE; tel. 0603 621414

Frank Roberts Herbal Dispensaries, 91 Newfoundland Road, Bristol BS2 9LT; tel. 0272 428704

Foresight (preconceptual care), The Old Vicarage, Church Lane, Witley, Godalming, Surrey GU8 5PN; tel. 0428 794500

Friends of the Earth, 26–28 Underwood Street, London N1 7QJ; tel. 071–490 1555

General Council and Register of Naturopaths, 6 Netherhall Gardens, London NW3 5RR; tel. 071–435 8728

Institute for Complementary Medicine (holds register of practitioners), Unit 4, Tavern Quay, Plough Way, Surrey Quays, London SE16 1AA; tel. 071–237 5165

Institute for Optimum Nutrition (training and therapy), Blades Court, Deodar Road, London SW15 2NU; tel. 081–877 9993

Larkhall/Green Farm (nutritional supplements by mail order), 225 Putney Bridge Road, London SW15 2PY; tel. 081–874 1130

London Lighthouse (Aids support), 111–117 Lancaster Road, London W11 1QT; tel. 071–792 1200

ME Action Campaign, PO Box 1302, Wells BA5 2WE; tel. 0749 670799

The Multiple Sclerosis Society, 25 Effie Road, London SW6 1EE; tel. 071–736 6267

National Asthma Campaign (list of nationwide support groups), Providence House, Providence Place, London N1 0NT; tel. 071–226 2260

National Eczema Society, Tavistock House East, Tavistock Square, London WC1H 9SR; tel. 071–388 4097

National Institute of Medical Herbalists (register of

practitioners), 9 Palace Gate, Exeter, Devon EX1 1JA; tel.
0392 426022

Nature's Best (health products), 1 Lamberts Road, Tunbridge
Wells, Kent TN2 3EQ; tel. 0892 539595 (enquiries); 0892
534143 (orders)

Neal's Yard Remedies (herbs by mail order), 5 Golden Cross,
Cornmarket Street, Oxford OX1 3EU; tel. 0865 245436

The Nutrition Society, 10 Cambridge Court, Shepherd's Bush
Road, London W12 7NG; tel. 071–602 0228

Nutri Centre (nutritional supplements), Hale Clinic, 7 Park
Crescent, London W1N 3HE; tel. 071–436 5122/071–631
0156

Relate (Marriage Guidance) – see local phone book or tel. 0788
573241

Relaxation for Living, 29 Burwood Park Road, Walton-on-
Thames, Surrey KT12 5LH

Society for the Promotion of Nutritional Therapy, The
Enterprise Centre, Station Parade, Eastbourne BN21 1BE;
tel. 0323 430203

The Soil Association (organic gardening), 86 Colston Street,
Bristol BS1 5BB; tel. 0272 290661

Women's Nutritional Advisory Service, PO Box 268, Lewes,
East Sussex BN7 2NQ; tel. 0273 487366

N.B. From 16 April 1995 all area codes starting with 0 will be 01.

Bibliography

General

Brown, Dr J. A. C. (rev. ed. Hastin-Bennett, Dr A. M.), *Pears Medical Encyclopaedia* (Sphere Books 1977, 1983)

Davies, Dr Stephen & Stewart, Dr Alan, *Nutritional Medicine* (Pan Books 1987).

Davis, Adelle, *Let's Eat Right To Keep Fit* (George Allen & Unwin 1966)

Davis, Adelle, *Let's Get Well* (Unwin Paperbacks 1974)

Davis, Adelle, *Let's Stay Healthy* (Unwin Paperbacks 1983)

Holford, Patrick, *The Family Nutrition Work Book* (Thorsons 1988)

Holford, Patrick, *Optimum Nutrition* (ION Press 1992)

Kirschmann, John D. (3rd ed. Dunne, Lavon J.), *Nutrition Almanac* (McGraw-Hill 1990)

Mackean, D. G. *Human Life* (John Murray 1988)

Pearce, Evelyn C., *Anatomy and Physiology for Nurses* (Wolfe 16th ed. 1975)

Peterson, Vicki, *Eat Your Way to Health* (Allen Lane 1981)

Quillin, Patrick, *Healing Nutrients* (Penguin 1989)

Werbach, Melvyn R., *Nutritional Influences on Illness* (Thorsons 1989)

Review Journals

International Clinical Nutrition Review ('Integrated Therapies', PO Box 370, Manly 2095, New South Wales, Australia)

Nutrition Abstracts and Reviews, Series A, Human and Experimental (Commonwealth Agricultural Bureau, Farnham Royal, Slough SL2 3BN)

Chapter 1

Cartwright, Frederick F., *Disease and History* (Rupert Hart-Davis 1972)

Cowie, Leonard W., *The Black Death and Peasants' Revolt* (Wayland 1972)

Kaufman, W., 'The use of vitamin therapy to reverse certain concomitants of aging', *Journal of the American Geriatric Society* (**3**: 927, 1955)

Lesser, Dr Michael, *Nutrition and Vitamin Therapy* (Thorsons 1985)

Chapter 2

Barnes, B. & Colquhoun, V., *The Hyperactive Child* (Thorsons 1984)

Birch, L., 'Children's preferences for high-fat foods', *Nutrition Reviews* (**50**, 9: 249–255, 1992)

Block, G., Patterson, B. & Subar, A., 'Fruit, vegetables and cancer prevention: a review of the epidemiological evidence', *Nutrition and Cancer* (**18**, 1: 1–29, 1992)

Boeing, H. et al, 'Dietary carcinogens and the risk for glioma and meningioma in Germany', *International Journal of Cancer* (**53**: 561–565, 1993)

Cannon, Geoffrey, *The Politics of Food* (Century Hutchinson 1987)

Diamond, Jared, *The Rise and Fall of the Third Chimpanzee* (Vintage 1992)

Keimis-Tavantzis, D. J. & White, A. A., 'Cardiovascular disease risk assessment among central Maine adolescents: blood lipids and lipoproteins', *Journal of Applied Nutrition* (**44**, 3/4: 22–34, 1992)

Murata, M., 'Nutrition for the young – its current problems', *Nutrition and Health* (**8**, 2/3: 143–152, 1992)

National Advisory Committee on Nutrition Education (NACNE), *Proposals for Nutritional Guidelines for Health Education in Britain* (Health Education Council 1983)

Nilsson, Lennart, *The Body Victorious* (Faber & Faber 1987)

Ponting, Clive, *A Green History of the World* (Penguin 1992)

Ross, Philip, E., 'Eloquent remains', *Scientific American* (May 1992)

Singh, R. B., et al., 'The diet and moderate exercise trial

(DAMET): results after 24 weeks', *Acta Cardiologica* (**47**, 6: 543–557, 1992)

UK Government White Paper, *The Health of the Nation* (HMSO 1993)

Vidailhet, M., 'Europe and the prevention of rickets', *Cahiers de Nutrition et de Diététique* (**28**, 4: 213–216, 1993)

Walker, Caroline & Cannon, Geoffrey, *The Food Scandal* (Century 1985)

Walker, Martin, *Dirty Medicine* (Slingshot 1993)

Chapter 3

Greer, Rita & Woodward, Robert, *The Good Nutrients Guide* (J. M. Dent & Sons Ltd 1985)

Jukes, Thomas H., 'Vitamins' in *Collier's Encyclopedia* (174–179, 1990)

Lappé, Frances Moore, *Diet for a Small Planet* (Ballantine 1971)

Mayer, Jean, 'Nutrition' in *World Book Encyclopedia* (630–636, 1990)

Mayes, Adrienne, *The A–Z of Nutritional Health* (Thorsons rev. ed. 1991)

Mindell, Earl, *The Vitamin Bible* (Arlington 2nd ed. 1985)

Ministry of Agriculture, Fisheries and Food, *Manual of Nutrition* (Her Majesty's Stationery Office 9th ed. 1985)

Newhouse, Sonia, *Complete Natural Food Facts* (Thorsons 1991)

Rose, Steven, *The Chemistry of Life* (Penguin 3rd ed. 1991)

Chapter 4

Birkin, Michael & Price, Brian, *C For Chemicals* (Green Print 1989)

Bjorneboc, A. & Gea, B., 'Antioxidant status and alcohol-related diseases', *Alcohol and Alcoholism* (**28**: 111–116, 1993)

British Medical Association, *The BMA Guide to Living With Risk* (Penguin 1990)

Ecoropa Information Sheet 20, 'Nuclear Power' (1992)

Eskelson, C. D. et al., 'Modulation of cancer growth by vitamin E and alcohol', *Alcohol and Alcoholism* (**28**: 117–125, 1993)

Friends of the Earth Factsheets: 'The Ozone Crisis' and 'Smokescreen on Air Pollution' (1992)

Holford, Patrick & Barlow, Dr Philip, *How to Protect Yourself from Pollution* (ION Press 1990)

Kenton, Leslie, *10 Day Clean-up Plan* (Vermilion 1992)

Lambert, Dr Barrie, *How Safe is Safe? Radiation Controversies Explained* (Unwin Paperbacks 1990)

Lang, Dr Tim & Clutterbuck, Dr Charlie, *P is for Pesticides* (Ebury Press 1991)

Langsteger, W. et al., 'The impact of geographical, clinical, dietary and radiation-induced features in epidemiology of thyroid cancer', *European Journal of Cancer* (**29**, 11: 1547–1553, 1993)

Lents, James M. & Kelly, William, J. 'Clearing the air in Los Angeles', *Scientific American* (**269**, 4: 18–25, 1993)

National Radiological Protection Board, 'Radon' (At-a-Glance Series 1990)

Odeleye, O. E. & Watson, R. R., 'Role of nutrition in alcoholism', *Journal of Applied Nutrition* (**44**, 1:50–62, 1992)

Rosen, J. F., 'Health effects of lead at low exposure levels', *American Journal of Diseases in Children* (**146**: 1278–1280, 1992)

Chapter 5

Bacon, Fiona, *Good Housekeeping Food Facts* (Ebury Press 1990)

Cartwright, Frederick F., *Disease and History* (Rupert Hart-Davis 1972)

Kenton, Leslie & Susannah, *Raw Energy* (Century Arrow, 1986)

Sanders, Dr Tom & Bazalgette, Peter, *The Food Revolution* (Bantam 1991)

Trickett, Jill, *The Prevention of Food Poisoning* (Stanley Thornes 2nd ed. 1986)

Chapter 6

Fielding, J. & Kehoe, M., 'Different dietary fibre formulations and the irritable bowel syndrome', *Irish Journal of Medical Science* (**153**: 178–180, 1984)

Hunter, J. O. & Alun Jones, V., *Food and the Gut* (Bailliere Tindall 1985)

Ippoliti, A. F. et al., 'The effect of various forms of milk on gastric-acid secretion', *Annals of International Medicine* (**84**: 286–289, 1976)

Kumar, N. et al., 'Effect of milk on patients with duodenal ulcers', *British Medical Journal* (**293**: 666, 1986)

Manning, A. P. et al., 'Wheat fibre and irritable bowel syndrome: a controlled trial', *Lancet* (**2**: 417–418, 1977)

Painter, J., *British Medical Journal* (**2**: 156, 1971)

Robinson, C. H., *Fundamentals of Normal Nutrition* (Macmillan 1978)

Scarfe, Christopher, *How to Improve Your Digestion and Absorption* (ION Press 1989)

Thijs, C. et al., 'Oral contraceptive use and the occurrence of gallstone disease – a case-controlled study', *Preventive Medicine* (**22**: 122–131, 1993)

Yudkin, J., 'Eating and ulcers' (Letter to the editor), *British Medical Journal* (16 Feb. 1980: 483–484)

Chapter 7

Brockis, J. G. et al., 'Vegetarians have 50–60% decreased risk of stones', *British Journal of Urology* (**54**, 6: 590–593, 1982)

Curhan, G. C. et al., 'A prospective study of dietary calcium and other nutrients and the risk of symptomatic kidney stones', *New England Journal of Medicine* (**328**, 12: 833–838, 1993)

Fisk, Dr Peter, *Pocket Guide to Cystitis* (Arlington 1982)

Robertson, W. G., Peacock, M. & Marshall, D. H., 'The prevalence of urinary stone disease in vegetarians', *European Urology* (**8**: 334, 1982)

Yudkin, J., Kang, S. S. & Bruckdorfer, K. R., 'The effects of high dietary sugar', *British Medical Journal* (**2**: 1396, 1980)

Chapter 8

Barboriak, J. J., et al., 'Vitamin E supplements and plasma high-density lipoprotein cholesterol', *American Journal of Clinical Pathology* (**77**: 371–372, 1982)

Belizan, J. M. et al., 'Reduction of blood pressure with calcium supplementation in young adults', *Journal of the American Medical Association* (**249**: 1161–1165, 1983)

Bell, L. et al., 'Cholesterol-lowering effects of calcium carbonate in patients with mild to moderate hypercholesterolemia', *Archives of Internal Medicine* (**152**, 12: 2441–2444, 1992)

Brown, J. J. et al., 'Salt and hypertension', *Lancet* (**i**: 456, 1984)

Burr, M. L., 'Fish and ischaemic heart disease', in *Nutrition and Fitness in Health and Disease* (ed. Simopoulos, A. P.) (49–60) (S. Karger AG, Switzerland 1993)

Durrington, P. N. et al., 'The effect of pectin on serum lipids and lipoproteins, whole-gut transit time and stool weight', *Lancet* (**ii**: 394–396, 1976)

Espinel, C. H., 'The Salt Step Test: its usage in the diagnosis of salt-sensitive hypertension and in the detection of the salt hypertension threshold', *Journal of the American College of Nutrition* (**11**, 5: 526–531, 1992)

Evbuomwan, M. L., 'Effect of garlic (Allium sativum) on the thrombogenic properties of blood on normal and hypercholesterolaemic rats, *Medical Science Research* (**21**: 25–26, 1993)

Goto, Y., 'Changing trends in dietary habits and cardiovascular disease in Japan: an overview', *Nutrition Reviews* (**50**, 12: 398–401, 1992)

Haga, H., 'Effects of dietary magnesium supplementation on diurnal variations of blood pressure and plasma Na+, K+-ATPase activity in essential hypertension', *Japanese Heart Journal* (**33**, 6: 785–801, 1992)

Jain, R. C., 'Onion and garlic in experimental atherosclerosis', *Lancet* (**i**: 1240, 1975)

Leaf, A. & Hallaq, H. A., 'The role of nutrition in the functioning of the cardiovascular system', *Nutrition Reviews* (**50**, 12: 402–406, 1992)

Ornish, D., 'Can lifestyle changes reverse coronary heart disease?' and *Nutrition and Fitness in Health and Disease* (ed. Simopoulos, A. P.) (S. Karger AG, Switzerland 1993)

Preuss, H. G., & Fournier, R. D., 'The effects of sucrose ingestion on blood pressure', *Life Sciences* (**30**: 879–886, 1982)

Rouse, I. L. et al., 'Blood-pressure lowering effect of a vegetarian diet: controlled trial in normotensive subjects', *Lancet* (**i**: 5–10, 1983)

Sabate, J., Fraser, G. E., Burke, K. et al., 'Effects of walnuts on serum lipid levels and blood pressure in normal men', *New England Journal of Medicine* (**328**: 603–607, 1993)

Sachet, P., 'Heart attack: the nutritional paradox of the French', *Revue Laitière Française* (**518**, 68: 1992)

Seltzer, C. C., 'The effect of smoking on blood pressure, *American Heart Journal* (**87**: 558–564, 1974)

Seppanen-Laakso, T. et al., 'Replacement of butter on bread by rapeseed oil and rapeseed-containing margarine: effects on plasma fatty acids composition and serum cholesterol', *British Journal of Nutrition* (**68**, 639–654, 1992)

Stein, P. P. & Black, H. R., 'The role of diet in the genesis and treatment of hypertension', *Medical Clinics of N. America* (**77**, 4: 831–847, 1993)

Chapter 9

Channel 4, *Take a Deep Breath* (Channel 4 Books 1993)

Horiba, F. et al., 'Screening of specific IGE antibodies in early infancy: early diagnosis of food allergy and prediction of bronchial asthma', *Japanese Journal of Pediatric Allergy and Clinical Immunology* (**7**, 1: 39–44, 1993)

Lean, Geoffrey, 'Asthma study may lead to curbs on cars', *Observer* (27 July 1993)

Mihill, Chris, 'Doctors warn of re-emerging threat of TB in inner cities', *Guardian* (29 July 1993)

Mohsenin, L. & Spannhake, R. et al., *American Review of Respiratory Disease* (**127**: 139 & 143, 1983)

Moisan-Petit, V. & Dutau, G., 'Association of dietary and pollen allergies in children', *Revue Française d'Allergologie et d'Immunologie Clinique* (**32**, 3: 129–133, 1992)

Moore, Pete, 'Out of Breath', *Guardian Education* (28 September 1993)

Royal College of Physicians, *Health or Smoking* (Pitmans Medical 1983)

Chapter 10

Anderson, J., *Diabetes – A Practical New Guide to Healthy Living* (Martin Dunitz 1983)

Anderson, R. A. et al., 'Chromium supplementation of humans with hypoglycaemia', *Federal Proceedings* (**43**: 471, 1984)

Budd, M., *Low Blood Sugar* (Thorsons 1983)

Collee, Dr John, 'Sugar's not so sweet', *Observer* (1992)

Quinn, S., 'Diabetes and diet: we are still learning', *Medical Clinics of N. America* (**77**, 4: 773–781, 1993)

Remer, T. & Manz, F., 'Assessment of the iodine status in children aged 2–3 years', *Zeitschrift für Ernährungswissenschaft* (**31**, 4: 278–282, 1992)

Shan, S. et al., 'Flat Glucose Tolerance Test: The significance of the flat G.T.T', *Journal of the Kansas Medical Society* (263–267, November 1975)

Vialettes, B. & Silvestre, P., 'Functional hypoglycaemias of the adult: role of diet in examination and treatment', *Cahiers de Nutrition et de Diététique* (**28**, 3: 173–175, 1993)

Chapter 11

Anderson, Roy M. and May, Robert M., 'Understanding the AIDS pandemic', *Scientific American* (**266**, 5: 20–26)

Berman, Dr Monty, 'Life in the balance: Aids – the neglect of nutrition's vital role', *Guardian* (21 August 1993)

Charles, Rachel, *Mind, Body and Immunity* (Cedar 1993)

Clifford, C. & Kramer, B., 'Diet as risk and therapy for cancer', *Medical Clinics of N. America* (**77**, 4: 725–744, 1993)

Cohen, L. A. et al., 'A hypothesis revisited. A rationale for dietary intervention in post-menopausal breast cancer patients: an update', *Nutrition and Cancer* (**19**: 1–10, 1993)

Corman, L. C., 'The role of diet in animal models of SLE: Possible implications for human lupus', *Seminars in Arthritis and Rheumatism* (**15**, 1: 61–69, 1985)

Crevel, R. W. R. & Saul, J. A. T., 'Review: Linoleic acid and the immune response', *European Journal of Clinical Nutrition* (**46**: 847–855, 1992)

Cuff, P. A., 'Aggressive nutrition support in AIDS', *Topics in Clinical Nutrition* (**7**, 2: 37–45, 1992)

Daniel, Dr Rosy, 'Cancer and Nutrition: The Scientific Evidence', Bristol Cancer Help Centre (1994)

Galland, L., 'Nutrition and candidiasis', *Journal of Orthomolecular Psychiatry* (**14**, 1: 50–60, 1985)

Glasziou, P. P. & Mackerras, E. E. M., 'Vitamin A supplementation in infectious diseases: a meta-analysis', *British Medical Journal* (**306**: 366–370, 1993)

Goodman, Dr Sandra, 'Nutrition and Cancer Database', Bristol Cancer Help Centre (1993)

Graf, E. & Eaton, J. W., 'Review: Suppression of colonic cancer by dietary phytic acid', *Nutrition and Cancer* (**19**, 1: 11–17, 1993)

Grimes, D. S., 'Refined carbohydrates, smooth-muscled spasm and disease of the colon', *Lancet* (**i**: 395–397, 1976)

Hawkes, Nigel, 'Vitamins clue to cancer treatment', *The Times* (15 September 1993)

Hodson, A. H., 'Empirical use of exclusion diets in chronic disorders: discussion paper', *Journal of the Royal Society of Medicine* (**85**: 556–559, 1992)

Holm, L. E. et al., 'Treatment failure and dietary habits in women with breast cancer', *Journal of the National Cancer Institute* (**85**: 32–36, 1993)

Kaplan, Jonathan, 'The curse of Aids cannot be forsworn', *Observer* (12 September 1993)

Keusch, G. T. & Thea, D. M., 'Malnutrition in AIDS', *Medical Clinics of N. America* (**77**, 4: 795–814, 1993)

Kochhar, R. et al., 'Lactose intolerance in idiopathic ulcerative colitis in north Indians', *Indian Journal of Medical Research, Section B* (**98**: 79–82, April 1993)

Nossal, Sir Gustav J. V., 'Life, death and the immune system', *Scientific American* (**269**, 3, 1993)

Prasad, K. N. & Edwards-Prasad, J., 'Vitamin E and cancer prevention: recent advances and future potentials', *Journal of the American College of Nutrition* (**11**, 5: 487–500, 1992)

Rohan, T. E. et al., 'Dietary fibre, vitamins A, C and E, and risk of breast cancer: a cohort study', *Cancer Causes and Control* (**4**, 1: 29–37, 1993)

Savilahti, E. & Kuitunen, M., 'Allergenicity of cow's milk proteins', *Journal of Pediatrics* (**121**: S12-S20, 1992)

Sofronion, Peter, 'HIV: Think positive', *Optimum Nutrition* (**6**, 3: 46–53, 1993)

Swank, R. L., *The Multiple Sclerosis Diet Book* (Doubleday 1977)

Terezhalmy, G. T. et al., 'The use of water soluble bioflavonoid-ascorbic acid complex in the treatment of recurrent herpes labialis', *Oral Surgery, Oral Medicine, Oral Pathology* (**45**: 56–62, 1978)

Thornton, J. R. et al., 'Diet and ulcerative colitis', *British Medical Journal* (293, 2 February 1980)

Vatten, L. J. et al., 'Polyunsaturated fatty acids in serum phospholipids and risk of breast cancer: A case-controlled study from the Janus Serum Bank in Norway', *European Journal of Cancer* (**29A**, 4: 532–538, 1993)

World Cancer Research Fund, *Dietary Guidelines to Lower Your Cancer Risk* (1993)

Chapter 12

Barton-Wright, C. E. & Elliott, W. A., 'The pantothenic acid metabolism of rheumatoid arthritis', *Lancet* (**2**: 862–863, 1963)

Bland, J. H. & Cooper, S. M., 'Osteoarthritis: A review of the cell biology involved and evidence for reversibility', *Seminars in Arthritis and Rheumatology* (**14**, 2: 106–133, 1984)

Chapuy, M. C. et al., 'Vitamin D_3 and calcium to prevent hip fractures in elderly women', *New England Journal of Medicine* (**327**: 1637–1642, 1992)

Darlington, L. G. & Ramsey, N. W., 'Review of dietary therapy for rheumatoid arthritis', *British Journal of Rheumatology* (**32**, 6: 507–514, 1993)

Emmerson, B. J., 'Therapeutics of hyperuricaemia and gout', *Medical Journal of Australia* (**141**: 31–36, 1984)

Goulding, A., Gold, E. & Campbell, A. J., 'Salty foods increase calcium requirements and are a potential risk factor for osteoporosis', *IDF News* (**138**: 16–19, 1993)

Hangarter, W., 'Copper salicylate in rheumatoid arthritis and rheumatism-like degenerative diseases', *Medizinischer Welt* (**31**: 1625, 1980)

Harward, M. P., 'Nutritive therapies for osteoporosis: the role of calcium', *Medical Clinics of N. America* (**77**, 4: 889–898, 1993)

Heaney, R. P. & Recker, R. R., 'Effects of nitrogen, phosphorus and caffeine on calcium balance in women', *Journal of Laboratory and Clinical Medicine* (**99**: 46–55, 1982)

Hernandez-Avila, M. et al., 'Caffeine and other predictors of bone density among pre- and perimenopausal women', *Epidemiology* (**4**, 2: 128–133, 1993)

Lucas, C. and Power, L., 'Dietary fat aggravates active rheumatoid arthritis', *Clinical Research* (**29**, 4: 754A, 1981)

Prince, R. L., 'The role of dietary calcium in the prevention of postmenopausal osteoporosis', *Proceedings of the Nutrition Society of Australia* (**17**: 125–129, 1992)

Schuette, S. A. et al., 'Studies on the mechanism of protein-induced hypercalciuria in older men and women', *Journal of Nutrition* (**110**: 305–315, 1980)

Skoldstam, L., 'Fasting and vegan diet in rheumatoid arthritis', *Scandinavian Journal of Rheumatology* (**15**, 2: 219–221, 1987)

Walker, W. R. & Keats, D. M., 'An investigation of the

therapeutic value of the copper bracelet', *Agents and Actions*
(**6**: 454, 1976)

Chapter 13

Burke, L. M. & Read, R. S. D., 'Dietary supplements in sport',
Sports Medicine (Auckland) (**15**, 1: 43–65, 1993)

Haynes, Antony, 'Peak performance', *Optimum Nutrition* (**7**, 1:
19–24, 1994)

Holt, W. S., Jr, 'Nutrition and athletes', *American Family Physician*
(**47**, 8: 1757–1764, 1993)

Probart, C. K. et al., 'Diet and athletic performance', *Medical
Clinics of N. America* (**77**, 4: 757–772, 1993)

Chapter 14

Campbell, A. J. & McEwen, G. C., 'Treatment of brittle nails and
dry eyes', *British Journal of Dermatology* (**105**: 113, 1981)

David, T. J., Wells, F. E., Sharpe, T. C. & Gibbs, A. C. C., 'Low
serum zinc in children with atopic eczema', *British Journal of
Dermatology* (**111**: 597–601, 1984)

Michaelsson, F., 'Zinc in relation to some skin diseases' in *Zinc
in Human Medicine – Symposium* (eds. Hambridge & Aggett)
(TIL Publications, 1984)

Wright, S. & Burton, J. L., 'Oral evening primrose oil improves
atopic eczema', *Lancet* (**2**: 1120–1122, 1982)

Young, E., 'Food and the skin', *British Nutrition Foundation
Nutrition Bulletin* (**17**, 66: 190–196, 1992)

Chapter 15

Birlouez-Aragon, I. et al., 'Disturbed galactose metabolism in
elderly and diabetic humans is associated with cataract
formation', *Journal of Nutrition* (**123**, 8: 1370–1376, 1993)

Farquharson, Marie (ed.), 'Eye openers', *Here's Health* (30–33,
April 1993)

Knekt, P. et al., 'Serum antioxidant vitamins and risk of cataract',
British Medical Journal (**305**: 1392–1394, 1992)

Whiteside, Dr Mike, 'Glue ear', *Here's Health* (68–69, November
1993)

Chapter 16

Boublik, J. H. et al., 'Coffee contains potent opiate receptor binding activity', *Nature* (**301**: 246–248, 1983)

Bouchard, C., 'Genetics of obesity and its prevention', in *Nutrition and Fitness in Health and Disease* (ed. Simopoulos, A. P.) (49–60) (S. Karger AG, Switzerland 1993)

Douglas, J. et al., 'Effects of a raw food diet on hypertension and obesity', *Southern Medical Journal* (**78**, 7: 841, 1985)

Edwards, K. I., 'Obesity, anorexia, and bulimia', *Medical Clinics of N. America* (**77**, 4: 899–909, 1993)

Gershon, Elliot S. & Reider, Ronald O., 'Major disorders of mind and brain', *Scientific American* (88–95, September 1992)

Holford, Patrick, 'Food for thought', *Optimum Nutrition* (**7**, 1: 48–53, 1994)

Howard, J. S., 'Folate deficiency in psychiatric practice', *Psychosomatics* (**16**: 112–115, 1975)

Hundleby, J. D. & Bourgouin, N. C., 'Generality in the errors of estimation of body image', *International Journal of Eating Disorders* (**13**, 1: 85–92, 1993)

Lissner, L. et al., 'Weight reduction diets and health promotion', *American Journal of Preventive Medicine* (**8**, 3: 154–158, 1992)

Lowndes, R. H. & Mansel, R. E., 'The effects of evening primrose oil on serum lipid levels of normal and obese subjects', *Clinical Uses of Essential Fatty Acids* (37–52, Eden Press, Montreal 1982)

Mahaja, A. N. & Bailey, J. M., 'A platelet phospholipase inhibitor from the medicinal herb feverfew (*tanacetum parthenium*)', *Prostaglandins, Leukortrienes and Medicine* (**8**: 653–660, 1982)

Mellin, L. M. et al., 'Prevalence of disordered eating in girls: a survey of middle-class children', *Journal of the American Dietetic Association* (**92**, 7: 871–853, 1992)

Mikkelsen, E. J., 'Caffeine and schizophrenia', *Behavioural Medicine* (December 1980)

Oski, F. A., 'Iron deficiency in infancy and childhood', *New England Journal of Medicine* (**329**, 3: 190–193, 1993)

Pattichis, K. et al., 'Phenolic substances in red wine and release of platelet 5-hydroxytryptamine', *Lancet* (**341**: 1108, 1993)

Ramchand, C. N. et al., 'RBC and serum folate concentrations in neuroleptic-treated and neuroleptic-free schizophrenic patients', *Journal of Nutritional Medicine* (**3**, 303–309, 1992)

Van Gaal, L. et al., 'Exploratory study of coenzyme Q_{10} in obesity', in Folkers & Yamamura (eds.), *Biomedical and Clinical Aspects of Coenzyme Q* (**4**: 369–373, Elsevier Scientific Publications, Amsterdam 1984)

Vasselli, J. R., 'Carbohydrate ingestion, hypoglycaemia and obesity', *Appetite* (**6**: 53–59, 1985)

Chapter 17

Abraham, G. E., 'Nutrition and the premenstrual tension syndrome', *Journal of Applied Nutrition* (**36**: 103–124, 1984)

Luhby, A. L. et al., 'Pyridoxine and oral contraceptives', *Lancet* (**ii**: 1083, 1970)

Piesse, J. W., 'Nutrition factors in premenstrual syndrome', *International Clinical Nutrition Review* (**4**: 54–81, 1984)

Rushton, Anna, 'Fertility rights', *Optimum Nutrition* (**7**, 1: 29–35, 1994)

Smith, C. J., 'Non-hormonal control of vaso-motor flushing in menopausal patients', *Chicago Journal of Medicine* (7 March 1964)

Chapter 18

Azais-Braesco, V., 'Hypervitaminosis A and teratogenesis. Incidence and mechanisms', *Cahiers de Nutrition et de Diététique* (**28**, 3: 143–150, 1993)

Bower, C., 'Folate and fetal abnormalities: the prevention of neural tube defects', *Proceedings of the Nutrition Society of Australia* (**17**: 198–201, 1992)

Davis, Adelle, (3rd rev. ed. Mandell, Marshall) *Let's Have Healthy Children* (Unwin Paperbacks, 1981)

Halliday, A., 'Infant feeding and neural development', *British Nutrition Foundation Nutrition Bulletin* (**18**: 11–12, 1993)

Hendricks, K. M. and Badruddin, S. H., 'Weaning recommendations: the scientific basis', *Nutrition Reviews* (**5**: 125–133, 1992)

Lawrence, R. A., 'Can we expect greater intelligence from human milk feeding?', *Birth* (**19**, 2: 105–106, 1992)

Neuringer, M., 'Cerebral cortex docosahexaenoic acid is lower in formula-fed than in breast-fed infants', *Nutrition Reviews* (**51**, 8: 238–241, 1993)

Silgur, U. et al., 'Faecal short-chain fatty acids in breast-fed and bottle-fed infants', *Acta Paediatrica* (**82**, 6/7: 536–538)

Simmer, K., 'Aluminium and infants', *Journal of Paediatric Child Health* (29: 80–81, 1993)

Spohr, H. L., 'Prenatal alcohol exposure and long-term developmental consequences', *Lancet* (**341**: 907–910, 1993)

Chapter 19

Castelli, W. P. et al., 'Lipids and risk of coronary heart disease: The Framingham Study', *Annals of Epidemiology* (**2**, 1/2: 23–28, 1992)

Edwardson, J. A. et al., 'Effect of silicon on gastrointestinal absorption of aluminium', *Lancet* (**342**: 211–212, 1993)

Fahn, S., 'A pilot trial of high-dose alpha-tocopherol and ascorbate in early Parkinson's disease', *Annals of Neurology* (**32**: S128-S132, 1992)

Johnson, K. & Kligman, E. W., 'Preventive nutrition: an "optimal" diet for older adults', *Geriatrics* (**47**, 10: 56–60, 1992)

Johnson, K. & Kligman, E. W., 'Preventive nutrition: disease-specific dietary interventions for older adults', *Geriatrics* (**47**, 11: 39–49, 1992)

Mimura, G. et al., 'Nutrition factors for longevity in Okinawa – present and future', *Nutrition and Health* (**8**, 2/3: 159–163, 1992)

Selcoe, Dennis J., 'Aging brain, aging mind', *Scientific American* (96–103, September 1992)

Welin, L. et al., 'Triglycerides and blood glucose are the major coronary risk factors in elderly Swedish men. The study of men born in 1913', *Annals of Epidemiology* (**2**, 1/2: 113–119, 1992)

Whitaker, R., 'Early stage Alzheimer's test', *Today's Life Sciences* (43–44, January 1993)

Chapter 20

Brown, Sarah, *Healthy Living Cookbook* (Dorling Kindersley 1985)

Cranks Restaurant, *The Cranks Recipe Book* (Orion 1993)

Forbes, Dr Alec, *The Bristol Diet* (Century Arrow 1986)

Hill, Diane, *Vegan Vitality* (Thorsons 1987)

Kenton, Leslie & Susannah, *Raw Energy* (Century Arrow 1984)

Mann, Dr Jim, *The Diabetics' Diet Book* (Martin Dunitz 1982)

Rippon, Sadhya, *The Bristol Recipe Book* (Century Hutchinson 1987)

Spoczynska, Joy O. I., *The Wild Foods Cookbook* (Robert Hale 1985)

Wakeman, Alan & Baskerville, Gordon, *The Vegan Cookbook* (Faber & Faber 1986)

Workman, E., Alun Jones, Dr V. & Hunter, Dr J., *The Food Intolerance Diet Book* (Martin Dunitz 1986)

Index

Page references in italics refer to tables and illustrations. Food entries with initial capitals denote recipes described in the book.

361

carnitine 217, 264; L-carnitine 140
carpal tunnel syndrome 212
carrots 31, 50, 51, 67, 235, 238; Carrot and Spinach Juice 320
cars 293; and pollution 77, 148
cartilage 64, 205
cashew nuts 62, 63, 64
cataracts 82, 235–6, 296, 320
catarrh 153, 309
catuaba 261–2
Cauliflower Curry 333
celery 67, 88; celery seeds 208; Celery Seed Tea 307
cells 34–6, 39, 43, 45, 54, 65, 68, 83, 130
cellulose 38, 49
cereals 23; whole 38, 65; see also whole grains
cerebral haemorrhage 296
cheese 41, 45, 46, 47, 48, 247; cottage 46; cream 52; minerals in 61, 63, 64, 65, 67, 68, 203; processed 25; vitamins in 51, 54, 55, 56, 57
chelated minerals 60; chelators 91
chemicals: in body 159–73; contaminating 83–6; household 69–74; garden 72
Chernobyl disaster 78, 79, 80
cherries, Acerola 57
chest pains 136–7, 249
chick peas 66
chicken: amino acids in 45, 46, 47, 48; chromium in 61; and salmonella 96; vitamin B_6 in 54; chicken liver 56
Chicory Tea 87, 113, 308; see also endive
chilblains 143–4
childbirth, labour in 285–6
children: and supplements 50; retarded 62, see also cretinism
chloride 61
chlorine 30, 35, 74, 101; in drinking water 59, 187
chlorofluorocarbons (CFCs) 82
chlorophyll 91, 136
chocolate 61, 86, 89, 247

362

cholecalciferol 58; see also vitamin D
cholera 94
cholesterol 25, 31, 39, 47, 53, 57, 68, 87, 137, 138
choline 245, 284, 298, 300
chromium 61, 141, 164, 165, 171, 217, 265
chromosomes 34, 37
cider vinegar 212
cigarettes see smoking
cinnamon 88, 340
circulation 130–1, 144
cirrhosis of the liver 22, 87, 122
citrus fruits 196
cleaning materials 70–1
cleft palate 280
clingfilm 100
Clostridium perfringens 95–6
cobalt 61–2
cocoa 63
cod 47, 84; see also fish oils
coeliac disease 59, 198
coenzyme Q 140, 259; coenzyme Q_{10} 217, 259, 297
coffee 25, 61, 63, 66, 87, 111, 124, 141, 208, 229, 246, 248; see also caffeine
colas 86
cold sores 11, 188–9
colds 11, 152, 309; see also coughs and colds
colic 197, 288
colitis 59, 194–5
collagen 57
colon 38, 332; see also intestine, large
coma, and diabetes 160, 162
Complementary Dairy 326–7
compounds 35
concentration: loss of 166, 167, 268, 298; enhanced 262
conception 263; nutritional guidelines 289–90; preparing for 276–8
confectionery see sweets
conjunctivitis 236–7
connective tissue 155

drugs 10, 12, 277; dependence on 46; *see also* antibiotics, anti-depressants, steroids, tranquillizers
dry-cleaning fluids 71
dry eye *see* xerophthalmia
duodenum 103; ulcers in 109
dyes, hair 231
dysmenorrhea 270–3
dyspepsia 111–12, 282

ears, problems and infections 196, 238–9
eating: disorders 256–9; process 305–6
echinacea 178
eclampsia 284
eczema 23, 56, 74, 225–6, 288
eggs 41, 74; amino acids in 45, 46, 47, 48; battery 299; minerals in 61, 62, 63, 66, 68; and salmonella 96; vitamins in 51, 52, 54, 56, 57, 58, 59
eicosapentaenoic acid (EPA) 137–8, 144, 185, 211
Eijkman, Christian 8
elderly 246–7, 292–301; food for 301–2
electro-magnetic fields 83
electrolytes 218, 245, 260, 315
embryo 275, 276
emphysema 46, 51, 78, 153–5, 333
'E' numbers 26, 150, 172; *see also* additives
encephalitis, viral 179
endive 56, 113; *see also* Chicory Tea
endocrine glands 159
endorphins 248, 252, 258
energy 36, 43, 56, 62, 63, 140, 146, 170; and carbohydrates 37, 52, 53; and fats 39; for muscles 215; and proteins 40
enzymes 36, 38, 43–4, 63, 64, 65, 67, 75, 101, 102, 103, 196, 297, 301; supplementary 44, 301
epilepsy 253–4
Epsom salts 150

ergocalciferol 58; *see also* vitamin D
essential fatty acids (EFAs) 23, 38, 39, 224, 255, 273, 279, 285, 286, 295–7
evening primrose oil: for acne 222–3; for Aids 182; and alcohol 88; for coronary heart disease 139; eczema 225; epilepsy, caution 254; for elderly 302; and hyperactivity 253; hypertension 135; at menopause 273; for migraine 248; multiple sclerosis 192; and nail problems 229; obesity 259; for premenstrual tension 271; in pregnancy 285; for psoriasis 227; and psychoses 255–6; for rheumatoid arthritis 210, 211
exercise 13, 89–90, 125, 161, 171, 252, 259, 300; aerobic 89
exhaustion *see* fatigue
eye 234; problems 71, 168, 233–8; sensitive, sore, tired 237–8; and vitamins 50, 51, 52, 320; *see also* blindness

faintness 166
fast food, dangers 16, 25
fatigue 47, 59, 64, 166, 182, 188, 192, 218, 246, 262
fats and oils 19, 26, 35, 39–40; and acne 222; animal, and pre-menstrual tension 272; and diseases 21, 22; mono-unsaturated 30; polyunsaturated 28, 30, 39, 58, 264, 287, 295, 305; rancid 45, 101; reduction of 28, 29, 152; saturated 14, 15, 17, 19, 24, 25, 39, 40, 105; *see also* essential fatty acids, transfatty acids
fennel seeds 64
fenugreek 165
ferritin 63
fertility 59, 320
fever 309
feverfew (*Tanacetum parthenium*) 211, 248, 307

fibre, dietary 14, 30, 105, 195, 311, 314, 318, 332, 335; importance 24, 38, 90, 115, 116, 117, 124, 142, 163, 170, 186; lack of *21, 22, 23*, 25

fibrocystic breast disease 25

fibrositis 219

figs 46, 47, 61, 63, 64, 66

fish 28, 41, 45, 101, 124, 145, 172, 186, 248, 302; polluted 84; Fish Terrine 325–6; *see also individual entries*

fish oils 9, 124, 135, 137–8, 144, 162, 182, 185, 192, 193, 207, 211, 235, 239, 284, 285; cod-liver oil 9, 51, 58; halibut-liver oil 51

fits, epileptic 253–4

flatulence 306, 337

flour, refined 7, 24, 26

flu *see* influenza

fluid retention *see* oedema

fluoridation 75–6

foetal alcohol syndrome *see* alcohol

folic acid (folacin) 22, 30, 31, 55, 56–7, 177, 255, 269, 281, 320, 332; deficiency 277, 279, 280, 283, 302

food contamination 83–6

food industry 17; attack on NACNE report 15

food intolerance *see* food sensitivity

food, nutritious 13

food poisoning 56, 94–8; natural remedies 98–9

food sensitivity 196–8; in babies 288; may aggravate: arthritis 209, 211; asthma 149; candida 188; colitis 195; cramps 219; depression 252, 256; eczema 225; glue ear 239; hay fever 151; headaches 247, 248; indigestion 111; irritable bowel syndrome 118; menstruation 272; mouth ulcers 108; multiple sclerosis 192; obesity 259; schizophrenia 256; smell, loss of 240

'food state' supplements 49

foods, convenience 28, 29, 293; packaged 21, 24, 25; *see also* junk foods

foods, detoxifying 90–2

forgetfulness, in old age 298–9

formaldehyde 72, 79

Fortified Soya Drink 156, 159, 182, 187, 310

free radicals: dangers of 58, 81, 101, 295–7, 305; and amino acids 47, 48

freezing of foods 29–30, 101; and vitamins 54, 59

French Dressing 323

fresh air 76–9

fructose 30, 37

fruit 6, 14, 28, 30, 38, 61; for arthritis 207; cancer 184–5, 186; and chemicals 84, 86; for healthy blood vessels 145; and lead poisoning 78; respiratory infections 152, 154; Fruit Cake, Special 330; *see also individual entries*

frying 51, 59, 305

Funk, Casimir 8

gallbladder *21*, 103, 112–13

gallstones 64, 112–13, 308

game, wild 19, 28

gamma-linolenic acid (GLA) 135, 211, 225

garlic: for asthma 150; candida 188; against cardiovascular disease 135–6, 141, 145; and diabetes 165; for infections 125–6, 127, 153, 240; Roast Garlic 331; and sex 262

gastric ulcers 109

gastritis 109

genes 37

ghee 305

gherkins 67

ginger 125, 135, 141, 239, 309; Ginger Brew 156, 309; Gingery Greens 332–3

Hunza apricots 313
hydrocarbons 70, 71, 73, 77
hydrochloric acid 46, 61, 102, 109, 110, 246, 301
hydrogen 35
hydrogenation of fats 40; in supplements 49
hygiene 93–101; poor and tuberculosis 157
hyperactivity 21, *23*, 252–3
hypertension 48, 131–6, 317, 324, 332; *see also* blood pressure, high
hyperthyroidism 51, 172–3
hypothyroidism 63
hypoglycaemia *23*, 46, 61, 66, 166–71, 244, 252, 254

immune-deficiency diseases 180–98
immune system 19, 72, 82, 147, 157, 174–98, 199, 287; boosting 11, 45, 54, 57, 66, 67, 152, 153, 176–7; foods for boosting 31, 32, 68, 177–8, 319; immunity, natural 20
impotence 266–7
indigestion 64, 111–12, 196
infant formulae 288
infants: protecting 286–7; weaning 288–9
infection, prevention of 57, 307, 321; infectious diseases 179–80
infertility 25, 263–6; and L-arginine 45; and zinc 68
inflammation 174
influenza 155–7, 309
infusions 307
inoculation 13
insomnia 60, 87, 166, 250–1, 298, 308
insulin 53, 61, 160–1, 168, 170, 337, 340
intelligence, and diet 14–15
international units (IU) 49–50
intestine: small 103, 113–15; large 105, 115–19
intrinsic factor 103
iodide/iodine 62–3, 81, 172, 286

ionizers 151
iron 21, 30, 57, 63, 74, 76, 87, 122, 171, 177, 208, 210, 231, 325; and anaemia 21, 63, 218, 245, 246, 282–3; and pregnancy 281; toxicity 63
irradiation of food 82
irritability 166, 246, 270
irritable bowel syndrome *21*, 117–19, 188
isoleucine 41
isothyocyanate 88
IU *see* international units

jams, avoidance 30
joints, pains in 188
juices, fruit 28; *see also* vegetable and fruit juices
juniper: berries 127, 307; oil 126
junk foods 16, 253, 277

kelp 59, 61, 66, 81, 172
kidney beans 57
kidney stones *22*, 57, 64, 123–5
kidneys (human) 120, 122, 161; and amino acids 45; cleansing action 89, 90–1; and minerals 61, 66
kippers 61, 67
kitchens, hygiene in 93–101
kiwi fruit 57; Kiwi Delight 339

labour (childbirth) 285–6
lactation 56
Lactobacillus acidophilus 91, 118, 179, 188
Lactobacillus bulgaricus 91
lactic acid 206, 215
lactose 37
lamb 28, 68; lamb's kidney 52, 54, 55; lamb's liver 52, 53, 54, 55, 235; minerals in 62, 65
laxatives 116–17
lead poisoning 77–8, 132, 136
learning difficulties 246
lecithin 113, 141, 193, 227, 298, 300
leeks 55, 56

metabolism 35, 37, 62, 65
methionine 41, 78, 91, 152; L-methionine 47, 78
microgram 49–50
migraine *23*, 47, 87, 188, 247–9, 268; and vitamins 53
milk, cow's 17, *23*, 24, 41, 53, 101, 203, 236, 253, 287; and amino acids 45, 48; dried 45, 48, 58; free, suspended 14; skimmed 28, 55, 58, 61, 67, 78; *see also* breast-feeding, goat's milk, soya milk
millet 43, 63; Millet Porridge 312–13; Millet Rissoles with Peanut Sauce 335–6
minerals 14, 35; and trace elements 59–68; chelated 60; in good diet 30
miscarriages 59, 278–80
miso 55, 67, 68, 186, 315; Miso and Onion Soup 156, 317–18
mitochondria 36, 217
molasses 63, 108, 178, 208, 229, 230, 246, 282–3, 328
molybdenum 65
mongongo nuts 18, 19
mononucleosis *see* glandular fever
monosodium glutamate 150
mood swings 166
morning sickness 54, 281–2
mouth, sore or cracked 52; *see also* ulcers, mouth
MS *see* multiple sclerosis
mucus 239
muesli 28, 30, 74, 145, 311–12
muirapuama 261
multiple sclerosis (MS) *23*, 191–3
mumps 179
muscles: cramps in 64, 67, 218–19, 311; feeding 45, 64, 65–6, *215*, 216–18, 332; problems with 188, 214–19
mushrooms 30, 53, 54, 66; Mushroom Pâté 324–5
mussel, green-lipped 209, 211
mustard seeds 88
myalgic encephalomyelitis (ME) *see* post-viral syndrome

myelin sheath 55, 191, 192

nails: problems with 68, 228–9; and vitamins 52
National Advisory Committee on Nutrition Education (NACNE) 14, 15, 25; table of medical conditions *21–2*
Nationwide Food Consumption Survey 27–8
nausea 54, 166
nervous system 242–60; and minerals 60, 64, 65, 67, 332; and vitamins 52, 53, 55, 56
Nettle Tea 307
neural tube defects *22*; *see also* spina bifida
neurological dysfunction 182
neurons 242–3; *see also* nervous system
neurotransmitters 46, 88, *243*, 244, 245, 298
niacin *see* vitamin B₃
night blindness 235
night cramps 54
nightshade family 209, 211
nitrates 74–5
nitrites 75
nitrogen 35
nitrogen dioxide 77
nitrosamines 75
N-nitroso compounds 25–6
nootropics 245
norepinephrine 298
nori seaweed 51, 52, 61, 81
nose 239–40
numbness 192
nutrients 10, 34–68, 130; eating of 305; protective 73–4
nutrition, orthomolecular 11
nutritional therapy 11–12
nuts: Nut Milk 326–7; Nut Roast 338; Nut Sausages 314–15; *see also* nuts and seeds
nuts and seeds, for protein 28, 30, 42–4, 145; storage of 101; *see also individual entries*
Nystatin 188

369

371

fertility 265; for healthy gums 107; hair 230; multiple sclerosis 192; in pregnancy 277; varicose veins 143

whole grains 14, 28, 43, 335; and blood sugar 170

wholemeal bread 29, 30, 38, 61, 62, 67, 73, 78

Wilson's disease 62

World Health Organisation: on Aids 181; aphrodisiacs 261; iodine 172; nitrates 75; on protein 41

wrinkles 296

xanthum gum 163

xerophthalmia 9, 233

yaws 19

yeast 194, 237, 260; and candidiasis 188; *see also* brewer's yeast

yeast extract 10, 55, 65, 67, 108, 178, 239, 247; *see also* Marmite

yoghurt: and amino acids 45, 46, 47, 48; athlete's foot 229; for beneficial bacteria 91, 116, 127, 179, 188, 301; cataracts 236; Yoghurt Dressing 323; and minerals 63, 203; Soya Yoghurt 326; and vitamins 59

zinc 30, 54, 62, 67–9, 76, 87; for acne 223; anaemia 246; anorexia 257; bronchitis 153; contraceptive pill 269; coughs and colds 153; cystic fibrosis 158; diabetes 165; eyes 233, 235; hair 230; herpes 189; hypoglycaemia 171; impotence 267; immune system 177, 178; infertility 264, 265; libido 262; at menopause 273; ME 190, 191; nails 229; in old age 299; against pollutants 73, 74, 78, 79, 88, 287; in pregnancy 277, 278–9, 281, 285; premenstrual tension 271; prostate gland 127; against radiation 81; for skin 226; affects taste 241